Volume II
The Foundations of Ethics
and Its Relationship
to Science

Knowledge Value and Belief

Edited by
H. Tristram Engelhardt, Jr.
and Daniel Callahan

THE HASTINGS CENTER
Institute of Society, Ethics and the Life Sciences

Institute of Society, Ethics and the Life Sciences
360 Broadway
Hastings-on-Hudson, New York 10706

Library of Congress Cataloging in Publication Data
Main entry under title:

Knowledge, value and belief.

  (Foundations of ethics and its relationship to science ; 2)
  Includes index.
  1. Ethics—Addresses, essays, lectures. 2. Medical ethics—Addresses, essays, lectures. I. Engelhardt, Hugo Tristram, 1941-   II. Callahan, Daniel, 1930-   III. Series.
BJ1012.K5   170   77-23033
ISBN 0-916558-02-9

Printed in the United States of America

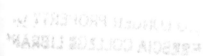

Contents

Contributors   v

Preface   viii

Introduction: Knowledge, Value and Belief   1
    H. Tristram Engelhardt, Jr.

Part A.

1. Can Medicine Dispense with a Theological Perspective on
    Human Nature?   25
    Alasdair MacIntyre

Commentary: Kant's Moral Theology or a Religious Ethics?   44
    Paul Ramsey

Commentary: A Rejoinder to a Rejoinder   75
    Alasdair MacIntyre

Commentary: Another Response to MacIntyre, Tragedy, Reason,
          Religion, and Ramsey   79
    Corinna Delkeskamp

Commentary: Morality and Religion   100
    Jack Bemporad

2. From System to Story: An Alternative Pattern for Rationality
    in Ethics   111
    David Burrell and *Stanley Hauerwas*

Commentary: Rationality, the Normative and the Narrative in
          the Philosophy of Morals   153
    E. D. Pellegrino

3. The Concept of Responsibility: An Inquiry into the
   Foundations of an Ethics for Our Age   169
   Hans Jonas
Commentary: Response to Hans Jonas   199
   Daniel Callahan

4. Toward an Evolutionary Ethic   207
   Bernard Towers

5. The Poverty of Scientism and the Promise of Structuralist
   Ethics   225
   Gunther S. Stent
Commentary: Deep Structures and an Evolutionary Ethic   247
   Patrick Heelan

6. The Meaning of Professionalism: Doctors' Ethics and
   Biomedical Science   254
   Stephen Toulmin
Commentary: The Fragmentation of Value   279
   Thomas Nagel

7. Error in Medicine   295
   Eric J. Cassell
Commentary: Errors in Medicine: Let Me Count Some Ways   310
   H. Tristram Engelhardt, Jr.

Part B
Preface   321
8. Interdisciplinarity: A Critical Appraisal   324
   Corinna Delkeskamp
9. How Does Interdisciplinary Work Get Done?   355
   Eric J. Cassell
Index   362

Contributors

JACK BEMPORAD is Rabbi of Temple Emanu-El, Dallas, Texas, and Adjunct Professor of Philosophy at Southern Methodist University.

DAVID BURRELL is Chairman of the Department of Theology at the University of Notre Dame. He received his Ph.D. in Philosophy at Yale University. He is the author, most recently, of *Exercises in Religious Understanding* and has completed a book on Thomas Aquinas.

DANIEL CALLAHAN is Director of the Institute of Society, Ethics and the Life Sciences. He received his B.A. at Yale and his Ph.D. in Philosophy at Harvard. He is the author, most recently, of *The Tyranny of Survival* and *Abortion: Law, Choice and Morality*. He is a member of the Institute of Medicine, National Academy of Sciences.

ERIC J. CASSELL, M.D., is Clinical Professor of Public Health at Cornell University Medical College and a Diplomate of Internal Medicine in private practice. For the past several years Dr. Cassell has been doing research and writing on the underlying bases of medical practice and the relationship between doctors, patients, and disease. He is the author of *The Healer's Art*.

CORINNA DELKESKAMP is Adjunct Assistant Professor, Department of Philosophy, Pennsylvania State University, University Park, Pennsylvania. She received her M.A. and Ph.D. (on David Hume) at Bonn University, and is presently working on the relation between science, religion and philosophy in the seventeenth century.

H. TRISTRAM ENGELHARDT, JR., Ph.D., M.D., is Rosemary Kennedy Professor of Medicine, Kennedy Institute, Center for Bioethics, Georgetown University. He is the author of *Mind-Body: A Categorial Relation* and co-editor of *Evaluation and Explanation in the Biomedical Sciences*, and *Philosophical Dimensions of the Neuro-Medical Sciences*.

v

STANLEY HAUERWAS is Associate Professor of Theological Ethics in the Department of Theology at the University of Notre Dame. He has previously published *Character and the Christian Life* and *Vision and Virtue*. Soon to be published is *Truthfulness and Tragedy: Further Investigations in Theological Ethics*.

PATRICK A. HEELAN is Acting Vice President for Liberal Studies and Professor of Philosophy at the State University of New York at Stony Brook. He has done research in physics and the philosophy of science and has lectured on the philosophy of medicine. He is the author of *Quantum Mechanics and Objectivity*.

HANS JONAS, Ph.D., D.H.L.h.c., D.L.L.h.c., D.theol.h.c., is Alvin Johnson Professor of Philosophy Emeritus at The New School for Social Research in New York. He is the author, most recently, of *Philosophical Essays: From Ancient Creed to Technological Man*. He is a Fellow of the American Academy of Arts and Sciences.

ALASDAIR MACINTYRE is University Professor of Philosophy and Political Science at Boston University. He is the author of *A Short History of Ethics* and *Against the Self-Images of the Age: Essays in Ideology and Philosophy*.

THOMAS NAGEL is Professor of Philosophy at Princeton University. He is the author of *The Possibility of Altruism* and an associate editor of *Philosophy & Public Affairs*.

EDMUND D. PELLEGRINO, M.D., is Professor of Medicine at the Yale University School of Medicine and President of the Yale-New Haven Medical Center. He is Director of the Institute for Human Values in Medicine and editor of the *Journal of Medicine and Philosophy*.

PAUL RAMSEY is Harrington Spear Paine Professor of Religion at Princeton University. His *Ethics at the Edges of Life: Medical and Legal Intersections* (Fall 1977) will be his fourth (the author vows, his last) book in the field of medical ethics.

GUNTHER S. STENT is Professor of Molecular Biology at the University of California, Berkeley. His current scientific research interest is the function and development of the nervous system. He is the author of *The Coming of the Golden Age* and of *Molecular Genetics. An Introductory Narrative*.

STEPHEN TOULMIN is Professor of the Committee on Social Thought, University of Chicago. He is the author of *Human Understanding, Wittgenstein's Vienna* (with Allan Janik) and *Knowing and Acting*.

BERNARD TOWERS is Professor of Pediatrics and Anatomy at the University of California at Los Angeles. He is President-elect of the Society for Health and Human Values, and the author of *Concerning Teilhard, and Other Writings on Science and Religion*.

Preface

FOR SOME YEARS NOW, The Hastings Center (Institute of Society, Ethics and the Life Sciences) has been devoted to studies of specific ethical dilemmas and problems arising out of advances in medicine and the life sciences. These studies have ranged from the very concrete—definition of death, the ethics of psychosurgery, mass genetic screening, for example—to the more general, such as justice and the distribution of medical care. Our work has always been conducted in an interdisciplinary way, but the main focus has been on attempting to find ways of resolving ethical dilemmas. In that sense, most of the Institute's work can be seen as applied ethics.

A few years ago, however, it became obvious that the Institute should also give some concerted attention to ethics in its own right. What is the present status of ethical theory and of different schools of thought? In particular, in what ways has contemporary science had an impact on ethical theory? If those were the very broad questions which seemed to require our attention, it seemed no less necessary that they should also be addressed by an interdisciplinary group. While it is tempting to see "ethics" as the special province of the philosopher or the theologian, such a view seems unduly restrictive. One does not have to spend much time observing our culture to see that the contribution of the moral philosopher or the moral theologian to ethical thought and practice is only one source of its values. A full inquiry into the foundations of ethics would also have to include the role of other fields and of other perspectives. In our particular case, it is the perspective of the scientist and the physician which is most pertinent. But it could well be argued that those perspectives are probably as crucial as any in the way our society perceives ethical issues.

The title of our project, "The Foundations of Ethics and Its Relationship to Science," expresses well, if very succinctly, exactly what we are after. This is the second volume to appear as the result of the program. The first, *Science, Ethics and Medicine*, made an initial stab at the topic, beginning where we know best how to begin, from within medicine. This volume, as the introduction by H. Tristram Engelhardt, Jr., will make evident, continues some general themes dealt with in Volume I. But it has, in addition, a special focus on theology and the foundations of ethics. It hardly needs to be noted that religious morality has been a major force in shaping the ethical and value structures of Western society. At the same time, of course, there has been for some centuries now a struggle between religious perspectives on morality and secular perspectives. A central feature of that struggle is debated in this volume by Paul Ramsey and Alasdair MacIntyre.

If we have, then, tried to take on some fundamental questions in ethics, we have also tried to do so in an interdisciplinary way. It has not been easy, not only because good interdisciplinary work is always difficult, but in this case because we are working at a level of abstraction and generality which makes it all the more difficult to talk across the usual disciplinary lines. It is not simply that disciplines have different subject matters, and different languages, and different methodologies. They also have different perspectives on the world, and their practitioners have different psychological sets as they work out of those perspectives. We have tried to cope with that problem and, in the process, reflect upon the very process of doing so. The second part of this volume presents some early conclusions in that respect.

Two further volumes are planned in this series. Just as we believe this volume represents an improvement on the first volume, we hope that the remaining volumes will reflect our own progress in grappling with the issues.

We are indebted to the National Endowment for the Humanities in making this research project possible. In particular, we wish to thank Richard Hedrich of the Endowment for his persistent interest and his just as persistent effort to keep us on target and to make of this project all that it should be.

Daniel Callahan
H. Tristram Engelhardt, Jr.

Introduction

Knowledge, Value and Belief

H. Tristram Engelhardt, Jr.

"Upon a deep green achmardi
she bore the perfection of paradise,
both root and branch.
That was a thing called the Grail,
which surpasses all earthly perfection."[1]

Parzival V. 235

THE HOLY GRAIL of modern Western thought has been objective truth untouched by uncertainty or value judgment, along with a secular account of values. This second in a series of four volumes is the product of analyses of the various elements of this quest. These analyses have been undertaken in order to become clearer about the nature of value theory, as well as about the interrelationships between the foundations of value theory and of science. A great number of the major figures in modern Western science and philosophy have undertaken this search. René Descartes, for example, sought to erect knowledge on certain and indubitable foundations. The first rule of his *Regulae ad directionem ingenii* was that "the end of study should be to direct the mind towards the enunciation of sound and true judgments on all matters that come before it."[2] Immanuel Kant, in attempting to liberate us from the seductions of a priori speculation, placed the sphere of practical action within the noumenal realm, severing the world of morality and free choice from the world of science.[3]

1

The logical positivists also attempted a rigorous reconstruction of the meaning of knowledge by accounting for the truth and falsity of theories, or of general statements about the world, in terms of sense experiences that verify or falsify them.

Such views of knowledge and reality led to portraying facts as value-free and to discounting values. One finds A. J. Ayer asserting that value judgments are as such simply ways of evincing one's emotions. Thus, "insofar as statements of value are significant, they are ordinary 'scientific' statements . . . and insofar as they are not scientific, they are not in the literal sense significant, but are simply expressions of emotion which can be neither true nor false."[4] As a result, "ethical philosophy consists simply in saying that ethical concepts are pseudo-concepts and therefore unanalyzable."[5] In short, science is disciplined knowledge, philosophy explains the grammar of knowledge, and ethics as a rational endeavor is an *ignis fatuus*.

In such accounts, the world of facts is the world of truth and falsity, and the world of values is the world of emotions. Science, accordingly, deals with the way things are. Ethics (here I will often, with some conceptual violence, use "ethics" expansively to include value judgments which to some extent fall outside of the moral realm *in sensu stricto*) portrays the constellations of ways we feel about the way things are. The mood of the early twentieth century, as reflected, for example, in behaviorism, suggested that science and technology were relatively free of moral ambiguity. Science was held not to raise questions about what one ought to do, but rather simply to portray the way things are. At most, moral issues would arise in the application of science.

Yet, some, with the noble naivete of a Parzival, have hoped that the grail of a value-free science would provide a true account of reality, as well as a sufficient structure for human life. This has led to a reappraisal of the quest leading to a hunger after a vision of the unity of ethics and science, of values and facts. Jacques Monod, for example, asserted that "The moment one makes objectivity the *conditio sine qua non* of true knowledge, a radical distinction, indispensable to the very search for truth, is established between the domains of ethics and of knowledge. Knowledge in itself is exclusive of all value judgment (all save that of 'epistemological value') whereas ethics, in essence nonobjective, is forever barred from the sphere of knowledge."[6] On the other hand, he acknowledged that

> True knowledge . . . cannot be grounded elsewhere than upon a value judgment, or rather upon an *axiomatic* value. It is obvious that the positing of objectivity as the condition of true knowledge *constitutes an ethical choice and not a judgment arrived at from knowledge, since, according to the postulate's own terms, there cannot have been any 'true' knowledge prior to this arbitral choice.* In order to establish the norm for knowledge the objectivity principle defines a *value*: that value is objective knowledge itself. Thus, assenting to the principle of objectivity one announces one's adherence to the basic statement of an ethical system, one asserts the *ethic of knowledge*.[7]

From this ethic of knowledge (which Monod takes to involve a commitment to a transcendent value of true knowledge!), Monod wished to derive a moral view of society and the world.

Other contemporaries such as Teilhard de Chardin attempted to show that the world of facts, the world of values, and in fact the world of religious beliefs are inextricably intertwined. Man and human values are not, according to Teilhard, mere accidents of nature or external to the meaning of reality. "In its present state, the world would not understand itself, and the presence in it of reflection would be incomprehensible, unless we supposed there to be a secret complicity between the infinite and the infinitesimal to warm, nourish and sustain to the very end—by dint of chance, contingencies and the exercise of free choice—the consciousness that has emerged between the two. It is upon this complicity that we may lay our base."[8] The world as portrayed by science, given an appeal to a religious belief (even if this religious appeal is attenuated to faith in an "Omega point"), is seen to be in a purposeful process that will develop, nourish, and support values.

Still, although the views of Monod and Teilhard conflict as atheistic and theistic, they agree regarding the importance of the quest for the ways in which science can ground the values we cherish. A gulf, though, remains of many dimensions between values and facts. In one sense, it is a cultural abyss separating what might be termed, in the idiom of C. P. Snow, two cultures.[9] There are, of course, more than the two cultures of the scientist and the humanist. There are the cultures of the physical scientist, the biological scientist, the social scientist, scholars in the arts, scholars in belles lettres, philosophers, theologians, technologists, biomedical scientists, among many others. After some Procrustean surgery, these may be reducible to the spheres of the scientists, the technologists, the secular humanists, and the theologians. In any event, one encounters a plethora of perspectives concerning what it means to study the world and to determine what is correct or proper conduct in it. Such heterogeneity calls for the search for a common ground among scientists, humanists, and theologians, assuming that such a fragmentation is neither desirable nor necessary. A serious person cannot view such a fragmented prospect upon reality and the nature of man without a certain disquietude. One cannot be concerned with the nurture of our culture without wishing to discover some underlying threads of unity or at least bases of cooperation which would place the power of science and technology within established constraints that reflect the values of life and freedom. One is brought, then, to address these gulfs among the cultures and to seek, if not for common fundamental commitments that will form bridges, then at least for a grammar of an interdisciplinary language.

But the issue is not simply one of communication. It has a metaphysical dimension as well. This dimension is expressed in questions such as: Are values ingredient in the nature of things? How does the nature of things influence the standing of human values? To some extent, questions such as these may concern what many have called (departing somewhat from G. E. Moore) the naturalistic fallacy—the attempt to conclude to value judgments from value-neutral descriptions of the world. But the issue is much broader, including the causal influence of states of affairs on evaluations. There is also an epistemological dimension. Both science and ethics are human artifacts and are surely not simply photograph-like presentations of facts and of values as they are in themselves. Science and ethics are constructed in terms of particular human goals and purposes. As a result, they cannot simply portray a hard and fast reality, but must at least in part reflect isolated constellations of human projects including the special concerns which structure each genre of ethics or science.

To bridge these various gulfs, philosophers, scientists, theologians, physicians, and historians have joined together to examine the foundations of ethics and the ways in which ethics and the sciences mutually presuppose and impregnate each other. The meetings that have led to the first two volumes of this series have produced papers fairly evenly divided between focusing on the foundations of ethics and analyzing areas of overlapping subject matter between ethics and the sciences. The result has been a rejection of the search for either a value-free science or an ethics independent of the sciences. In fact, questions raised in understanding the foundations of ethics have led to issues important in understanding the sciences and human reason more generally. To return to the image of Parzival, by examining the roots and branches of the grail we have sought to identify ways in which basic issues in the foundations of ethics bear upon the sciences, or presuppose concepts found in the sciences. And the converse has been pursued as well—the ways in which the sciences presuppose basic concepts from ethics.

The first year's set of meetings (embodied in the first volume of this series) provided five general conclusions concerning the foundations of ethics and its relationship to the sciences:

1. The images and metaphors of ethics are often borrowed from and influenced by theories of science and knowledge.
2. The sciences, in particular those sciences bearing on the human condition, are structured by value judgments concerning what humans should be like and should be able to do.
3. Science and ethics, though conceptually distinguishable, are in fact inseparable due to a web of interdependent concepts and ideas.
4. It is necessary to place the activities of science within the broader scope of human activities in general.
5. Ethics, in order to guide conduct successfully in this world, must be attentive to the deliverances of the empirical sciences.[10]

These five points indicate an overlap both of subject matter and of key concepts so that a clear line cannot be drawn between evaluation and explanation.[11] Valuing the world presupposes certain descriptive and explanatory accounts of the world. Further, descriptive and explanatory accounts cannot be pursued while eschewing all evaluations of the world or appeals to values generally, nor are such accounts value-free in either their perspective or their purpose. In short, the first year of analyses showed that there are important interdependencies between ethics and the sciences. It showed as well the fruitfulness of an interdisciplinary exploration of these interconnections.   .

The second year of these explorations which produced this volume has pressed these issues further. It addressed: (1) whether adequate accounts of ethics require an appeal either to a transcendent value or power (e.g., God), or to a special value possessed by processes in the world (e.g., evolution), or particular levels of life in the world (e.g., mankind or sentient beings); (2) whether rationality is of one fabric or is necessarily fragmented into many incommensurable accounts of reality; (3) how professions secure a special set of values and assume a particular set of obligations; and (4) which interdisciplinary discussions can succeed in giving a coherent and unitary overview of science and the humanities. Each of these four points addresses, in its own way, the coherence or synoptic possibilities of rationality. In order for science and ethics to share foundations, they must constitute elements of a general enterprise of giving reasons, testing premises, and framing coherent arguments. To the extent there are incommensurable rational enterprises, ethics and science may be radically different and nonintegrable endeavors. In fact, there will be the possibility of radically different ethics or sciences. This volume addresses these issues with special reference to beliefs in God.

In the modern West, God was more than simply a hypothesis; an appeal to God offered an insurance against such possible fragmentation. That is, God offered a hypothetical viewpoint in terms of which reality and ethics could be judged. Though there might be views of reality peculiar to various species of sentient beings, or even different cultures, the deity's view of reality and of values was privileged. Though other accounts of reality might bear a subscript (e.g., reality $_{human}$ or reality $_{modern\ Western\ thought}$), God's viewpoint was taken to be absolute. Thus, in the rationalist systems of Spinoza and Leibniz, God's view of the universe was the way the universe was and all other views simply deviated through ignorance or failure to perceive clearly and distinctly. But the insurance provided by this viewpoint has generally lapsed. The contemporary world view has been characterized by fewer appeals to God as a guarantor of knowledge and values. In addition, not only have absolute space and absolute time as the sensoria of God lost credibility, but absolute space and time have ceased to be absolute as well.

The first set of papers by Alasdair MacIntyre, Paul Ramsey, Corinna Delkeskamp, and Jack Bemporad explore the role of appeal to the existence of God in the foundations of ethics, especially with regard to the motivation for acting ethically. They investigate the matrix of knowledge, value, and belief. Professor MacIntyre presents the dilemma of contemporary moral theory. On the one hand, moral obligation presents itself as unconditional. On the other hand, nontheistic accounts of the motivation to act upon moral obligation, even to the point of self-sacrifice, are less than convincing. MacIntyre focuses upon Kant's account of morals, and its dependence upon an appeal to God. MacIntyre rejects Kant's argument on the basis of the implausibility of the existence of God, and suggests that the *summum bonum* sufficient to motivate moral action would be a commitment to history as a moral progression:

> Kant makes the significance of history depend on the moral progress of individuals rather than *vice versa*. . . . Hence also God is required as a power to give that moral form to the events in the after-life of individuals which Kant sees as lacking in the events of their mortal life. Kant's thesis that moral obligation necessarily presupposes teleology turns out to be correct; his thesis that teleology necessarily presupposes theology turns out to be incorrect. Hence the incredibility of Christian theology need not endanger belief in moral obligation after all. (MacIntyre, p. 41)

In order to supply the motivation for self-sacrifice that belief in God offered, MacIntyre argues that:

> If sacrifice is to be an intelligible notion, the individual has to be understood as a participant in the larger history of a group or an institution: the house of Atreus, the people of Israel, the city of Rome, the revolutionary proletariat. . . . The most basic moral question for each agent is therefore: of what histories am I a part? (MacIntyre, p. 39-40)

As the reader will discover, the issue of moral histories and how one may choose among them will be raised by other authors in this volume. Here, MacIntyre simply wishes to advance the general lineaments of what he might term a secular "grail legend" (MacIntyre, p. 34) in order to provide a *summum bonum* to motivate self-sacrifice when obligatory.

Professor Paul Ramsey responds that MacIntyre has misconstrued the nature and the force of Kant's argument. Ramsey argues that MacIntyre's acceptance of the notion of unconditional obligation should, as Kant contended, force him to acknowledge the existence of God at least as a practical postulate. (Ramsey, p. 54) Professor Ramsey then proceeds to sketch a view of moral conduct which has the source of its moral norms "within the religious dimension itself. God is worthy of worship because of who he is and his actions among men, and not because he incorporates in his commands the judgments men are capable of making without knowledge and acknowledgment of him." (Ramsey, p. 59) Ramsey argues, in short, that an appeal to God and religious commitments is required for a full view of ethics. Thus, Ramsey concludes by suggesting that MacIntyre "may have to follow Voltaire's advice to get himself crucified and found a religious movement in order to halt the onward march of utilitarianism." (Ramsey, p. 72)

In a spirited rejoinder, MacIntyre suggests that Paul Ramsey, if his faith commitment is not to be arbitrary, is in the predicament of having to appeal beyond religion to general ethical norms in order to establish the superior appeal of a commitment to, say, Christianity, rather than to Naziism. As MacIntyre puts it, "when faith meets faith, how are we to judge between them, if not in the light of an ethics which is not subordinated to the very religion it is required to judge?" (MacIntyre, p. 77) It is important to note, though, that in making this rejoinder, MacIntyre acknowledges "we do not as yet know how to provide the kind of warrant that ethics needs." (MacIntyre, p. 77) In short, MacIntyre's response to Ramsey's rejoinder suggests that we should understand his paper as a negative, not as a positive, critique of ethical theory.

In response to both MacIntyre and Ramsey, Corinna Delkeskamp sketches the one-sidedness of either a religious or secular foundation to ethics. In criticism of Ramsey, she reiterates the dilemma that MacIntyre forwards:

> Either the word of God defines what is morally good, or it is acceptable as the word of God only because it agrees with an independently known morality. If the first, no convincing basis can be conceived for deciding which religious (or ideological) pronouncement of morality to choose. Yet it is just such a choice between the pronouncements of Jahweh and those of the Führer to which the quest for a fortified morality commits one. If the second, an independent standard of morality is acknowledged. Yet then religion cannot be the ground of morality. (Delkeskamp, p. 79)

Against MacIntyre, Delkeskamp suggests that an appeal to history opens individuals to being sacrificed by others for the sake of history. It does not simply provide a motivation for one's own self-sacrifice on behalf of moral obligation. "History is the stuff from which dramas are made; for MacIntyre that drama is entrusted to history. Who, then, can restrain Robespierre and St. Just from wishing to *play* the ancient Romans and also claiming that it is *real*?" (Delkeskamp, p. 93) In short, to avoid the tyranny of an aesthetic appeal to history, one must maintain, so Delkeskamp argues, the moral distinctions ingredient in the notion of obligation. Otherwise, one may be tempted to create a beautiful history at the expense of moral obligation.

Finally, in the first section of this volume, Rabbi Jack Bemporad proffers grounds for accepting a religious attitude. He argues that the senses of hope, despair, and awe point beyond the merely moral order. In fact, ideas of repentance and forgiveness go beyond the moral sphere. For example, who but God could forgive a person of the murder of an innocent? The moral significance of self-sacrifice and the moral roots of forgiveness appear to transcend the ethical order. Bemporad agrees with Kant that coherence of the moral life and of experience requires at least a regulative appeal to a mutual ground for both the ethical and the factual order, for a reconciliation of the kingdoms of Grace and of Nature. He finds such a ground in God. Knowledge and values are grounded in a religious belief.

The papers of MacIntyre, Ramsey, Delkeskamp, and Bemporad thus raise three general issues regarding whether: (1) ethics requires an appeal to transcendent values; (2) rational grounds exist for decisions among various faith commitments (e.g., being a Marxist, a Christian, a Fascist, etc.); (3) ethics has a priority vis-a-vis religious claims insofar as its principles play a role in the choice among faith commitments or general ways of life. These issues, it should be noted, are basic to understanding the scope and unity of rationality. If ethical claims can be established independently of appeals to transcendent powers, then one can, as Abraham, remind God of the strictures of justice in His dealings with Sodom and Gomorrah: "Peradventure there be fifty righteous within the city: wilt thou also destroy and not spare the place for the fifty righteous that *are* therein: That be far from thee to do after this manner, to slay the righteous with the wicked: and that the righteous should be as the wicked, that be far from thee: Shall not the Judge of all the earth do right?" (Gen. 18:24-25) In fact, the Western religious tradition (as Rabbi Bemporad indicated in the unrecorded discussion of the papers of this volume) contains a strong strain of commitment to the priority of rationality in the religious life. This commitment ranges from a certitude that God is bound by strictures of logic to the position that humans should appeal to rationality, not the miraculous, in framing the religious life. One of the best examples of the latter is found in the Talmud where it is contended that one should rely on common agreement on the basis of rational arguments and exegesis, not on the basis of appeals to supernatural events.

> On that day R. Eliezer brought forward every imaginable argument, but they did not accept them. Said he to them: "If the *halachah* agrees with me, let this carob-tree prove it!" Thereupon the carob-tree was torn a hundred cubits out of its place—others affirm four hundred cubits. "No proof can be brought from a carob-tree," they retorted. Again he said to them: "If the *halachah* agrees with me, let the stream of water prove it!" Whereupon the stream of water flowed backwards. "No proof can be brought from a stream of water," they rejoined. Again he urged: "If the *halachah* agrees with me, let the walls of the schoolhouse prove it," whereupon the walls inclined to fall. But R. Joshua rebuked them, saying: "When scholars are engaged in a *halachic* dispute,

what have ye to interfere?" Hence they did not fall, in honour of R. Joshua, nor did they resume the upright, in honour of R. Eliezer; and they are still standing thus inclined. Again he said to them: "If the *halachah* agrees with me, let it be proved from Heaven!" Whereupon a Heavenly Voice cried out: "Why do ye dispute with R. Eliezer, seeing that in all matters the *halachah* agrees with him!" But R. Joshua arose and exclaimed: "*It is not in heaven.*" What did he mean by this—Said R. Jeremiah: That the Torah had already been given at Mount Sinai; we pay no attention to a Heavenly Voice, because Thou hast long since written in the Torah at Mount Sinai. *After the majority must one incline.*

R. Nathan met Elijah and asked him: What did the Holy One, Blessed be He, do in that hour?—He laughed [with joy], he replied, saying, "My sons have defeated Me, My sons have defeated Me."[12]

This passage is significant in its reliance upon general canons of rationality for the development of a way of life, even a religious way of life. It, in short, suggests that there is a unity and univocal character to rationality—a monorationality, as it were, binding on all persons.

The papers by Professor Burrell and Hauerwas challenge this view of rationality, especially with regard to ethics. They argue that in attempting to find a rational foundation for morality, contemporary ethical theory ignores the significance of narrative and, therefore, fails to give a convincing account of moral character, moral virtues, or the grounds for assuming particular moral roles (e.g., as a physician, mother, Christian, American, husband). Moreover, they wish to argue against viewing ethics primarily as an endeavor to solve moral quandaries. To pervert a metaphor from Thomas Kuhn, they are seeking a normal, rather than a crisis ethics, one that solves the everyday problems of moral virtue and character, not the crisis issues of the inter-paradigmatic conflicts of basic ethical principles.[13] Further, like Kuhn's science, Burrell and Hauerwas's ethics is contextual. It has its sense and purpose within the ambience of a particular moral story or account of the world. Moral arguments, thus, have the inconclusiveness, so they suggest, of a discussion between a member of the Palestine Liberation Organization and an Israeli about "whether an attack on a village is unjustified terrorism. They both know the same 'facts' but the issue turns on the story each holds, and within which those 'facts' are known." (Burrell/Hauerwas, p. 120) Against those who would hold that there are general moral considerations to decide what would count as justified or unjustified terrorism, the authors suggest that no unambiguous answer is forthcoming. Rather, the questions and their answers are bound within the rich texture of particular moral narratives concerning the human condition. Burrell and Hauerwas recognize that:

> the standard account is motivated by the interest of securing moral truthfulness. But it mistakenly assumes that truthfulness is possible only if we judge ourselves and others from the position of complete (or as complete as possible) disinterest. . . . Far from assuring truthfulness, a species of rationality which prizes objectivity to the neglect of particular stories distorts moral reasoning by the way it omits the stories of character formation. If truthfulness (and the selflessness characteristic of moral behavior) is to be found, it will have to occur in and through the stories that we find tie the contingencies of our life together. (Burrell/Hauerwas, p. 123)

Burrell and Hauerwas present the foundations of ethics as in part surd. One does not, according to them, choose to conform to the moral point of view. It is rather a gift consequent upon being part of a particular moral narrative. Still, Burrell and Hauerwas presuppose at least some canons for critics of such stories, so that they can test each story in terms of the sort of person it shapes. (Burrell/Hauerwas, p. 136)

> Any story which we adopt, or allow to adopt us, will have to display:
>
> (1) power to release us from destructive alternatives
>
> (2) ways of seeing through current distortions
>
> (3) room to keep us from having to resort to violence
>
> (4) a sense for the tragic: how meaning transcends power. (Burrell/Hauerwas, p. 137)

The authors hold that these criteria should not be taken as features which a story must display; they are not lineaments of a standard account in terms of which a disinterested observer could judge the merit of a particular rational life plan. In a somewhat Wittgensteinian fashion, Burrell and Hauerwas suggest that each story has its own grammar, while denying that there is a grammar of grammars. Yet, their discussion appears to presuppose at least an attenuated grammar of grammars, or story of stories.

In commentary upon Burrell and Hauerwas, Pellegrino argues that their account of ethics fails to guard against ethical subjectivism or relativism. Given their account, Pellegrino is concerned that we will be confined within our particular moral narratives without the ability to decide which narratives are morally superior. "Every narrative has its own justification simply because it reveals a unique set of moral events. Without insistence on some elements of objectivism, we easily confuse coherence and plausibility with something very different—namely, moral truth." (Pellegrino, p. 164) The point raised by Pellegrino is similar to Delkeskamp's critique of MacIntyre's appeal to history. There is a danger of reducing ethical values to the aesthetic values of a plausible narrative. As Pellegrino puts it, "they recommend a form of rationality 'especially appropriate to ethics,' which is based on an ordering principle itself unpredictable in its operations." (Pellegrino, p. 157) Pellegrino is, in short, concerned with the unity of the rational enterprise. While, on the one hand, he recognizes with Burrell and Hauerwas that ethics is more than a process of solving quandaries or problems, and that any fully developed account of ethics must include moral narratives in order to make the nuances of the moral life comprehensible, still he fears that an overemphasis upon moral context and ambience will undercut the senses of obligation and duty which are foundational concerns of ethics.

The papers by Hans Jonas, Gunther Stent, and Bernard Towers, along with the commentaries by Daniel Callahan and Patrick Heelan, concern attempts to provide generally compelling accounts of the ethical order. They are concerned with the provision of what Burrell and Hauerwas have called a standard account—a view of the world which a disinterested observer should be able to achieve and use in resolving moral quandaries, and in directing his or her moral life. Professor Jonas addresses "The Concept of Responsibility: Its Place in an Ethical Theory for the Technological Age." He argues that there are two basic moral responsibilities. The first and the most overriding is that mankind continue to exist, and the second is that men live a life of quality. The first obligation Professor Jonas takes to be an ontological imperative—the responsibility to maintain the existence of our species. "The possibility of there being responsibility in the world which is bound to the existence of men, is of all objects of responsibility, the first." (Jonas, p. 182) In Professor Jonas's account it is human existence itself which is the primary or fundamental object of responsibility, whether in a natural or contractual ethical context, whether in the case of a parent or in the case of a statesman. The intent of this argument is very similar to one forwarded by Kant against suicide,[14] except in this case it is explicitly focused against species' suicide, or even death through negligence. And, unlike Kant who constructed his argument in terms of the conditions for coherent moral action, Jonas's argument has a metaphysical structure. The very existence of humans produces this obligation. Moreover, the weight of this ontological imperative increases as knowledge and technological power (and thus their influence upon the survival of humans) increase. (Jonas, p. 189).

As Daniel Callahan stresses, the view forwarded by Professor Jonas has implications for an ethics of technology. One is, in particular, forced to determine (1) what obligations now exist for those who possess scientific and technological power; (2) whether the archetype of parent-child responsibility, which Professor Jonas employs, can be applied to the responsibility of technologists and scientists; and (3) whether the ontological imperative is sufficient even though "there appear to be no goals toward which human life should strive." (Callahan, p. 201) Still, Callahan holds that Jonas provides an accurate diagnosis of the current moral predicament especially if mankind, because of scarce resources, population pressures, and insufficient food, becomes radically dependent upon science and technology for survival. Under such conditions, Jonas's parent-child model for responsibility may well apply in part to the relationship between the scientific and technological community and mankind generally. (Callahan, p. 203) In any event, Jonas offers a foundation for a standard account of moral responsibility based on an ontological imperative enhanced by a special focus upon the contemporary obligations of technologists and scientists.

Bernard Towers in "Toward an Evolutionary Ethic" offers a *telos* for Jonas's ontological imperative. He accepts Teilhard de Chardin's argument that the evolutionary development of complexity in biological organization is tied to increasing complexity of consciousness. He, then, holds that the place of evolution as a central fact of existence provides the warrant for modern science; in particular, he sees the science of biological evolution as laying "the groundwork for, and [establishing] the mode of modern ethics." (Towers, p. 212) Science should, so Towers argues, provide the central foundations of ethics. "The bioethicist must first discover, and learn, and inwardly digest, what it is that the biological scientist and the medical practitioner have to tell him about the way things move in nature, rather than attempt to instruct him, on the basis of some ethical theory or other (whether normative, utilitarian, formalist, situationist or whatever), about how things are or how they ought to be." (Towers, p. 212) Towers holds that science, by providing an account of evolution, gives a warrant for human moral responsibility. "At the human level we find not only the power but the responsibility to continue the trend towards increased complexity-consciousness. The *power* is clearly there in nature, as it has always been. The *responsibility* comes because, for all that *we* are utterly dependent on *nature* for survival, yet nevertheless, because of the power over nature that we have already achieved, many parts of *nature* are utterly dependent upon us, upon our conscious reflection, upon that 'love' which Teilhard saw as the ultimate manifestation of the force that draws things together." (Towers, p. 218) Towers, thus, forwards a scientific account of the foundations of ethics: (1) science discloses the evolutionary character of reality; (2) natural processes have a goal and purpose; and (3) humans are held to be obliged to support and nourish that goal and purpose—the nourishment and increase of consciousness through evolution.

In contrast, Gunther Stent rejects as hard-core scientism the argument advanced by Professor Towers. Stent argues that one cannot, given the strictures of the naturalistic fallacy, infer moral obligations from states of affairs. That evolution leads to more

complex forms of consciousness does not imply anything ethically, i.e., that it *should* lead to higher forms of consciousness
or that humans are morally obliged to support such progress.
More than simply descriptive premises are needed. Science,
though, can make a contribution to the foundations of ethics
through a structuralist account of ethics. Just as Kant argued that
one brings certain forms of intuition to one's experience of the
world, so Stent wishes to argue that there is a biologically innate
deep structure to all human ethical activity. "In addition to being
fully consonant with modern evolutionary thought, the notion of
a Kantian a priori, and its latter-day, neo-Kantian structuralist
elaboration, finds support from recent neurological findings which
indicate that, in accord with those tenets, information about the
world reaches the brain not as raw data but as highly processed
structures that are generated by a set of stepwise, preconscious
informational transformations of the sensory input." (Stent, p.
238-9) In this fashion, Stent provides a biological account of
obligation as a fact of reason, "or rather of the nearly universal
phenomenon of a feeling of obligation to obey moral principles."
(Stent, p. 241) Particular moral judgments would "arise by a
generative process involving transformational operations on a
subconscious mental deep structure." (Stent, p. 242) Stent is,
thus, giving a causal account of ethics, realizing that even if
science cannot justify moral values it can give an account of their
biological basis. (Stent, p. 241)

As the commentary by Patrick Heelan indicates, Bernard Towers and Gunther Stent contribute a number of useful insights to
the bearing of science on the foundations of ethics. On the one
hand, Towers's account shows the importance of distinguishing
between scientific images which are not goal-oriented or person-
oriented, and manifest images which describe things in terms of
their intended functions or moral roles. Heelan suggests the need
for Towers to be clear whether his account of evolution falls
strictly within the austere scientific image, or whether it is elaborated with goal-oriented, manifest images. Heelan argues that
Towers requires the second to have his argument succeed; that is,
ethics must march hand-in-hand with science, not follow science,
in order to sustain the conclusions that Towers forwards. Moreover, in order to insure "the emergence of the eschatological

global society" (Heelan, p. 247) of Teilhard and Towers, some appeal to a transcendent power, or at least a divine force, seems to be needed. "I do not then believe one can be a Towers without being a Teilhard all the way." (Heelan, p. 251) Such a religious appeal is required, so Heelan holds, if not to warrant the value of evolution, then at least to insure its "success." Towers's binding of knowledge and values requires, so Heelan contends, an appeal to a religious belief. As to Stent, Heelan underlines his disclaimer: a scientific account of ethics can provide a causal explanation of ethical activity but it cannot warrant the content of any ethical system. Though a biological deep structure for ethical behavior "would influence the form of ethical conduct," it would not determine its content. (Heelan, p. 253) Moreover, the existence of such a deep structure would not validate or disqualify any particular ethical system.

Still, knowledge of the character of the development of the world (e.g., the presence of evolution and the existence of deep structures to account for ethical activity) can help in understanding the nature of the ethical enterprise. Though science cannot validate particular ethical systems, it may be able to indicate the ease or difficulty of acting upon particular moral obligations. The character of the world we live in must, at the very least, be taken into account when developing a theory of ethics. Science provides, if not the foundations of ethics, at least an understanding of the ambience and context of ethics, and of the nature of humans as moral agents. Finally, science contributes a large part of the narrative of our general story about ourselves. This contribution can be decisive in varying measure as (1) Burrell and Hauerwas succeed in establishing the importance of moral narrative; or (2) MacIntyre succeeds in making historical moral progression the *summum bonum* to motivate moral obligation; or (3) Towers endows Jonas's ontological imperative with a *telos*; or (4) Stent gives an account of our biological predilections as moral agents. Each of these indicates the historical, context-bound nature of human values. Moreover, one of the characteristics of our contemporary world culture is that its narrative is in an important and inextricable way fashioned and shaped by science and technology. Science and technology contribute in a singular fashion to what ethics is and to our understanding of the foundations of ethics. They fashion our standard narrative, if not our standard account.

The concept of moral narratives or regional ethics is addressed as well by Stephen Toulmin and Thomas Nagel in their consideration of the meaning of professionalism. Toulmin discusses three features of professions: (1) professionals engage in their activities for a living rather than for diversion; (2) there is a recognized body of skills communicated through a special form of instruction often accompanied by accreditation; and (3) statutory bodies confer special privileges attaching to the exercise of those skills. (Toulmin, pp. 256) Particular "professions" may satisfy one or more of these conditions. In addition, professions support a particular set of values, and as a result assume special obligations. Moreover, these obligations are often potentially at variance. For example, the obligation of a lawyer to maintain client-attorney privilege or to be the advocate of his or her client may conflict with the obligation to be an officer of the court. Similar conflicts exist between a physician's responsibility to report certain infectious diseases and to maintain physician-patient confidentiality. Toulmin argues that there is no escape from such conflicts.

These conflicts are likely to become more acute as more physicians assume a second role of conducting human experimentation. They will have assumed obligations of developing knowledge, which obligations may often be in conflict with their obligations to the patients whom they are treating. Insofar as physicians protect their patients from the power of death and disease, as attorneys protect their clients from the power of the state, this additional role of researcher will increase the traditional tension between a physician's obligations to his patients and those to "the art." In addition to exacerbating the inherent ethical conflicts in medicine, assumption of the role of researcher will tend to subordinate a physician's legally responsible role to a "legally irresponsible one as a scientist." That is, unlike physicians, scientists do not satisfy the third condition of a professional—being regulated by statutory bodies. Though Toulmin does not hold that one should license scientists as one licenses physicians, he stresses that one should recognize that biomedical science is a profession and a legitimate area for social concern and public involvement—as reflected in lay community representation on Institutional Review Boards. (Toulmin, p. 277)

In considering Toulmin's account, Thomas Nagel suggests that such conflicts between disparate values, claims, and interests are not limited to the professions. Nagel is, also, not sanguine about developing a system of priorities which would allow resolution of such conflicts. Instead, he holds that there are five fundamental types of value and that their different claims are the sources of our moral conflicts. They are: (1) specific obligations to other people or institutions; (2) constraints upon action deriving from general rights of persons; (3) issues of utility; (4) claims of perfectionist aims or values; and (5) commitments to one's own projects or undertakings. These obligations, rights, utilities, perfectionist ends, and private commitments generate basically irresolvable moral conflicts. Faced with such complexity, Nagel suggests that we pursue as systematic an ethics as possible, realizing that a completely unitary account will never be forthcoming, and that one will always have to appeal to something like the practical wisdom of Aristotle in making moral judgments.

The function of such practical wisdom or moral judgment comes to the fore in Eric Cassell's account of medical error. The physician makes judgments in intrinsically ambiguous situations. Moreover, so Cassell argues, the individuals and circumstances involved in health care are interdependent in such an intricate fashion that an account of an error by any one of them requires a reference to the situation as a whole. "Each case, whether error is present or not, is like a stage play. A setting, an audience, a disease whose story is told, and a set of actors. Only by examining that piece of theatre—medicine's individual—can one gain understanding of error—or even of cure or care." (Cassell, p. 309) Any thorough account of error in medicine is contextual and complex. On the basis of this view, Cassell provides a rich catalogue of: (1) error in medicine; (2) the functions of compensation for medical malpractice; (3) the ways in which false understandings of medicine generate particular views of medical error; and (4) the ways in which concepts and connotations of disease guide medical practice. In doing so, the paper displays the role of the physician as scientist, as technologist, and as a member of a particular culture with its own account of the physician's role and abilities. The web of errors that can be identified in medicine reflects the maze of the varying understandings of the meaning and status of medicine; what counts as error in medicine is dependent in large part upon the view of the science and technology of medicine. An account of the foundations of medical ethics must, as Eric Cassell obliquely suggests, take into consideration the status of the science and technology of medicine. The analyses become unavoidably interdisciplinary.

As this volume shows, this interdisciplinary enterprise has employed conceptual, symbolic, and causally-oriented analyses of the interplay of the foundations of ethics and science by focusing on: (1) conceptual interdependencies; (2) ways in which symbols and general constellations of meaning influence human practices such as ethics; and (3) the ways in which states of affairs influence ethics (thus opening ways for the sciences to make contributions to the understanding of the foundations of ethics). The question of the appropriate methodologies for the study of the relation of the foundations of ethics to the sciences, as well as the kinds of conclusions that can be forthcoming from such analysis, raises further issues regarding the nature of interdisciplinary investigations. Consequently, a major portion of the discussions of this last year were themselves given over to an analysis of the interdisciplinary enterprise. In her essay, Corinna Delkeskamp examines whether there are good grounds for holding that transdisciplinary projects are likely to be fruitful. As she indicates, at least three sorts of arguments are given for interdisciplinary activities: (1) arguments from the object of study— that since one can construct an intelligible overview of various disciplinary enterprises, the fragmentation of scholarship into specialized departments is inappropriate (this, though, can lead one to conclude falsely that various subject matters have a unity from the fact that one can construct an intelligible overview); (2) an argument from social concerns—that the urgency of some societal issues, which transcend particular disciplines, requires a super-disciplinary systems-theory approach to those issues (this, though, often runs the risk of an ideological determination of what will count as "useful" scholarship); (3) an existential argument—that human life in modern society is fragmented into unconnected activities (though any "whole" view will be interesting only if there is a complexity of human activity to bring together); and (4) an ethical argument that specialization within the university has traded humanism for technical skills (with the consequence that such interdisciplinarity often lacks substance and rigor).

Delkeskamp then proceeds to survey the first two years of discussions in this series. In particular, she addresses the extent to which an interdisciplinary endeavor can remain usefully interdisciplinary without itself becoming a separate discipline (as, for example, bioethics has become a separate enterprise). After reviewing the interdisciplinary character of these first volumes, she suggests that there are three phases that occur in interdisciplinary endeavors: an initial phase of external criticism in which experts from various fields learn how their fields are viewed by others, a second phase of internal criticism in which each specialist uncovers areas where foreign concepts can be applied to his or her own discipline, and a third phase where each participant develops a modified self-interpretation of the other's discipline. This leads finally to a self-conscious reappraisal of one's own discipline. In short, what is achieved is a quasi-philosophical reflexivity, arguing for the central and special interdisciplinary role of philosophy.

Finally, Eric Cassell sketches ways in which the personal appreciation of one's own discipline and that of others is transformed in the course of a successful interdisciplinary undertaking. In particular, he stresses the ways in which an interdisciplinary common language is developed, allowing a reappraisal of one's own discipline, as well as an appreciation of its context among other enterprises. In short, both Delkeskamp and Cassell indicate the dialectical nature of interdisciplinary endeavors. In attempting to appreciate the underlying or overarching common themes among disciplines, those disciplines themselves are altered. One unexpectedly comes to see that the foundations of ethics and the sciences share issues in common and share common difficulties, and as a result fashion each other.

In reviewing the analyses offered by the second year of these meetings, a set of tentative conclusions, as well as basic methodologies, emerges. To begin with, there are basic interplays between the foundations of ethics and the sciences:

1. Reasoning in ethics and in science has a contextual dimension which is in part historical. Though this volume has explored this issue with a focus on ethics, last year's volume and next year's extend this search to the sciences.[15] Moral and scientific rationality has in part a narrative character—science and ethics are guided by the metaphorical suggestiveness, not simply the conceptual force, of their basic notions, and these notions display a historical development. Both the Burrell/Hauerwas account of moral narrative and the Bernard Towers account of the moral significance of evolution fall under this rubric.

2. Ethics can be divided into normal and crisis ethics, to abuse a Kuhnian image. Burrell and Hauerwas can fruitfully be viewed as arguing for a normal ethics (i.e., the development of character and virtue within established paradigms of ethical conduct), while decrying crisis or quandary ethics which tests basic ethical principles. Even if one may not wish to accept the fragmentation of moral reasoning that Burrell, Hauerwas, and Kuhn want to witness, still there may be a heuristic merit in exploring the similarities between moral narratives or moral enterprises, and scientific paradigms or research programs.

3. Science may provide important insights into the ways in which we build ethical systems. Though science cannot justify an ethics, it may be able to predict and causally explain certain ethical behaviors and interests in ethics. Though values may not be inferable from facts, states of affairs may cause evaluations (compare how a pre-adolescent male and a post-adolescent male value females).

4. The power given to humans by modern science and technology expands human responsibility (see the essay in this volume by Hans Jonas).

5. Professions bring together various, usually potentially conflicting, moral obligations. Such tensions are compounded when professions overlap, as in the case of physician-scientists. This point is similar to the first above—science and technology can only be understood contextually—here in terms of the special social allocation of roles to particular professions with the conse-

quent tensions this engenders. As a result, any coherent account of science or medicine as a profession will require an analysis of the constellations of values which shape their conduct, and the conflicts which that can engender.

These discussions and analyses have proceeded by an analysis of: (1) conceptual, (2) symbolic, and (3) causal connections between ethics and the sciences. What has emerged is the need to distinguish among these three analytic leitmotifs. For example, it is important to distinguish between a causally-oriented methodology as forwarded by Gunther Stent, and a conceptually-oriented methodology as forwarded by Edmund Pellegrino. Both of these are to be distinguished from accounts such as that offered by Burrell and Hauerwas, which look to narratives for guidance, recognizing that they do not afford the notional clarity and universality of concepts.

In sum, we have come, on the one hand, to see overlapping areas of subject matter and competence between ethics and the sciences. On the other hand, we have come to isolate dimensions of analysis or methodological approach central to understanding the relationships between the foundations of ethics and the sciences. In short, there has been progress, if only of a tentative fashion, in coming to address this global yet fundamental intellectual quest. The grail myth is perhaps helpful here—one must, like Parzival, learn when to ask questions and what questions to ask. After all, because of his failure to understand the proper use of questions, Parzival postponed his acquisition of the grail while causing Titurel to continue in agonizing pain. Though we, unlike Titurel, may not suffer with a wound in our privy parts while waiting for Parzival to cure us with the right questions, still the issue of understanding the bearing of ethics upon the sciences, or the sciences upon ethics, is central to any unified view of our culture and of reality. The pain is, to say the least, intellectual. Insofar as it bears upon our competent use of science and the technologies, the pain may be quite similar to the physical pain of Titurel.

NOTES

1. Wolfram von Eschenbach, *Parzival,* trans. H. Mustard and C. Passage (New York: Vintage Books, 1961), p. 129.

2. René Descartes, *The Philosophical Works of Descartes*, trans. E. Haldane and G. Ross (Cambridge: Cambridge University Press, 1967), vol. I, p. 1.

3. Immanuel Kant, *Grundlegung zur Metaphysik der Sitten*, in *Kants Werke* (Akademie Textausgabe), Band IV, p. 452.

4. Alfred J. Ayer, *Language, Truth and Logic* (New York: Dover Publications, Inc., 1946), pp. 102-3.

5. Ibid., p. 112.

6. Jacques Monod, *Chance and Necessity* (New York: Alfred A. Knopf, Inc., 1971), p. 174.

7. Ibid., p. 176.

8. Teilhard de Chardin, *The Phenomenon of Man*, trans. Bernard Wall (New York: Harper Torchbooks, 1959), p. 276.

9. C. P. Snow, *The Two Cultures: And a Second Look* (Cambridge: Cambridge University Press, 1959).

10. H. Tristram Engelhardt, Jr. and Daniel Callahan, eds., *The Foundations of Ethics and Its Relationship to Science, vol. I: Science, Ethics and Medicine* (Hastings-on-Hudson, N. Y.: Institute of Society, Ethics and the Life Sciences, 1976), p. 12.

11. H. Tristram Engelhardt, Jr. and Stuart F. Spicker, *Evaluation and Explanation in the Biomedical Sciences* (Dordrecht, Holland: D. Reidel Publishing Company, 1975).

12. *Babylonian Talmud, Baba Mezia*, 59b, Soncino Edition.

13. Thomas S. Kuhn, *The Structure of Scientific Revolutions* (Chicago: University of Chicago Press, 1962).

14. Immanuel Kant, *Grundlegung zur Metaphysik der Sitten*, in *Kants Werke* (Akademie Textausgabe), Band IV, pp. 423-24.

15. I have in mind here Toulmin's article, "Ethics and 'Social Functioning': The Organic Theory Reconsidered," as well as Lester King's "Values in Medicine," and Marx Wartofsky's "The Mind's Eye and the Hand's Brain: Toward an Historical Epistemology of Medicine" in *The Foundations of Ethics and Its Relationship to Science, vol. I: Science, Ethics and Medicine*, ed. H. Tristram Engelhardt, Jr. and Daniel Callahan (Hastings-on-Hudson: Institute of Society, Ethics and the Life Sciences, 1976). One will also find suggestive remarks on this issue in the paper by Eric Cassell in this present volume.

1

Can Medicine Dispense with a Theological Perspective on Human Nature?

Alasdair MacIntyre

I

"THE OFFICES OF T-4 prepared a questionnaire which was sent to all mental hospitals and psychiatric clinics in Germany. On the basis of the completed questionnaire . . . a committee of three experts, chosen from among the doctors connected with T-4, made a decision. If this long-distance diagnosis was unfavorable, the patient was sent to an 'observation station' . . . unless there was a contrary diagnosis by the director of the 'observation station,' he was transferred to a euthanasia establishment proper . . . when doctors were placed at the head of these establishments, more efficient methods were introduced. . . . The method they devised was asphyxiation by carbon monoxide gas. . . . Patients were generally rendered somnolent by being given morphine, scopolamine injections or narcotic tablets before being taken, in groups of ten, to the gas chamber. . . . Families were advised of the patient's death by form letters which stated that the patient had succumbed to 'heart failure' or 'pneumonia.' "[1]

Poliakov is describing the euthanasia program introduced in Germany by government decree on September 1, 1939. Two features of the episode deserve to be noticed. The first is that, as Poliakov shows, the euthanasia program for the mentally feeble and the insane was an important prelude to the extermination program for the Jews. The second is that there was no difficulty at all in recruiting distinguished and able members of the German medical profession first to the euthanasia program and then to the extermination program. It is no part of my intention to suggest that Germans have a peculiarly horrifying lack of moral capacity or that physicians are peculiarly corruptible; quite the opposite. It is, in fact, precisely because the German medical profession in pre-Nazi Germany honored the Hippocratic Oath with apparently the same degree of sincerity, conviction, and moral capacity with which it is honored by our own medical men that the ready participation of such professors of psychiatry as Heyde, Nietzsche, and Pfannmüller in the euthanasia program, and of such professors of medicine as Clauberg and Kremer at Auschwitz and Ravensbruck, puts us too to the question.

Discussions of medical ethics usually focus upon what has now become problematic for physicians and surgeons. I want to attend instead to what is still taken for granted, namely, the unconditional and absolute character of certain of the doctor's obligations to his patients. The German example shows how fragile commitment to this absolute and unconditional character may be; it is all the more important, therefore, to enquire what grounds we have for such commitment. If we omit from view all the areas about which there is now argument and debate—voluntary euthanasia, abortion, continuation of life by extraordinary means—there remains that large and central area of medical practice in which the doctor is required to treat the life of the patient as an object of unconditional regard and concern—it seems natural to say that he is required to treat the life of the patient as sacred. This kind of requirement is, of course, central to *all* morality: the same unconditional character is embodied in the student's obligation not to cheat in an examination, the patriot soldier's (as contrasted with the mercenary's) obligation to accept death rather than dishonor, the obligation on us all not to engage in malicious gossip—and, most strikingly, the simple obligation upon all of us to give up our lives rather than allow certain evils of Auschwitz and Ravensbruck. Any account of morality which does not allow for the fact that my death may be required of me at any moment is thereby an inadequate account.

When someone says truly, "I ought to do so-and-so," he or she is not, of course, always acknowledging such a requirement. What discriminates the occasions on which such an obligation or requirement is acknowledged from those in which it is not? Kant believed that the two occasions could be distinguished by a reference to what he took to be the logical form of the sentence uttered. Only a categorical sentence, one containing no explicit or implied "if" clause, could express such a requirement. But on this Kant is clearly wrong. For although he was right to exclude such "if" clauses as "if I want to be happy" or "if I want to reach Boston within the hour" from such utterances, there may be other "if" clauses that are not only compatible with the expression of such an obligation or requirement, but that may throw light on its nature. They seem to fall into two classes.

The first class refers to the consequences for the agent him- or herself. "I ought to do so-and-so, if I am not to incur guilt," where guilt is to be contrasted with both regret and shame. If I merely regret doing something, then my concern is only for myself; if I feel shame, then my concern is for how I may be regarded by others. But if I acknowledge guilt, I understand myself to be in the wrong, to be a person whom others ought to view in a radically different light from previously, an outlaw from the moral order. (It may be that in using the words "regret," "shame," and "guilt" to mark these distinctions I am not using them in a way entirely consistent with ordinary usage, but I doubt if ordinary usage is itself internally consistent on these topics.) Thus guilt presupposes a moral order with which I can be at one or at variance.

Closely connected with this presupposition is the way in which an acknowledgment of guilt entails an admission of liability to repair in any way possible the wrong that has been done, to compensate, to make the world as nearly as possible what it was before I did evil. "I acknowledge my guilt, but I admit no obligation to make reparation," is, if "guilt" is being used as I am using it, self-contradictory. The discussion of guilt, shame, and regret has been of course clouded by the modern tendency to view them primarily as states of feeling. But although there are indeed feelings of guilt, shame, and regret, these may be appropriate or inappropriate, and they are appropriate only where an agent truthfully can acknowledge guilt or shame or regret, where the acknowledgment is of a concern or an obligation and not of a feeling. Thus the feeling states are secondary phenomena.

The second class of "if" clauses, which may occur in the expression of an absolute obligation or requirement of morality, refers to the consequences for the moral order which will be violated if the obligation or requirement in question is not upheld. They are of the form "if evil is not to enter the world." The concept of evil involved is the concept of that which is absolutely prohibited. No reason of any kind can justify or excuse the doing of evil. This, however, does not settle the question whether it may not on occasion be necessary to do evil in order, for example, to prevent a greater evil. But even if this is ever right, the moral agent who made this choice would not thereby be excused from the charge of having done evil. He would still need to acknowledge guilt, to receive forgiveness, to be reconciled. For the moral order is not necessarily a coherent one; demands may be made upon us such that we cannot meet them all and yet all are required of us, absolutely and unconditionally.

II

The accounts of this absolute and unconditional character given by moral philosophers all seem to encounter the following dilemma: *either* they distort and misrepresent it *or* they render it unintelligible. Teleological moralists characteristically end up by distorting and misrepresenting. For they begin with a notion of moral rules as specifying how we are to behave if we are to achieve certain ends, perhaps *the* end for man, the *summum bonum*. If I break such rules I shall fail to achieve some human good and will thereby be frustrated and impoverished. Virtues are dispositions, the cultivation of which will enable men to achieve the good, and defects in virtue are marks of a failure to achieve it. This is a scheme embodied in one way in Aristotle's moral theory, in another in J.S. Mill's.

There are two closely connected inadequacies in any account

which remains within the limits imposed by such a teleological scheme. The first is that it suggests that moral failure is like, say, educational failure. I set myself to get a degree in medieval literature, but I find Italian difficult and I give up temporarily or permanently. I am the poorer for not being able to read Dante in the original, and I am forced to recognize that my knowledge and taste are less adequate than they might be. But it would be parodying morality to suggest that my temporary or permanent failure to become truthful is a failure of the same kind as my failure to learn Italian; what is wrong with a grossly untruthful person is not that he has a less rich and achieved personality than a truthful man. The appropriate attitude to my own educational failure is regret, perhaps deep regret; the appropriate attitude to my own acts of untruthfulness is guilt.

Secondly what was wrong with the German professors and physicians at Auschwitz was not that they were not good enough, that they had not progressed far enough towards the *summum bonum*. It was that they were positively evil. Aristotelians characteristically treat indulgence in vices as failure to be virtuous; utilitarians characteristically treat goodness and badness as defined by one continuous scale so that "the bad" is simply "the less good." Evil is nothing other for both than an absence or deprivation of good. But the cruelties of the camps cannot be characterized as failures to be kind or sensitive. What the Nazis set up was a systematic inversion of the moral order in which virtues appeared as vices. "The new measures are so convincing," wrote Dr. F. Hölzel of the German euthanasia program in 1940, "that I had hoped to be able to discard all personal considerations. But it is one thing to approve state measures with conviction, and another to carry them out yourself down to the last consequences. . . . If this leads you to put the children's home in other hands, it would mean a painful loss for me. However, I prefer to see clearly and to recognize that I am too gentle for this work. . . . Heil Hitler!"[2]

An evil person is not just someone who has not yet approached the good closely enough; he or she is someone engaged in an attempt to disrupt the whole moral order by setting him- or herself and others to move in the opposite direction, in a positive cultivation of wickedness. It is complicity with positive evil that requires guilt and repentance, and for which regret is clearly inadequate.

Yet, those moral philosophers who have understood the inadequacies of teleological ethics—thinkers as various as Kant, Bradley, and Prichard—have tended to present the unconditional and absolute character of the central requirements of morality in a way which makes it difficult to understand their precise character. For Kant, the requirements of morality are requirements of practical reason; this makes it easy to understand why Kant tries to use a criterion of *consistent* universalizability to discriminate genuine categorical imperatives from false pretenders to that status, but very hard to understand the connection that he makes with the conception of *law* and of the respect required by law. For since "moral principles are not based on properties of human nature,"[3] since all positive knowledge is irrelevant, we cannot build up our conception of the moral law by any analogy with positive law, whether human or divine. Hence the concept of a moral *law* derives its absolute and unconditional character from elsewhere; indeed the movement in Kant's own thought is from the requirements of the moral law to those of positive law and not *vice versa*.

When later philosophers discarded Kant's theory, but retained his notion of the special character of moral duties, the character of this absolute and unconditional requirement of morality became even less intelligible. In Prichard's writing, for example, the claim is that there is a distinctive sense of the word "ought" which expresses the distinctive demand that morality makes of us. What is this demand? Prichard speaks of a feeling of imperativeness, but he only characterizes this imperativeness as that which morality makes us feel. Indeed it is clear that Prichard believes that we all know perfectly well what "ought" means in its distinctive moral sense and that it cannot be further explicated without circularity. Why is this so unsatisfactory?

Elsewhere,[4] I have compared the "ought" discussed by Prichard with "taboo" as used in the late eighteenth century in the Pacific Islands. Captain Cook and his sailors were told that men and women could not eat together, because it was *taboo*. But when they enquired what that meant, they could learn nothing except that it was an absolute and unconditional requirement which could not be further explained. We do not take *taboo* seriously; why then should we take seriously Kant's or Prichard's *ought*?

The dilemma, which I suggested earlier, can now be framed more clearly. Either we try to place the absolute requirement of morality in a teleological framework or we do not. If we do so place it, however, we find ourselves dictating and misrepresenting its character, as Aristotle and J. S. Mill do; if we do not, we find ourselves unable to discriminate this requirement from irrational demands for absolute obedience of a superstitious or neurotic kind. The relevance of this dilemma to contemporary discussions of medical ethics is clear. At the one extreme we have the warm partisans of voluntary euthanasia or of a pregnant woman's unlimited right to an abortion, at least within the first three months of pregnancy; at the other, those equally warmly opposed. The latter party see the first as having moved the obligations of the physicians on to shifting ground. If each particular case can be decided on its merits, no matter by whom, we lose the notion of an unconditional requirement on all human beings to abide by some general rule; and once we have abandoned that we shall have lost our hold on the central concept of morality. Hence, their fear, which appears so unreasonable to their opponents, that, if certain types of practice are permitted, in time anything will be permitted. Their opponents, in turn, see those opposed to liberal permissiveness in areas such as abortion and euthanasia as the victims of a superstitious fetishism, who are able to give no further *rational* ground for their moral appeal.

To understand that these contending groups reincarnate in their controversy a continuing dilemma of moral philosophy may make us a little more sympathetic to their stances. But it also suggests that to secure a reasonable consensus in medical ethics may require a solution to the problem posed by this dilemma. Where should we begin to look for such a solution? It is worth noticing at this point that Kant himself felt the pressure of some of the considerations which I have been arguing. I therefore turn from the Kant of the *Fundamental Principles* to the Kant of the second *Critique* and of *Religion Within the Bounds of Reason Alone* to consider Kant's own solution.

III

In Book II of the second *Critique*, Kant argues that if I seriously consider what is involved in the requirements of morality, I shall find that they commit me to a belief not only in freedom, but also in God and in immortality. Modern moral philosophers have, therefore, often wanted to detach Book I from Book II, following Heine in seeing the introduction of theological notions as essentially arbitrary. It appears to me that the introduction of these notions is much less arbitrary than is commonly supposed, because in understanding Kant's arguments a key step is passed over. Kant argues that it is a requirement of practical reason to pursue the *summum bonum*; that the *summum bonum* consists not merely of moral perfection, but of moral perfection crowned with happiness; that practical reason cannot require the impossible; and that the affixing of happiness to a completed virtue is possible only beyond this present world and by divine power. It is possible to quarrel with any of the first three stages in this argument. Some existentialist writers have suggested that precisely the impossible is required of us—hence the applicability of the myth of Sisyphus; and the very conception of a *summum bonum* has been put in question radically enough to make both the first and second steps doubtful. But most critics have not given sufficient emphasis to what is the key concept here, that of a moral progress.

Kant's conception of moral progress is inseparable from his conception of the radical evil in human nature. Men are not merely frail and so desirous of satisfying certain inclinations that they often act with mixed motives; their depravity lies in their deliberately preferring other maxims to those of morality. It is the universality of this depravity in the human species which leads Kant to speak of it as natural to man. And since Kant speaks of nature as that which is to be contrasted with the realm of freedom, the realm in which the maxims of the categorical imperative find their application, we may treat Kant's account of radical evil as in some sense empirical. Certainly he finds it easy to cite examples of moral evil; whereas he allows that we cannot be certain that there is even one actual case in which the maxims of the categorical imperative have been obeyed simply for the motive of duty. But if Kant's thesis is empirical we have not far to look for evidence.

Not one of the subjects in Milgram's famous experiments[5] refused to continue intensifying what they took to be electrical shocks administered to the body of a subject in a learning experiment before the level labelled *Intense Shock* (300 volts). Most went beyond this; and more than half to the limit. Milgram's sample of postal clerks, high school teachers, salesmen, engineers, and workers suggests what seemed also to emerge from denazification proceedings: that there was nothing psychologically extraordinary in the vast majority of concentration camp guards or S.S. men. The capacity for positive evil is indeed normally both restrained and disguised by social and institutional practice; it seems clear that what enabled Milgram's subjects to behave as they did was a definition of the social situation—that of a scientific experiment—that legitimated behavior not normally permitted; just as a definition of a situation as *a war* legitimates forms of behavior that individuals do not normally permit themselves. But this first crude sketch of a possible sociological explanation for such changes in behavior does nothing to displace the moral question: why and how to create social structures which do not distract agents from the unconditional requirements at the heart of morality.

How does the presence of radical evil in the world connect with the notion of moral progress? Underlying Kant's account of morality, concealed from view almost altogether in the *Fundamental Principles*, obtruding in the second *Critique*, and manifesting itself much more clearly not only in *Religion Within the Bounds of Reason Alone* but also and especially in the writings on history, is a crucial metaphor, that of the life of the individual and also of that of the human race as a journey toward a goal. This journey has two aspects. There is the progress toward creating the external conditions for the achievement of moral perfection by individuals: "with advancing civilization reason grows pragmatically in its capacity to realize ideas of law. But at the same time the culpability for the transgression also grows."[6] Within the framework of law and civility the individual progresses toward moral perfection, a progress "directed to a goal infinitely remote." It follows that the significance of a particular moral action does not lie solely in its conformity to the moral law; it marks a stage in that journey the carrying through of which confers significance on the individual's life. Thus a link does exist between the acts of duty and the *summum bonum* conceived as the goal of the individual's journey. Radical evil provides the obstacles both to the progress of the race and that of the individual. Without radical evil there would be no progress, no journey, for there would be nothing to overcome; without the *summum bonum* there would be no goal to reach by overcoming the obstacles.

Kant's moral philosophy thus has kinship to a whole family of narrative portrayals of human life, of which the Grail legends are prime examples. Human life is a quest in which a variety of dangers and harms may befall me; unless I am prepared to sacrifice my life on occasion I cannot achieve that which I seek. To fail to sacrifice my life, necessarily will be to fail as a man. The themes are originally perhaps Pythagorean and Orphic; they reappear in Plato's myths as well as in his attitude to the death of Socrates and they are crucial to Jewish and to Christian theology. In both Platonic and Judeo-Christian versions it turns out to be the case that *only* if I am prepared to—in some versions only if I do—sacrifice my life can I achieve the goal. Only if I place my own physical survival lower on the scale of values than other goods, can my self be perfected. Teleology has thus been restored but in a form very alien to either Aristotle's thought or Mill's. It is no wonder that Kant finds in Greek ethics no adequate conceptual scheme for the representation of morality, but views Christianity as providing just such a scheme.

So the basic thesis of Book II of the second *Critique* and of *Religion Within the Bounds of Reason Alone* can now be restated. Our moral experience presupposes the form of a progress toward a goal never to be achieved in this present world; but this in turn presupposes that the moral agent has a more than earthly identity, and that there is a power in the universe able to sustain our progress toward the goal in and after the earthly life. Morality thus does presuppose our own life after death and the existence of a power that we may call divine. Since the whole point of this power's activity, as belief in it is presupposed by us, is to bring about moral perfection and the *summum bonum*, we cannot, if we see rightly, see our duty as in any way different from the precepts of such a power. We must see our duties as divine commands.

This brief and compressed outline of Kant's account of the presuppositions of pure practical reason, highly inadequate although it is, suggests that the connection between Kant's conception of morality and his theological commitments is a great deal more plausible than is usually supposed. To put the matter crudely, it is beginning to seem that if you take Kant's account of morality seriously then you may find that *either* your position has to move steadily toward that of Prichard *or* it has to retain something uncomfortably like Kant's philosophy of religion. Most modern commentators on Kant have thought it deeply implausible that belief in the unconditional character of the absolute and unconditional requirements of morality should commit the agent to belief in God; but once it is seen that the choice is between God and Prichard, God may appear the less daunting prospect.

IV

Yet theologians will be ill-advised to seize upon this conclusion too eagerly. Every deductive argument is reversible. If I discover that my well-established belief that *p* logically presupposes a previously unaccepted and taken to be unacceptable belief that *q*, instead of accepting a commitment to *q* as well as to *p*, I may decide that the rational course is to reject *p* as well as *q*. The argument may move in either direction and I must find sure reasons for moving in one rather than the other. Moreover, we may be reminded at this point of the parallels between the concept of *moral obligation* as specified by Prichard and the concept of *taboo* as encountered by Captain Cook. That concept presupposed a more complex background of beliefs, but to recover that connection would not make belief in *taboos* more warrantable. We should merely understand how both background beliefs and the concept of *taboo* had to be rejected together. Perhaps in a parallel way belief in the absolute and unconditional character of certain moral requirements is discredited by its presupposing belief in something akin to Kant's philosophy of religion, rather than the latter made more credible by this presupposition.

What might lead toward this conclusion is the *arbitrariness* which the premises of all theological argument now seem to possess to those who do not already accept them. This sense of arbitrariness does not derive from the reading of skeptics, such as Voltaire and Russell, so much as from reading widely in contemporary theology. For the theologian in a secularized world finds himself in the following difficulty: *either* he is able to present his position in terms which are intelligible within that secularized world *or* he is not. If he is so able, then he may find himself in one of two difficulties. For either his assertions will conflict with some of the body of secular beliefs or they will not. The former possibility is less often realized these days than formerly; theologians no longer usually claim that certain features of the natural world require explanation in terms of the divine. But the latter possibility is all too real. A Bultmann decodes Christianity and what is left is—Heidegger's philosophy; a van Buren decodes it and what is left is. . . . To decode turns out to be to destroy.

It is the theologians who have resisted all decoding who preserve Christianity; and they do so by insisting that the secular world must accept Christianity on its terms and not on the terms of a secularized universe. It is no accident that Karl Barth is the greatest of modern theologians and that he characterizes the problem for the man who confronts Christianity as: "He has to speak about something of which no man can speak."[8] Or to put matters less dramatically, he has first to believe in order to be able to come to terms with belief—part of the message of Barth's book on Anselm. The theological universe depends on epistemological circularities. To this the rejoinder may be—it was the rejoinder of Raphael Demos, for example[9]—that the natural sciences also involve epistemological circularities, that the interpretations of the theologian raise no more grounds for unbelief than do the problems of induction. The force of this rejoinder ought not to be underrated, but it does not meet what is in fact the central difficulty.

The difficulty is that we all, including contemporary theologians, inhabit an intellectual universe in which the natural sciences are at home and theology is not. The believer has not only to make theological claims about the existence and nature of God, but he also has to make special epistemological claims about the character of his theological claims, if he wants to be heard. The unbeliever equally has to decide what grounds he might have for giving credibility of any kind to the theologian's interpretations. For both parties, the question of what would settle the argument has characteristically become unclear in a way in which it was not unclear either for medieval theologians or for eighteenth-century materialists. Hence the interesting irrelevance of unbelievers who focus their attack on the theses of the Middle Ages or the Reformation and of theologians who believe as though what they had to rebut was the atheism of the eighteenth or nineteenth centuries. Yet just because the argument between theologians and unbelievers is in this peculiarly contemporary state of unclarity, we may be brought back to something very like Kant's own position. For Kant's account of the limits of theoretical reason clearly excluded the possibility of finding good reasons for theological beliefs by means of theoretical enquiry. In other words, the *only* ground, according to Kant, for theological belief arises from the way in which morality presupposes a belief in God and in immortality. But this seems to be the outcome of the present argument too. Hence we may seem to be free not merely to reject theology, but to have no reason not to accept *both* such a dismissal *and* a concomitant dismissal of any absolute and unconditional requirement in morality. But is this really so? Do the absolute and unconditional requirements of morality and theological presuppositions of a Kantian kind really stand or fall together?

It is certainly worth noting that, as a matter of sociological fact, theological beliefs may not prove supportive of this central part of morality. Or they may assist in seeing as sacred and absolute obligations which are, on occasion, subversive of morality. There is no doubt that German Lutheranism did at least as much (to put matters charitably) to hallow the German officers' oath of allegiance to the Führer, and the German people's definition of their situation as one in which obedience to authority was paramount, as it did to underpin the resistance of the Confessional Church. Heydrich had a Lutheran upbringing; Himmler, Goebbels and Hoess came from strict Catholic families. Such considerations make the question of the last paragraph the more urgent.

V

I argued earlier that Kant's moral philosophy does have more of a teleological framework than is usually recognized, and I suggested that his teleology is less distorting to moral experience than Aristotle's or Mill's. I now need to amplify this point. I shall begin by considering two other defects in Aristotelian ethics.

The first is the dreadful banality of the true end for man when its content is finally made known. All those remarkable virtues are to be practiced, all that judgment and prudence is to be exercised so that we may become—upper middle class Athenian gentlemen devoted to metaphysical enquiry. What matters here is not just the unintendedly comic character of Aristotle's conclusion; any attempt to specify the true end for man by describing some state of affairs, the achievement of which will constitute that end, is bound to fail in a parallel way. That is why descriptions of heaven or of earthly Utopias, such as the communist society that Marx envisaged at the end of history, are seldom, if ever, convincing.

A closely related defect in Aristotle's view is that he is forced to take an entirely negative attitude to suffering and death. Hence his revulsion at the *Republic*'s description of the wholly good man suffering from calumny and torture and finally put to death. For Aristotle, as for utilitarianism, my death, if it comes too soon, simply frustrates the moral quest. For I will be deprived by death or suffering of achieving that state of affairs that constitutes *eudaimonia* or *the-greatest-possible-happiness-for-me-and-for-others* or whatever. It is then paradoxical that at the heart of morality there should be an absolute and unconditional requirement which may demand of me that I give up my life to prevent certain evils. For those who obey this demand are likely to be the very people who are frustrated thereby in the moral quest.

This is, of course, far more than an objection to Aristotle or Mill. It is a problem about the character of morality, not about the particular doctrines of any moral philosopher. On the one hand it seems difficult to make sense of morality except within some teleological framework; yet, on the other hand, at the heart of morality there lies this absolute demand so incompatible with most and perhaps all teleological theories of any power. Prichard, faced with this fact, separated moral obligation entirely from the exercise of virtues. The right and the good lose all connection. And this too seems thoroughly implausible.

What I want to suggest is that the mistake at the heart of most teleological doctrines lies in understanding the true end for man as a state of affairs. Christian teleology, as in Augustine or Aquinas, begins to approach nearer to the truth with its recognition that in this life we are always *in via*. But it retains the notion of a state of affairs in some other world as constituting man's true end; and it bequeaths this notion to Kant. Yet perhaps this too both can and ought to be expelled from our moral teleology. Perhaps we are *in via* in a more radical sense than even Christianity supposes. Consider the following possibility: that a crucial part of moral progress consists in learning how to transform our notion of moral progress, that the meaning of a particular life does not lie in attaining any particular state of affairs but in the agent's having traversed a course which is part of a larger moral history in which death and suffering are not merely negative deprivations. Indeed, it is at those moments at which risking death is morally required that an individual life is most clearly seen to have significance in the context of a larger history.

What kind of history could this be? The *Orestes* and the *Antigone* provide one type of example; the story of Abraham another; Livy a third; Guiccardini a fourth; the Marxist tradition a fifth. Such histories present human life as enacted dramatic narrative. The death of Iphigenia, the demand upon Abraham to take Isaac's life, the stand of the Horatii, the struggle of the Paris commune show that a conception central to such narratives is that of *sacrifice*, a notion totally alien to Aristotle or to Mill. If sacrifice is to be an intelligible notion, the individual has to be understood as a participant in the larger history of a group or an institution: the house of Atreus, the people of Israel, the city of Rome, the revolutionary proletariat. The enacted narrative of the individual's life derives its point from its place in the enacted narrative of the group or the institution. And this, in turn, may derive its significance from some more extended narrative. The most basic moral question for each agent is, therefore: of what histories am I a part?

How is such a question to be answered? Any acceptable answer must meet at least three requirements. First, only *true* stories are acceptable. Hence for us the interpretation of our historical existence cannot be mythological. The question of the criteria of truth for extended historical narratives is notoriously complex, and there may well be periods in which the conflicting claims of rival historical interpretations cannot be put to a finally decisive test. Secondly, the history of which I am a part must belong to some identifiable genre. The narrative that constitutes my life[10]—and not merely the reward of my life—may be tragic, comic, or of many other kinds. But as a narrative it must have some generic shape. The implicit assumption of many of our contemporaries is that the genre to which their lives belong is that to which Beckett's *End Game* also belongs.

Thirdly, any acceptable answer must do justice to the facts of moral complexity and more especially to the tragic character of human existence. This tragic character is inseparable from the relationship of the absolute and unconditional requirements of morality to guilt and evil. It puts the vulnerability and the failures of moral agents at the center of the moral picture. But it insists also upon giving a significance to that vulnerability and that failure of a kind that is implicitly denied in much contemporary writing about morality, both philosophical and practical. It is also worth noting that in a tragic perspective the activities of praising and blaming, of passing moral judgments, so central to so much contemporary moralizing, themselves become ambiguous activities about which we ought to practice a certain asceticism. For the individual who knows himself to be part of a moral history whose outcome is as yet unsettled may be less likely to claim prematurely that title of universal moral legislator that Kant bestowed on all rational agents and which has had such great effects on the character of moral activity.

At the heart of the difference in outlooks between, on the one hand, that perspective according to which the individual only has his moral identity as part of a larger history and, on the other hand, the prevailing moral views of our own culture, lie the individualist assumptions which have dominated both our social life and our moral philosophy since the early years of the bourgeois age. It was his reliance on such individualist assumptions which was responsible for the defects in Kant's treatment of the relationship between moral obligation and teleology. For Kant makes the significance of history depend on the moral progress of individuals rather than *vice versa*. Hence, death must be for him merely a negative boundary, and individual immortality is required for the only significant events that can take place after any individual's death. Hence, also, God is required as a power to give that moral form to the events in the after-life of individuals that Kant sees as lacking in the events of their mortal life. Kant's thesis that moral obligation necessarily presupposes teleology turns out to be correct; his thesis that teleology necessarily presupposes theology turns out to be incorrect. Hence the incredibility of Christian theology need not endanger belief in moral obligation after all.

VI

But what kind of teleology does the absolute character of moral obligation require? One apt immediate comment on my examples of moral histories would be that they are an exceptionally heterogeneous and various collection. Clearly, the moral structure of Greek tragic drama differs radically from that of early Hebrew narrative and so do both from the histories of ancient Rome or of renascence Italy. Yet these very different histories themselves stand in an important historical and moral relationship to each other; there is a larger moral history of which all these histories are themselves a part—and it is this that we inherit, or fail to inherit.

Kant's moral philosophy is itself yet another episode in this larger history and a peculiarly significant one. For in the seventeenth, eighteenth, and early nineteenth centuries, two rival currents of thought coexist uneasily in our predecessor culture. Both express reactions to the destruction of the classical or theistic view of the world; both inherit fragments from that view. The classical and theistic view of the world from its place in a cosmic order; the destruction of belief in that order seemed to some thinkers to reveal that human society was nothing but a set of isolated individuals. The task of philosophy was to show how, out of the experiences of such individuals, justified belief in an objective world could be constructed. Kant's genius was to show the impossibility of fulfilling this program either by rationalist or by empiricist methods. Rational belief in persons or objects cannot find its only basis in individual experiences; rational belief in moral precepts cannot find its only basis in individual feelings or goals. But Kant's great negative demonstrations of these truths were accompanied, in the name of individualist autonomy, by a divorce of morality from any social and historical context and a treatment of the social and historical as part of the realm of value-free fact. From which arises his difficulty in making absolute and unconditional obligation intelligible.

Yet counter to this development of thought, which moves from rationalists and empiricists through Kant to neoKantianism and empiricism, was the development of a quite different type of reaction to the loss of the classical and theistic world view. Its founder is Vico and it has later representatives in thinkers as different as Herder and Hegel. One of the most important theses shared by these thinkers is that individualism itself is most illuminatingly to be viewed as an episode in an enacted dramatic narrative, and that the moral history of individualism is, in fact, one in which the quest for individual autonomy is continuously frustrated. But if this is so, then the dilemmas within which the controversialists over absolute obligation in the realm of medical ethics have been imprisoned may be the outcome of viewing the problems of absolute obligation within an individualist framework. We could hope to escape those dilemmas, not by any attempt to find a theological solution—although as long as the problems remain in their present state there will be a recurrent temptation to seek such solutions—but only by a renewed criticism of the individualist framework and of the social institutions that sustain it and are sustained by it. More fruitful work in medical ethics requires new initiatives in general moral and political theory and in the philosophy of history.

NOTES

1. Leon Poliakov, *Harvest of Hate* (Philadelphia: Jewish Publication Society, 1954), pp. 185-6.
2. Ibid., pp. 186-7.
3. T. K. Abbott, *Kant's Critique of Practical Reason and other works on the theory of ethics* (London: Longmans, Green, 1873), p. 27.
4. Alasdair MacIntyre, *Against the Self-Images of the Age: Essays in Ideology and Philosophy* (London: Duckworth, 1971), p. 166.
5. Stanley Milgram, *Obedience to Authority* (New York: Harper & Row, 1974).
6. Immanuel Kant, *Perpetual Peace*, Appendix I. Professor Ramsey appears to think that Kant's moral philosophy is incompatible with any belief in moral progress in time and history. He can only do so by ignoring what Kant actually wrote about this and especially *An Old Question Raised Again: Is The Human Race Constantly Progressing?* (Both works cited in Lewis White Beck, ed., *On History*, [Indianapolis: Bobbs Merrill, 1963]).
7. Abbot, *Kant's Critique*, p. 220.
8. Karl Barth, *Römerbrief*, 2d ed. (Munich, 1922), p. 128.
9. S. Hook, ed., *Religious Experience and Truth* (New York: Collier, 1961).
10. Alasdair MacIntyre, *Epistemology and Dramatic Narrative* in *After Virtue* (forthcoming).

Commentary

Kant's Moral Theology or A Religious Ethics?

Paul Ramsey

I

THE FIRST TITLE GIVEN US for this conference was "Does Medical Ethics Need a Basis in Theological Ethics?" or ". . . Theological Ethics as a Foundation?" Whether under that head or under Alasdair MacIntyre's more limited title, I want first to indicate what a proper theologian should never attempt to demonstrate about the bearing of religion or theology on sorts of human activity other than the religious (or in particular on medical practice).

My sweeping disavowal, which brackets all of my following discussion, can best be expressed in three favorite quotations of mine which with increasing clarity and exactitude express the initial point I wish to make.

The first are the words of Paul Weiss in an article entitled "The True, the Good and the Jew,"[1] where he wrote: "It is desirable that religious men endorse and encourage the ethical life, but they have lost their religion when they forget that ethics must play a subordinate role. Ethics should, from the perspective of religion, stand to religion as the lower to the higher, the easier to the harder, the negative to the positive, commands to avoid to commands to do."

The second is Soren Kierkegaard's assertion[2] that "in our age speculative philosophy has arrogated to itself such authority that it has almost tempted God to feel uncertain of Himself, like a king who awaits anxiously to learn whether the Constitutional Assembly will make him an absolute or a limited monarch."

Best of all is the view of true religion obliquely voiced by C. S. Lewis's Screwtape, an archdemon, giving advice to his nephew Wormwood on how most shrewdly to tempt mankind into the service of "our Father below."

> . . . We do want, and want very much [wrote Screwtape] to make men treat Christianity as a means; preferably as a means to their own advantage, but, failing that, as a means to anything—even social justice. . . . For the Enemy [God] will not be used as a convenience. Men or nations who think they can revive the Faith in order to make a good society might just as well think they can use the stairs of Heaven as a short cut to the nearest chemist's shop. Fortunately it is easy to coax humans around this little corner.

I introduce Screwtape's advice into our present concern about the foundations of ethics not simply because of its pertinent medical reference to short cuts to the nearest chemist's shop. Its appropriateness is rather to be found in Screwtape's further enforcement of Wormwood's mission on earth in the service of "our Father below." He continues:

> Only today I have found a passage in a Christian writer where he recommends his own version of Christianity on the ground that "only such a faith can outlast the death of old cultures and the birth of new civilizations." [Then directly to Wormwood:] You see the little rift?[3]

The internal quotation is from one of Reinhold Niebuhr's early books entitled *Does Civilization Need Religion?* Which brings us back to our topic, Does Medical Ethics Need Religious Backing? Or foundation and warrant in theological perspectives?

If this brief introduction means anything, it means that as a theological ethicist I approach grappling with MacIntyre's essay with a certain divine nonchalance about the outcome. If Christian ethics exerted a shaping influence to date on our extant medical ethics (which no doubt it did), it was not because Christianity or Christian theological ethics took that to be one among its primary tasks. The same must be said about shoring up the shaking foundations of medical ethics today. To a religious man or to an authentically religious age it will seem self-evident that religion as a vocation, or rather as *the* vocation, of humankind should not be used as a convenience for anything else or anything less. If anyone needs religion in order to sleep soundly at night, or to endure the journey of life between drugstores, or as an engine behind extremely worthwhile social causes, or as enabling power to support already-known moral principles needing help, or to save civilization, or to undergird a physician's absolute loyalty to his patient—that is his problem. In any such situation, an authentically religious man will rightly suspect he is being asked to lend the dwindling allurements of religious platitudes to support worthwhile but weak or threatened earthly causes. A theological ethicist will know he is being asked to justify faith in God in terms of some other *plus ultra*. He has, properly, little interest in the success or defeat of Kant's enterprise, to which MacIntyre narrowed the question. I shall not join in treating God as a fool, not even to secure foundation for medical ethics. That explains my title.

II

"Medical ethics" can mean a number of things. So also does "theological perspective." These are the obvious variables. The Jehovah's Witness medical ethics in regard to blood transfusion certainly cannot dispense with a particular theological perspective. Medical practice can dispense with both, while leaving room for the right of a believing Witness to refuse treatment. On the other hand, the medical ethics produced by utilitarianism, cost/benefit analysis, or a teleological outlook that at no time finds good reason for preferring a righteous death to survival certainly needs no background justification in theological perspectives. Indeed, medical ethics in general may need certain theological perspectives in order to withstand the coming triumph of these viewpoints. Jewish medical ethics and Christian medical ethics in some of their features seem *prima facie* to require distinctive theological outlooks. The ethics and the theology were twin-born; they may also be Siamese, so bound together that they are destined to perish together.

There is, however, a third variable, namely, how justifying reasons found in theological perspectives are alleged to sustain or warrant the cardinal principles of a particular religious ethics or unconditional obligation. Kant's view is only one among many ways of relating unconditional moral requirements to a religious philosophy or outlook.

I propose, therefore, in this paper, first, to make a few comments on MacIntyre's chapter. These remarks concern points I judge worthy of note or needing further debate or clarification, and questions that remain at the end of his post-Kantian[4] critique of Kant. Then I shall simply set down a view of theological ethics that gives authorizing reasons for unconditional imperatives alongside of Kant's (and alongside the position MacIntyre develops by retaining a version of Kant's unconditional imperative and his view of radical evil enfolded into a philosophy of history that only by stipulation or as a consequence of future intellectual labors can, it is hoped, provide authorizing ground for such obligations).

1. MacIntyre clearly identifies the chief canon of medical ethics he means to espouse, namely, "the unconditional and absolute character of the doctor's obligations to his patients." If the doctor is required to treat the life of the patient as an object of unconditional regard and concern, MacIntyre observes that "it seems natural to say that he is required to treat the life of the patient as sacred." That canon of medical ethics is only a special case of the moral point of view in general. It rests upon "the simple obligation upon all of us to give up our lives rather than allow certain evils to occur; . . . any account of morality which does not allow for the fact that my death may be required of me at any moment is thereby an inadequate account."

Even here it is worth noting that MacIntyre speaks only of "certain" of a doctor's obligations to his patient. In any ethics, of course, only certain obligations are unconditional; others may not be. In this instance, however, MacIntyre stipulates that "we *omit* from view *all* the areas about which there is *now* argument and debate—voluntary euthanasia, abortion," etc. (italics added).

Then there "remains" a core of medical ethics that requires treating the life of the patient as an object of unconditional concern. The admission of cultural conditioning, the "now" looming historicism which triumphs in the end of the paper (along with collectivism over individualism in our approach to ethics) makes it a fair question to ask what future times may deem fit issues to omit. Peeling off the layers of a physician's obligation to his patient may, as in *Peer Gynt*, disclose that the onion has no core. This is only to say that if we reject the authorization Kant proposed for an unconditional obligation, along with more adequate accounts of a theological perspective, we need clear and crucial justifications to put in their place.

2. Clearly MacIntyre peels off very little. It is important for us "to enquire what grounds we have for such a commitment," I should say, not only because the German example shows how fragile medical commitment is, but also because of the absoluteness of the moral demand itself. MacIntyre's medical ethics seems on its face to be a prime example of an ethics needing theological justification, one that cannot dispense with any backing that anyone have good reason to believe forthcoming from theological perspective. For this cause also, the author pursues the question assiduously. For my part, I must say that MacIntyre is brilliant in criticizing what he rejects; obscure and futuristic when he tries himself to state the context of, or authorization for, unconditional obligation which he affirms to replace that of Kant or any other theological perspective.

3. MacIntyre's anti-theological feet are showing when he draws up the security of the warm blanket of the *facticity* of the modern world view around his neck. He speaks of "*arbitrariness* which the premises of all theological argument now seem to possess to those who do not readily accept them." That reads to me rather like a definition of *felt* arbitrariness. He basically assumes that we "inhabit an intellectual universe in which the natural sciences are at home and theology is not." He believes it is "certainly worth noting that *as a matter of sociological fact* theological beliefs may *not* prove supportive" of a central core of unconditional morality (italics added). MacIntyre suggests that we are equally free to reject theological justifications or to "accept a

concomitant dismissal of any absolute and unconditional requirement in morality." He states, *factually*, that "most modern commentaries on Kant have thought it deeply implausible that belief
in the unconditional character of the absolute and unconditional
requirements of morality should commit the agent to belief in
God . . ." That argument he expresses in *p's* and *q's*—as is the
custom among philosophers. "Every deductive argument is reversible," he writes. "If I discover that my well established belief
that *p* logically presupposes a previously unacceptable . . . belief
that *q*, instead of accepting a commitment to *q* as well as to *p*, I
may decide that the rational course is to reject *p* as well as *q*."

Concerning that, it must simply be said that MacIntyre has no
intention of abandoning *p*. He does not weaken the moral imperative. Therefore his statement that "*theologians* will be ill advised
to seize upon this conclusion too eagerly" (italics added) is a
statement binding him to establish *p* firmly on some other foundation than *q*. His warning to theologians that they not cite
theological perspectives as authorizing grounds for unconditional
obligation (for fear that their contemporaries are more likely to
abandon such an understanding of certain of their moral obligations) sounds like a threat or special pleading, and, moreover,
one MacIntyre is not entitled to use in good faith, since he
himself does not believe it permissible to abandon that moral
point of view (*p*).

The foregoing quotations from MacIntyre, however, do focus
our attention on "burden of proof" arguments. I do not suppose
that MacIntyre meant to count noses to settle intellectual questions, i.e., the number of persons now moldering in their graves
who believed the medieval religious world view against the number of moderns, living or dead, who believe the contrary. If not,
then what?

The claimed rational situation is as follows. Suppose someone
fifty years ago put forth the claim that parallel lines meet. He
would have borne the burden to show that was the case. A
properly operative "conservative" principle on the part of adherents of euclidean geometry rightly placed on him the burden of
proof. So it must be to a similar and proper conservative principle to which MacIntyre must appeal when he generally believes

that in our time and place theology has the task of making itself credible, and concludes that it fails.[5]

If MacIntyre's is not a nose-count argument, but more like the Quine/Ullian "conservative" principle, we still must ask: How should one in a secular age attempt to counter the burden-of-proof argument? One way to proceed is to contend that the original *casting* of the burden of proof on a religious view as against the secular view was a mistake.

Here for brevity's sake I simply appeal to my distinguished former colleague Walter T. Stace.[6] Concerning the world history of the seventeenth-century scientific revolution, Stace asserts that "no single discovery was made, no idea was put forward which, from the point of view of logic, should have had the slightest effect in the way of destroying belief in God. And yet the scientific revolution actually did have such an effect." That revolution produced a devastating effect upon the central beliefs of religion only because of "non-logical transitions due to suggestion and association."[7] ". . . The scientific picture of the world has penetrated the marrow of our minds. It has become an unconscious background of all human thinking." ". . . A view of the world as having no purpose, is not a logical transition. . . . Nevertheless the modern mind has made the illogical jump." The burden of proof placed on a religious perspective was simply a mistake.

That can, I think, be said while not forgetting that the *sort* of religious perspective Stace made room for was quite unlike the explanations and justification procedures for unconditional morality that are at home in Judaism or Christianity.

Moreover, there are sociological facts that are sufficient explanations of MacIntyre's sociological facts to which appeal may be made to explain the mistaken *casting* of the burden of proof upon a religious outlook in the modern age. One need not appeal only to erroneous extrapolations from "the world history of the seventeenth-century scientific revolution," as Stace does. That may have been only a ripple upon the modern mind in comparison to what C. S. Lewis believed was the most significant division in western history—"that which divides the present from, say, the age of Jane Austen and Scott"—namely, the machine and industrial civilization.[8] That presents a vast and overwhelming problem for, say, Christian apologetics; but it *ought* not to determine the "premises" upon which an intellectual builds his theological or philosophical edifice.

4. MacIntyre takes from Kant a notion of moral progress. (Below, I question this interpretation of Kant.) He affirms that "the significance of a particular moral action does not lie solely in its conformity to the moral law; it marks a stage in that journey the carrying through of which confers significance on the individual's life." Radical evil makes that journey significant; the *summum bonum* sets for Kant the goal. But MacIntyre objects to the notion of "moral perfection *crowned* with happiness" (italics added). He rejects Kant's "*affixing* of happiness to a completed virtue . . . possible only beyond this present world and by divine power" (italics added). Below we shall look at the account of moral progress MacIntyre endorses instead of Kant's.

Here my comment is directed to MacIntyre's understanding of Christian theological ethics which, he says, bequeathed to Kant the *addendum* of happiness to virtue, yet (MacIntyre acknowledges) held a more radical notion of *homo viator*.

MacIntyre's point is that Kant appealed to a "state of affairs," beyond all family resemblance to states of affairs we know, which would support our doing our duty to death. This is also his view of a defect in the Christian world view. He calls for a more radical understanding of *homo viator* than either the Christian or the Kantian expectation of a future, confirmatory "state of affairs" allows. Therefore, MacIntyre objects not only to some teleological doctrines because they mistake "the true end for man to be a state of affairs." This is also his objection to the Kantian appeal to the *summum bonum* and to ordinary Christian appeals to an ultimate congruence of duty with blessednesss. He wants to construe our moral lives to be always *in via*, radicalizing both Kantianism and Christianity.

While MacIntyre is correct when he says that the mistake at the heart of some religious teachings lies in understanding the true end of man as a state of affairs, he could go further than he has in disassociating Christian theology from such a view. That in this life we are always *in via* is a truth he takes from Christian theology. He then is left with a journey having no goal; mankind's moral history having no eventuality in a state of affairs.

But the goal need not be a state of affairs, or Kant's addendum of the *summum bonum* to a virtuous life. I grant, of course, not only that in popular Christian beliefs heaven is portrayed as a place where rewards are given to faithful persons.[9] I grant also that this is a prominent element in the portrayal of great theologians and religious literature such as the *Revelation of St. John* (all addressed, MacIntyre is correct, to sustaining the "patient endurance" of humankind *in via*). Still, a deeper comprehension of Christian theology will show, I think, that its great representatives have not been as trivial as Kant. Of course, I grant "the dreadful banality of the true end for man when its content is finally made known"—if that end is a state of affairs simply added to the Way thereto. However, the blessedness of heaven is *not* in happiness added, but simply and only the perfection of virtue, the completion of holiness, the achievement and gift of perfect love to God and love for one another in God. *That's* the happiness of it; no additional state of affairs needed. So here we have a journey with a goal whose goal is part of the journey. The Way participates in the End, and the End is the Way.

It is true that Christian theology spoke more often of the good than of obligation. So Augustine spoke of the enjoyment of God (fruition) and of the enjoyment of one another (fruition) in God as the supreme good or end of humankind. But that is also the good here and now.

5. In the end MacIntyre's position is a teleology without end. ". . . A crucial part of moral progress," he writes, "consists in learning how to transform our notion of moral progress." By that he means learning that an individual's moral progress is not located on the way toward an individual goal but rather "the agent's having traversed a course which is part of a larger moral history in which death and suffering are not merely negative deprivations. Indeed, it is at those moments at which risking death is morally required that an individual life is most clearly seen to have significance in the context of a larger history."

So a man may die for his country, but his country does not die for him. So also a physician may refuse to train Green Beret aidmen in medical arts, because he locates his life within a different moral history for which he is willing to suffer imprisonment rather than participate in evil-doing. Thus, in general, an individual's life "derives its point from its place in the enacted narrative of the group or institution." Those enacted narratives, in turn, derive significance from "some more extended narrative." Presumably, that more extended narrative is the moral history of mankind. But I do not know that this is MacIntyre's position, since at this point his paper ends with a summons.

One characteristic of an account of that larger moral history, of which all these histories are a part, seems clear. It must be a moral history "whose outcome is as yet unsettled." It must be a Way without End, which we inherit or fail to inherit. As likely as not that will mean making moral progress by, slowly over the decades, eroding certain unconditional moral obligations as we learn how to transform our notion of moral progress. For this reason, in an earlier version of my response, I said that MacIntyre must have a Cartesian "seeing eye" by which he perceives clearly and distinctly the validity of a physician's unconditional concern for the life of his patient. That must be a self-justifying claim. At least MacIntyre has not given us the authorizing context. He has called for one.

I am left with the feeling Soren Kierkegaard expressed about Lessing's conclusion, that if God held all truth [the extended history in which unconditional moral obligation finds authorizing reasons] in his right hand, and in his left the lifelong pursuit of it, he would choose the left hand.[10] Kierkegaard's comment[11] was: "When Lessing wrote these words the System was presumably not finished; alas! and now Lessing is dead." Likewise, MacIntyre sets out on the path of replacing superstitious fetishisms by rational ground for their moral appeal. In his case, however, it is stipulated that the outcome of our most encompassing narrative moral history remain unsettled.

By Jove, I do believe the watered-down Kantianism of R. M. Hare is to be preferred. Hare writes that the world must be believed to be such that the moral life is not pointless or futile.[12] He could have added (as Aquinas said at the end of each of his "five ways" of proving the existence of God): "and that men call God." Hare says something that seems reasonable and necessary to affirm, but casts it not in terms of "future states." He says not how; but yet there is an appeal beyond self-justifying moral grounds to the ultimate nature of the universe in which we live that prevents stringent moral requirements from being illusions or nonsense or arbitrarily terminal or threatened by erosion over the course of time. Indeed, I hold that all references to future "states of affairs" are only imaged or imaginative overflows from assertions about the present relation of reality to our moral obligations.

Alas! however, MacIntyre is still alive to rebut me.

6. We noted above that, when MacIntyre issued his warning to theologians, he stated that "every deductive argument is reversible." One can simply withhold his commitment to an unconditional obligation if belief in God or the *summum bonum* follows as a conclusion. I had not thought it proper to characterize Kant's method as "deductive." Instead, Kant's critical philosophy in-states a "presuppositional" method. The question of the First Critique, for example, was: What are the *conditions of the possibility* of scientific knowledge? Empiricism (induction) and rationalism (deduction) had failed to explain how knowledge of universal laws of the physical universe is possible. Kant took scientific knowledge to be possible and argued that any *necessary* presuppositions of that knowledge had to be equally valid.

The same holds for reason in its practical employment (moral reasoning). Having established (he believed) that moral reason legislates an unconditional obligation, Kant then asks: What are the *necessary* presuppositions and postulates of the categorical imperative? Not just any presuppositions or postulates that can be thought of or used in support of duty, but necessary conditions. Moral reasoning, as it were, must move on to religious reasoning, or else deny the undeniable. Kant's move is not reversible. His is *not* a hypothetical syllogism "*If p*, then *q*," where one is rationally free to deny the consequence *q* and then go back and call *p* into question. There is no "if-ness" about *p* in the first place. Moreover, "then *q*" refers to a class of assertions (by necessary presupposition) about the ultimate (noumenal) nature of the self, the world, and God that nothing observable in the phenomenal world could prove or refute. Indeed, antinomies or contradiction within reason in its pure or objective employment point to these unities as "ideals of pure reason" that are nevertheless unknowable to pure reason itself. So the way is open for the move from moral reason to the necessary presuppositions and postulates of religious reason. One must deny and then refute Kant's argument; it is not, I believe, simply reversible.

Parenthetically, we may ask why MacIntyre concentrates on God, immortality, and the *summum bonum*, and says nothing about freedom. The self's freedom is no less a necessary presupposition and postulate of moral reason (unconditional obligation). Kant's "I ought, therefore I can" is not a deductive argument (despite the "therefore" in that shorthand expression). Nor is it a hypothetical syllogism ("If I categorically ought, then I am free") which could be disconfirmed by scientific knowledge about the phenomenal self or the phenomenal world. Someone who has a distaste for human freedom (*q*), or who believes science rules it out, is not rationally at liberty to go back and deny *p* (unconditional obligation) since, according to Kant, that has already been firmly established by moral reason.

7. I have argued that Kant took from his upbringing in Lutheran pietism an inadequate notion of the *summum bonum* as a state of affairs "affixed" to a virtuous life. The blessedness of heaven, I said, lies essentially in the completion or perfection of the good or righteous wills of persons on the way there. What is the good now is the good then.

Still, Kant's understanding that happiness is only "added to" the good will reflects a paradox at the heart of Christian eschatology and ethics from the New Testament onward, namely, that blessedness is given only to those who love God for his own sake and love one another in God, with no motive arising from hope for happiness or any other reward. "Blessed are they who are persecuted for righteousness' sake [who do their duty for duty's sake, a physician's unconditional care for the preciousness of his patient's life, our simple obligation to give up our lives rather than allow certain evils to occur], for they *shall be* comforted" collapses into impurity of will if that comfort is in any measure the objective of our moral wills and actions. Indeed, the latter comes close to being Kant's definition of the radical evil in the human will, as it is also Luther's heavenly-oriented mercenary spirit for which there is no hope of reward.

In addition to Kant's answers to the question, What can we know? and to the question, What ought we to do?, the *summum bonum* provides the answer to his third question, What may we hope? Still that hope is not a goal to be morally willed; it is not pursued. Whoever seeks a life of happiness congruent with virtue shall lose it.

MacIntyre's rejection of Kant's "added" state of affairs, strangely enough, brings him closer to the narrative account of our moral histories contained in Christian and other religious outlooks (which he wishes to radicalize still further), and at the same time propels him further away from the Christian *homo viator* than Kant was. MacIntyre's radicalization of our human moral pilgrimage does more violence to (at least) the Christian story than Kant did. I also believe that he gives an inaccurate account of Kant's views, or at least that his rendition of Kant's meaning is a free, modern translation in which the original sense has been lost.

So we read that for Kant "it is a requirement of practical reason *to pursue* [italics added] the *summum bonum*," to seek moral perfection *crowned with happiness*. Heretofore, I have supposed that Kant taught that while we can pursue our neighbor's happiness but not his virtue, only moral perfection is the objective of our own moral wills, not our happiness. Again we read, in MacIntyre's rendition, that "the significance of a particular moral action does not lie solely in its conformity to the moral law; it marks a stage in that journey the carrying through of which confers significance on the individual's life." The latter expression, however eloquent a rendition, is obscure until we are told in the next sentence that "thus a link does exist between the acts of duty and the *summum bonum* conceived of as *the goal of the individual's journey*" (italics added).

How can this be? How can this be Kant? In the same paragraph Kant is quoted to the effect that "with advancing civilization reason grows pragmatically in its capacity to realize ideas of law. But at the same time the culpability for the transgression also grows." That would seem to be a stand-off, admitting no temporal moral progress at all. Still, MacIntyre assures us that within "the framework of law and civility the individual progresses toward moral perfection—a progress 'directed toward a goal infinitely remote.' " The latter internal quotation, I suppose, is from Kant. But MacIntyre transfers to the empirical, phenomenal world, and flattens out temporally, Kant's meaning of "infinitely remote" in order to ascribe to Kant or to derive from him some notion of historical moral progress. The same has to be said about MacIntyre's rendering of Kant as believing that "the life of the individual and also of that of the human race [is] a journey towards a goal."

How can this be? How can this be Kant? The word "journey" entails temporality, and we all know that, for Kant, time was a form of perception of the phenomenal world, not the world in which moral reason dwells.

Quite decisive is MacIntyre's admission that, while Kant's account of radical evil is in some sense empirical and abundant examples of moral evil can be accumulated from the moral history of humankind, "we cannot be certain that there is even one actual case in which the maxims of the categorical imperative have been obeyed simply from the motive of duty." If there is no actual case in the observable historical world or its institutions of which we can truthfully say that a moral agent obeyed the unconditional imperative simply from the motive of duty, how is it possible for anyone to appraise moral action by anything other than its interior conformity to the moral law? How could any moral agent locate any moral action, his own or another's, along the stages of a journey or a narrative history, or esteem any moral action because of its place in historical moral progress? How can anyone or how can social institutions learn in time how to apportion happiness to virtue if we can never detect a genuine moral act, if there is no way to infer from phenomenal actions to noumenal dispositions?

I draw two conclusions from the foregoing, one concerning Kant, the other concerning *tendencies* inherent in MacIntyre's position to which he certainly does not subscribe.

For Kant, there is no such thing as moral progress in temporal history. Moral progress conferring significance on an individual's life takes place only in the noumenal world. In that ultimately real world, a moral agent who acts in accord with his unconditional obligation can be described as someone who is now being righteous (he does his duty for duty's sake) and as someone who is now being made happy (by a scientifically unknowable "causality" not his own that "affixes" the *summum bonum* to his righteous moral will). Moreover, MacIntyre's charge that Kant is too individualistic is untrue. In the noumenal world, where alone moral progress is possible, the individual is a member of a "kingdom of ends."

MacIntyre, however, has transposed Kant's "link" between acts of duty and the *summum bonum* to the temporal, observable, phenomenal world. He has made the *summum bonum* something to be instituted and pursued by human moral agents.

There in the phenomenal world the pursuit of "moral perfection crowned by happiness" can only mean the pursuit of happiness—since there is no phenomenally evident case of moral obedience to the unconditional moral imperative simply from the motive of duty. If that is too strong a claim, let me suggest simply that, in aiming at the *summum bonum* in human history, one of its ingredients (happiness) is bound to prove more and more evidently able to be pursued than the other (unconditional obligation) in social history and institutions. This is especially the case if the "kingdom of ends" is shifted to the historical plane. MacIntyre's restoration of teleology may at first yield the perfection of the self by placing one's own physical survival lower on the scale of values than other goods. I venture to suggest *contra* MacIntyre that—if those are historical goods and goals—the yield is apt to be placing the preciousness of someone else's life also lower in some scale of values. The reader of this "debate" should at least be troubled by these possible consequences, since MacIntyre nowhere gives us the grounds or warrants for the unconditional obligation to which he subscribes, and his chapter ends in a summons.

I must, therefore, say that MacIntyre's reiterated allegiance to an unconditional moral obligation—as things now stand—is rhetoric only, or seeks its ground in a philosophy of history that, in any present moment, is not yet finished. This being the case, his summons that "a crucial part of moral progress consists in learning how to transform our notion of moral progress" seems apt to lead to peeling off more layers of the onion of unconditional moral obligation in pursuit of the temporally overriding happiness-aspect of the *summum bonum*. This is the more likely consequence of MacIntyre's location of moral progress in historical time where Kant located it not.

III

In this section I shall undertake to exhibit the religious perspective common and uncommon to Judaism and Christianity. My purpose is to show the appeals, warrants, outlooks that the Judeo-Christian tradition understands to be needed in explanation and justification of, say, a doctor's unconditional obligation to his patient. This will be to say more about that story, or extended narrative account, in which individual moral histories are set; the story of God's dealings with humankind that may require suffering or even martyrdom of us rather than complicity in evil-doing.

The view I mean to explain and espouse contains the source of its own moral norms within the religious dimension itself. God is worthy of worship because of who he is and his actions among men, and not because he incorporates in his commands the judgments men are capable of making without knowledge and acknowledgment of him. I do not deny the importance of the relation of Jewish and Christian ethics to natural morality. Indeed, for a complete ethics a Jew or Christian also needs judgments based on man's sense of justice or injustice. That, however, is not the concern of this paper. Instead, I want to explore the strictly theological ethics of Christianity (and of Judaism, so far as I may partially understand it[13]); and to show how religion is ethics and ethics is religion, without waiting for the addition of a natural or rational morality (however necessary the latter may also be). Such a view does not make morality *depend* on or *derive* from religion, or religion *depend* on or *derive* from morality. Neither is secondary to the other. Instead, the two are not at all separate things. The question simply does not arise whether God is worthy of honor and worship because his will and purposes are good, or his claims upon us and his purposes for us are right because he is good, in terms of antecedent or autonomous human conceptions of "goodness." The latter may, I have said, be also *needed* in a religious ethics.

The covenantal religious and the covenantal moral categories of the Bible are a way of saying that men "faith" in all their doing, and in all their doing, they and their communities "faith." The will of God constitutes the meaning, the cardinal content of morality; he is not simply the sanction of a morality that may be fashioned and fashionable apart from his righteousness. Nor is he there simply to "affix" happiness to virtue. Such is the common heritage of our three western religions, Judaism, Catholicism, and Protestantism.

My thesis is that the Jewish people and the Christian community in all ages are standing "metaethical" communities of discourse about substantive moral matters; they propose to shape and fashion how that discourse should proceed. This may be the way to understand Karl Barth's "Dogmatics as Ethics," Ethics as Dogmatics,[14] a program he executes everywhere in his systematic theology. There is no theological statement that is not at the same time an ethical claim, no ethical statement that does not indicate its theological reason. The metaethics function of religious faith and community, I suggest, is the way to understand statements like those of Emil Brunner: "What God does and wills is good; all that opposes the will of God is bad" and "The Good is that which God does; the goodness of man can be no other than letting himself be placed within the activity of God."[15] Suchlike theological ethical statements are first to be understood as meta-ethical *definitions* of the good.

In order to explain this thesis I shall make use of what Professor William K. Frankena has written about metaethics. Since "performative language analysis" is a proper and the most profound way to understand the covenantal *normative* ethics of the Bible, I shall also draw upon that school of thought. My use of these philosophical positions requires no "decoding"; quite the contrary. Only for brevity's sake need these philosophers be invoked at all. In what follows, I hope simply to enable the reader to follow Wittgenstein's counsel to "look and see" the use to which religious ethical concepts are put.

In trying to understand theology (and behind every theological formulation, the faith-ing of religious men) to function as a metaethics, we need to learn from what Frankena has written concerning a "*normative* metaethics" in distinction from a simply descriptive, elucidatory or reportive type of metaethics.[16] The latter analyzes the meaning that "right," "good," and other ethical terms have in ordinary moral discourse, how they function in *the* or in *an* extant moral language. Reportive metaethics attempts "to lay bare what we actually mean when we judge that something is good or right."[17] But behind every descriptive or elucidatory metaethics, Frankena contends, there is a *normative* metaethics, i.e., a proposal for how ethical terms *should* be used. This may be hidden from view, because the *normative* metaethics behind a number of elucidatory analyses of moral discourse is a *conservative* one, i.e., a proposal that moral terms should continue to be used in the way and with the meaning described as being the case. It is only when someone or some community of men come forward with a *revisionary* proposal, a reforming normative metaethics, that the distinction between normative and descriptive metaethics becomes quite evident.

There are a plurality of universes of moral discourse. Within each of these a descriptive account can attempt to lay bare what "we" actually mean when "we" judge that something is good and right. Such descriptions of the meaning of ethical terms have already the force of a *normative* metaethical statement, i.e., that we ought readily to conclude that what "we" mean "men" mean (or should mean) when they judge that something is good and right. Among normative metaethical communities, for example, is one that would *reduce* the meaning of ethical terms to nonmoral meanings, whether by shouting silence in a loud metaethical voice, or by recommending that the terms continue to be used but henceforth only with the meaning some science gives to them. ("An 'onlook which rejects onlooks,' " Evans writes, "is perhaps what some people have called 'the scientific attitude.' "[18]) Most contemporary philosophers do not subscribe to such a normative metaethics.

Also among the plurality of universes of moral discourse are the world's living religious communities. Philosophers do not seem to be able to take the language of these communities with utmost seriousness, even though they generally have concluded that there is more than one meaning for a term, and that one must simply listen to hear what is meant. At the center of every congregation of church and synagogue, men and women are continually giving themselves, renewing and enforcing, from the faith that has brought them together, the meanings that are appropriately to be used in making moral appraisals.

A report that the world's living religious communities are among extant *normative* metaethical proposals may be simply to

report mankind's ethical division at its deepest level. Nevertheless, a religious community that is living from the past through
the present into the future is surely engaged continually in recommending or conveying its view of what should be the meaning of
the terms of future moral discourse.

Its reasons for doing so are at bottom religious or theological
reasons, or else it has slipped from being religion. There is
nothing wrong with offering theological considerations as good
reasons for moral meanings. Frankena can be called to testify to
that, in his contention that a good reason in support of a normative metaethics may be either a good *moral* reason or a good
reason of some other sort. ". . . An inquiry into the meaning and
logic of moral discourse may be normative without being moral.
Normative judgements and proposals [in metaethics] are not necessarily moral."[19] The judgment, for example, that we should in
normative metaethics presume that revisions are not to be advo-
cated unless necessary (which goes to support our continuing to
use ethical terms with the meaning they currently have among
some groups of human beings) may not itself be a *moral* reason.
Likewise, a "people of God," a people in the service of God,
proposes to understand the righteousness by which it judges
performances among men according to the measure of the righteousness it believes God displayed in his word-deeds intervening
in times past in men's deeds and moral talk. Such a community
of moral discourse is, formally, like any other under the sun, in
this case plainly giving non-moral, i.e., religious, warrants for its
"first order" moral meanings.

Frankena formulates the place in normative metaethics that
Christian theological ethics, faithful to its task, must occupy.
There are statements at the heart of any theological ethics that
refer for the meaning of "good" or "right" to "the will of God"
or to "how God brought us up out of the house of bondage" or
"how God first loved us." These religious acknowledgments or
faith commitments refer the "correlative performative force" of
man's obligation to a "divine performance." "[A] human utterance concerning this divine performative is a self-involving acknowledgment which has correlative performative force."[20] A
believing community affirms that it is placed under obligation by
the actions of another (as in gift-giving). Performative language

analysis in ethics need not be limited to *human* word-deeds (which is the usual understanding of this school of thought).

Such statements are usually objected to in ordinary language analysis on the ground that one cannot derive an Ought from an Is. This reply takes classically the form of "the open question" argument. That is to say, the rejoinder in the case of any alleged theological ultimate will be, "But is 'the will of God' or that divine performative action *good*?" Frankena contends, and I think rightly, that the objector can only riposte a *like* normative meta-ethical statement; he can say "surely this is not a desirable use of words,"[21] or the meaning that should be assigned the terms "good" or "right" or "obligatory." It is perfectly proper for a normative metaethics (e.g., Jewish or Christian theological ethics) to appeal to reasons that are not themselves intrinsically moral. One appeals rather to God's word-deeds in the extended narrative moral history of our lives.

Good reasons in Jewish or Christian normative metaethics cannot without circularity themselves fall within the system of Jewish or Christian normative ethics (e.g., forgiveness is good). Nor can such good reasons be drawn from *another* normative metaethics with its *prescriptions* as to what moral terms must mean and how be used. That would simply show the dissolution of church or synagogue. There is no need for Jew or Christian— either in normative ethics or in normative metaethics—to be "frightened out of our wits by the relativists, subjectivists, and sceptics,"[22] or by MacIntyre's appeal to an as yet uncompleted moral history of mankind, when they are only explaining the reasons they affirm to be good ones in support of a certain use of moral terms, and appealing to the religious foundations in which they believe unconditional moral obligations to be grounded. Frankena concludes (in language that itself shows, verbally at least, the influence of Christianity functioning as a standing meta-ethical community by going beyond laying bare the meaning of ordinary morality and undertaking to affect what men shall mean by "good," etc.): ". . . Perhaps we may now roll away the stone from before the tomb in which naturalism [and also what is called 'supernaturalism'] has lain ever since that day when the earth trembled under the naturalistic fallacy and the rocks were rent by the open question."[23] Those objections to Jewish or

Christian theological ethics (even in the mind of a philosopher who himself does not undertake its task) fall before the simple realization that "No metaethical Ought can logically be derived from any metaethical Is alone."[24] It is perfectly proper for the synagogue or the Christian church throughout history to have proposed the meanings it intends to assign to certain primary ethical terms, and to have tried to influence men to come and do likewise, on grounds not all of which are already intrinsically moral, i.e., falling within the Judeo-Christian system of ethics or borrowed from some other.

So much is at stake in saying that Our Father in heaven is the Name from whom the meaning of all performatives (like all fatherhood) in heaven or in earth is taken. This I suppose can be more simply stated by saying that Jewish and Christian ethics makes ultimate appeal to a divine performance, making prototypical use of something that is also said in the analysis of human performatives, namely, that it is not only one's own committing action that creates an obligation; one can also be put under obligation by another's conduct rather than by one's own,[25] as when a beggar asks us for help or in claims upon our hospitality or in the so-called "Good Samaritan" principle in our law. This does not mean that God is good because he is a father; but the claim is that from the measure of his steadfastness we know something of the meaning to assign to "good" fatherhood. It does not mean that God's performative actions are to be acknowledged because they have a moral quality gathered from men's committals, but rather that from the nature of his self-involvement with us in our history we know something of the self-involvement men should display in their elected and their nonelected covenants of life with life. If, as Helen Oppenheimer writes, "to marry, to become a parent, to make friends, is to put oneself morally into a distinct situation," then ". . . a fortiori, to be made God's children by adoption and grace can be understood as a change of status capable of transforming one's elementary categories."[26]

It is not at all necessary to prove first by a general or autonomous ethical investigation the correctness of such normative ethical statements as that we should be thankful to all who benefit us or that we should forgive others because others have forgiven us;

or that one should obey God's ordinances because it is "right" to do so or that God's will is "good" according to tests for this that have arisen in some other community of moral discourse, or according to an elucidatory metaethics that describes the meanings and logic and what men mean by good in some other "ordinary language." This is not necessary even though there are good reasons for some or many of these statements in a good many systems of normative ethics. It is not necessary because all these are statements of *normative* Christian metaethics (and, I venture to say, normative Jewish metaethics as well). Those statements express what Jews and Christians mean and are resolved to mean by the right and the good among men. Synagogue and church propose to inculcate an entire "symbolic form," "type of discourse," or "realm of meaning."[27]

Whether this means a *revisionist* or a *conservative* normative metaethics can scarcely be decided. It is conservative in the sense that there are these standing metaethical communities whose moral discourse can simply be elucidated or described in these terms, plus the recommendation that these moral meanings and this logic of ethics continue to be fostered and used. It is *revisionist* in the sense that, amid the pluralism of discourse today about ethics, these understandings of the elements of ethics would cut athwart many an all-too-ordinary language or rival normative metaethics—so much so that the Christian language and logic of ethics is hardly understandable today to a good many notable intelligences, including some who are by denomination "Jewish" or "Christian."

In any case, Jews and Christians mean or should mean in ethics to say that there are correlative performative understandings of moral acts, relations, and situations that arise from their faith-commitment or acknowledgment of God's performance and his mandates. This they mean to say in some sense also of all men and their good always. This they express when they say, "I look on all men as brothers whom God made to be one," or "I look on each man as a brother for whom Christ died."[28] In these primary "norms," which are controlling, certainly, in a Christian ethical system, there is appeal to the performative force of God's "verdictives"; and then there follows for the Christian ethicist the task of living the meaning of this in all his rational reflection, and of elaborating and deepening every one of its requirements.

This, I suppose, is not far from Frankena's meaning when he speaks of adopting an "appropriate mode of expressing oneself when one is taking a cognative point of view and meaning to be rational within it"; or when he writes that in making a normative ethical judgment, we mean to suggest "that there are good reasons for a certain action or attitude, and we usually have in mind more or less clearly a certain type of reason, that is, we are taking a certain point of view and claiming that one who is rational from that point of view would or would not have that attitude or perform that action."[29] If one *begins* in Christian normative ethics with some such statement as "Look on all men as brothers for whom Christ died," or "Be grateful to the Lord who made us his covenant people," and if all moral reasoning is then reasoning from these "premises," then the ultimate warrant for moral norms must be an appeal to what the Lord of heaven and earth is believed to have been doing and to be doing in enacting and establishing his covenant with us and all mankind, in all the estates and orders and relations of life to which we have been called. These performative actions, the final authorizing reasons for normative ethics, are celebrated in the action and worship of synagogue and church through all ages. This is what makes a religious community a standing normative metaethical community. Within the larger setting of these narrative histories, it is proposed to show our children's children (if not our children) what should be the meaning of "righteousness" and "faithfulness" among men.

Church and synagogue are communities of adoration, remembrance, celebration, worship, and praise. These communities engage in faith-ing whenever by common liturgical action or procession they say forth their faith by doing; or when by song, recital, confession, reading, or preaching they, by saying, do. These acts-speech and speech-acts are understood to be human performatives in response to a divine performative. Each of these faith-acts and faith-statements of a congregation is at the same time a way of talking about ethical talk, a way of conveying and fostering what the community means to mean by righteousness.

Doubtless, religious folk also belong to other communities of moral discourse; this does not concern us here. Insofar as they have religion in exercise, however, they are also saying how they want to say the ethical thing, how they want the ethical thing to be said in their midst, in society generally, and in the future, how they want their moral behavior and that of other men finally to be judged. They nurture meanings in the ethical terms they use. They transmit from generation to generation "second order" instruction in what *should be* the "first order" meaning, out of faith in and love to God, of the terms used in ethical deliberations and moral decisions and actions.

If the question is how one should treat a wanderer, the answer terminates not in the proposition that wanderers should be cared for for their manhood's sake, but in: "A wandering Aramean was my father, yet the Lord called him" and made something of us. If the question is how to treat strangers, righteousness takes its measure from, "You know the heart of a stranger, since you were strangers and sojourners in the land of Egypt; and the Lord your God acted rightly by you when he brought you up by a mighty hand, and so rightwised your dealings with every stranger." In *giving* that meaning to "righteousness," Judaism in its normative metaethics does not need to go further and reduce its religious reasons to generally valid ethical statements, like: Be grateful for gifts of rescue. "Hear, O Israel, the Lord thy God is one God, extending his steadfast love (*hesed*) to thousands of generations, and thou shalt love the lord your God with all your heart, soul, mind and strength" is sufficient in itself to convey the meaning of fidelity to every covenant.

"Love one another *as I have loved you*," "Have this mind in you which was also in Christ Jesus . . ." and "God shows his love for us in that while we were yet sinners, helpless, his unreconciled enemies, Christ died for us" may be outlandish proposals for the meaning of "charity" and its primacy in moral discourse; but there is no formal reason requiring anyone to give up using the term in that way or trace it home to another moral meaning having greater currency. If the question is "Why look on each man as a brother for whom Christ died?" the answer need not be "Because that is 'good.' " The answer can perfectly well be, "Because he *is* a man for whom Christ died and that's the rock-bottom meaning we mean and shall continue to mean by 'righteousness' and 'fidelity' to the 'good' for him" (whatever source there may be for getting to know needed additional and the more specific meaning these claims have).

In this way Jewish and Christian ethics makes ultimate appeal to a divine performance as the ground for and the source of the core-content of men's correlative obligations to one another. The theology of the Exodus is at the same time an Exodus morality. A Christocentric theology is at the same time a Christo-*nomos* and a Christo-*didacti* in ethics. Jewish or Christian ethics would no more propose to establish themselves upon the foundation of men's general moral insights or judgments, than Jewish theology propose to prove the God of Abraham, Isaac and Jacob or Christian theology propose to prove Jesus Christ worthy of lordship because he measures up to men's general knowledge of God. In either case, if that were so, men should simply resort at once to that other knowledge of God and to that other lead given to morality. The Judeo-Christian knowledge *into God* and the knowledge *into ethics* in these religions would, by such a procedure, be simply bypassed or rendered dubious in ostensible certification of them.

The vitality of church-community has a great deal to do with what we in our generation and the generations to come shall mean by righteousness, justice, and injustice. What Christians owe to Christians and to all men, because they look upon men as brothers for whom Christ died, has also some degree of influence upon what men acknowledge to be the claims of mankind upon them. (The same can be said of every "high" or universal religion.) The actions of church and synagogue as communities of adoration, celebration, worship, and praise constitute a wellspring of ethical terms and judgment having the highest significance for human actions and relations. Where they have not made themselves a convenience—an engine behind other communities of moral discourse—synagogue and church are normative metaethical communities existing through time. From faith's apprehension of the chief end of man, its pursuit of the highest and universal vocation of man, its narrative account of the moral history our lives inherit or fail to inherit, and its vision of reality flow substantive moral claims. Any "faith-ing" serves to intervene in any talk about the normative ethical terms men should be using in every substantive moral deliberation.

In our pluralistic society there are, of course, many communities having moral significance. But this simply means that every man must decide the community of moral discourse to which he belongs, and whose continuation into the future he seeks. Each of us has to decide how he wants the ethical thing to be said in our society, by what standards of righteousness or faithfulness he is willing for his own action and those of other men to be judged. In faith-communities of all sorts is laid bare what men finally mean when they judge something to be good or right. We form our consciences and shape our behavior in accord with some community of ultimate reference in terms of which we understand what we should mean by the right and the good. This establishes a community of moral discourse in which these meanings are enlivened and renewed and transmitted to future generations of mankind. By a person's answering religious performances to the verdicts or performances of the God confessed, his status, role in life, basic moral standards undergo significant alteration.

To repeat the foregoing in another way. N. Fotion argues[30] that a speaker may include in the content portion of a language act the form and character of his speech to follow. Then that was a Master Speech Act, like: Come, let us reason together; hereby other language acts are given a certain ordering. Variations in the content portion of a spoken formula can control important aspects of the use of language to which we are thereafter committed. There are Master Speech Acts that do a job for subordinate speech acts. Something is said that applies to a whole conversation, discussion, book—or a realm of moral discourse—that follows. Master Speech Acts generate, control, or have jurisdiction over new and subsequent speech acts. They do not simply *report* what the following speech acts are or will be; they *express* forcefully what the following speech acts *should* be. A Master Speech Act is therefore indivisibly connected with those speech acts over which it has jurisdiction; the reasoning-together announced is not a separate or another thing from reasoning-together in execution. Subsequent speech acts are "in" or "out" of character according to the meaning set by the content portion of the Master Speech Act.

Fotion's analysis can be extended from performative language to actions that speak. That is the meaning of "liturgy." In liturgy, the synagogue or church by saying do, and by doing say. Not only can a *speaker* control the character of his subsequent language acts. Also a speech-*actor*, by master acts of non-verbal religious acknowledgment, exercises command over his subordinate (moral) performative word-deeds. Faith-acts or religious acknowledgments of divine performances are Master Speech Acts, whether of a religious individual or a religious community. The "content portion" of the verbal or non-verbal "faith-ing" of men and of communities varies. It varies according to the divine performance or according to the nature and character of the god confessed. Subsequent acts are "in" or "out" of character with that.

Whoever *acknowledges* with Abraham Lincoln, "Four score and seven years ago *our fathers* brought forth on this continent a new nation conceived in liberty and dedicated to the proposition . . .," thereby dedicates himself to future performatives of like character. (He derives, if some say so, an "ought" from an "is.") Likewise—if men may be obligated by the action of another—whoever says with the prophet Hosea, "When Israel was a child [when *we* were children], then I [the Lord, *our* God] loved him, and called my son out of Egypt. . . . I taught Ephraim also to walk, taking them by their arms. . . . I drew them with cords of a man, with bands of love . . ." (11:1, 3a, 4a), whoever acknowledges and adheres to this divine performance, whoever "faiths" in this way, dedicates himself to future performatives of like character (thereby deriving, if some say so, an "ought" from an "is").

One might argue, of course, that statements of the religious warrants are not value-free, that the "content portion" of statements about a divine performance or the divine nature, or in the narrative account of our histories are not value-free; and that consequent statements of men's correlative beliefs are not simple statements of (theological) fact. One can search for a prescription in there somewhere. Thus one might avoid saying that religious ethics derives ought-statements from is-statements strictly construed. It is more correct, however, and more forthcoming, simply to deny that the supernaturalistic fallacy is a fallacy.

It is better, in explanation of religious ethics, forthrightly to appeal beyond all human righteousness to a divine performance in which the righteousness of God was revealed "from faith to faith" for us men and for our salvation—and for men's judgments and appraisals, too. Only then will one find himself discussing theological ethics or even the *possibility* of a religious ethics, and not something else.

IV

One final word about the account of religious ethics outlined above. In a religious ethics, the "justifying reasons" are at the same time the "exciting reasons" (Francis Hucheson).[31] MacIntyre may doubt my view that his unconditional moral obligation, no less than Kant's, needs theological authorization. In any case, I think it cannot be denied that neither view of obligation is explicable historically, culturally, or in point of origin without reference to some sort of "divine command" account of the moral life or a theological perspective upon human beings as created in the "image of God." The source of an unconditional obligation, tested by suffering and giving up one's life rather than to do or to allow evil to be done, is to be found in the web of authorizing and exciting reasons that once were the fabric of our civilization. In numerous works of philosophical ethics today after "the moral point of view" has been fully set forth, there is yet another chapter called for, one usually entitled "Why Be Moral?" Given the univocity of the authorizing and the exciting reasons in religious ethics, no such chapter is needed.

As philosophy bakes no bread, it also rarely produces a cultural movement capable of shaping moral practice to the standard of stern moral laws. The Presocratic philosophers were often the founders of a quasi-cult. This Justice Blackman noted when he called the Hippocratic Oath a "Pythagorean manifesto,"[32] in its condemnation of abortion uncharacteristic of Greco-Roman medicine, which Christianity happened to take up and use to influence Western civilization (no mention made of the fact that pre-Christian morality also condemned neither the exposure of infants nor sports spectaculars in which gladiators killed one another).

There are, of course, other philosophies which, like the great religions, have shaped the moral thinking and behavior of masses of mankind. The chief example in modern times is utilitarianism (which MacIntyre regards as quite incapable of producing an authentic moral point of view) and Marxism (which I doubt can be credited with sustaining MacIntyre's belief that the moral history of mankind—and within that history, the moral history of individual agents—is more important than its medical or economic history).

MacIntyre may have to follow Voltaire's advice to get himself crucified and found a religious movement in order to halt the onward march of utilitarianism as a dominant influence upon medical and moral practice (however philosophically discredited that position may be). So also, Hans Jonas's ontology of purposive being's absolute obligation to protect purposive being into the future, against all the pre-mortem threats of modern technology, reflects along every vein and sinew the Biblical outlook of a Fackenheim who says that—for all the problematic of believing in God after the Holocaust—we Jews ought not to give Hitler a posthumous victory. So across the Holocaust the generations pick up again the story of God's dealings with them.

There seems to me to be good authorizing and exciting reasons for going beyond what MacIntyre and Jonas regard as the terminus in philosophical justification. That, I suggest, seems to be a sufficient terminal justification only because of precedent religious or cultural movements. And I am certain that, if MacIntyre and Jonas are concerned that their views influence a professional practice, they have good reason to appeal to an existing movement which is the bearer of such absolute moral claims, or they must set about creating their own cults in the hope that they will grow to have general influence in contemporary cultures. One thing that will not do the job is MacIntyre's appeal to a philosophy of history yet to be completed.

NOTES

1. *Commentary*, 2, no. 4 (October 1946), p. 316.
2. Soren Kierkegaard, *The Concept of Dread* (Princeton, N.J.: Princeton University Press, 1944), p. 134n.
3. C. S. Lewis, *The Screwtape Letters* (New York: The Macmillan Co., 1944), pp. 119-20.
4. I use this term because it is more neutral than "Hegelian" or "Marxist" or "historicist."
5. See W. V. Quine and J. S. Ullian, *The Web of Belief* (New York: Random House, 1970), p. 43ff, for an account of the conservative principle: an hypothesis proposed for our belief "may have to conflict with some of our previous beliefs; but the fewer the better."
6. *Religion and the Modern Mind* (New York: Lippincott, 1960), pp. 90, 94, 107, 109.
7. For example, "the terrible gulfs of time which have elapsed since God made himself manifest in the world chill our minds and numb our hearts. This train of thought, of course, is not logic. But logic has little to do with human thinking" (p. 98).
8. C. S. Lewis, "De Descriptione Temorum." Inaugural Lecture at Cambridge. Walter Hopper, ed., *Selected Literary Essays* (Cambridge University Press, 1969), p. 7.
9. Paradoxically, in Christian eschatology, e.g., in Luther, rewards are given only to the pure in heart, i.e., only to those who serve God for his own sake with no motive arising from hope for reward. Moral progress is not measured by approximation to a future state of affairs.
10. Lessing, *Werke* (Maltzahn's ed.) X, p. 53.
11. Soren Kierkegaard, *Concluding Scientific Postscript* (Princeton, N.J.: Princeton University Press, 1941), p. 97.
12. R. M. Hare, "The Simple Believer," in Gene Outka and John P. Reeder, Jr., eds., *Religion and Morality* (Garden City, N.Y.: Doubleday Anchor Book, 1973), pp. 393-427.
13. I believe I am not mistaken in what I affirm about Jewish ethics. My account, however, is clearly inadequate in what I omit: the role of law and the tradition of rabbinical interpretation.
14. Karl Barth, *Church Dogmatics*, I/2 (Edinburgh: T & T Clark, 1956), p. 782-96.
15. Emil Brunner, *The Divine Imperative* (London: The Lutterworth Press, 1932), pp. 53, 55.
16. William K. Frankena, "On Saying the Ethical Thing," Presidential

address delivered before the Sixty-Fourth Annual Meeting of the Western Division of the American Philosophical Association in Minneapolis, Minnesota, May 5-7, 1966. *Proceedings and Addresses of the American Philosophical Association*, 1965-6 (Yellow Springs, Ohio: The Antioch Press, 1966), 39, pp. 21-42.

17. Ibid., p. 22.
18. Donald Evans, *The Language of Self-Involvement* (London: SCM Press, 1963), p. 254.
19. Frankena, "On Saying the Ethical Thing," p. 23.
20. Evans, *The Language of Self-Involvement*, p. 77. The reader's attention should be directed to the fact that, in the text above, this point and this point alone is used in elucidating the nature of a religious ethics. Here I am not concerned with other aspects of the performative language school of ethics as developed by Austin and Evans.
21. Frankena, "On Saying the Ethical Thing," p. 25.
22. Ibid., p. 32.
23. Ibid., p. 33.
24. Ibid., p. 25.
25. John Lemmon: "Moral Dilemmas," in Ian T. Ramsey, ed., *Christian Ethics and Contemporary Philosophy* (New York and London: The Macmillan Co., 1966), p. 264.
26. Helen Oppenheimer, "Moral Choice and Divine Authority," in Ian T. Ramsey, ed., *op. cit.*, p. 231.
27. See Frankena, "On Saying the Ethical Thing," p. 26.
28. See Evans, *The Language of Self-Involvement*, p. 129; and the entire section on "Onlooks," pp. 124ff.
29. Frankena, "On Saying the Ethical Thing," pp. 37, 39. As for the claim that, among the rivalry of *normative* metaethics, the Christian outlook and consequent ethical onlook may in some sense be true for all men, the reader might ponder Frankena's remark on p. 41: "At any rate, so long as the case against the absolutist claim is not better established than it is, we may still make that claim; it may take some temerity, but it is not unreasonable. As for me and my house, therefore, we will continue to serve the Lord—or, as others may prefer to say, the Ideal Observer."
30. N. Fotion, "Master Speech Acts" (unpublished paper).
31. In L. A. Selby-Biggs, *British Moralists* (Oxford: Clarendon Press, 1897,) I, pp. 403ff.
32. *Roe* v. *Wade*, 410 U.S. 113 (1973).

Commentary

A Rejoinder to a Rejoinder

Alasdair MacIntyre

I

I CAN DISCOVER ONLY ONE POINT OF AGREEMENT between myself and Professor Paul Ramsey. Of course it is true that, as a matter of history, belief in the unconditional requirements of morality was originally rooted in a religious view of the world—provided, for example, we recognize Sophocles as a religious writer, just as much as the author of Deuteronomy. But Ramsey's contention that belief in morality's unconditional demands requires (both for logical warrant and that it may have practical effect) some kind of theological belief is much less precise than Kant's. Ramsey says (p. 66) "that the ultimate warrant for moral norms must be an appeal to what the Lord of heaven and earth is believed to have been doing and to be doing in enacting and establishing his covenant with us and with all mankind. . . ." A little earlier he puts the word "premises" into quotes, thus casting some doubt on what exactly he means by using the word "warrant." Either, I take it, the beliefs that he cites function as premises in an argument, thus providing a putative warrant, or they do not. If Ramsey's claim is not that such beliefs function as premises, then his use of such expressions as "warrant" and "premises" is still not clear enough to discuss; if his claim is that they do so function, then his argument encounters an obvious difficulty.

For how do we derive any norms detailed enough to guide us in medical ethics, say, from *any* account of what the Lord of heaven and earth was or is doing? The biblical accounts of what the Lord of heaven and earth did and does belong to the pre-modern world in which most of our contemporary issues just did not arise; and the Lord of heaven and earth carefully refrained from giving guidance on any issues except those engaging those contemporary with the biblical revelation. How then to extrapolate? I know how the Catholic church extrapolates; I know how John Calvin extrapolated. But Ramsey gives us no clue at all as to where he stands. Rome and Geneva spoke and speak clearly enough for it to be possible to disbelieve what they say; but Princeton does not as yet provide anything clear enough even to disbelieve.

Let me put the challenge in this way. Let Ramsey provide one decisive position on a question disputed in contemporary medical ethics; let him provide one belief about the Lord of heaven and earth; and then let him show us how the former is derived from the latter. Until he does this, what he is asserting will remain quite unclear.

Two final points in this initial section: Ramsey claims that the theological beliefs that he cites function as "a normative metaethics" (p. 62), citing Frankena in support. But no one, including Frankena, has as yet made clear to me the meaning of that barbarous neologism "metaethics." The notion of a metalanguage has a clear and precise meaning in the context of formal logic; outside that context it seems at best a metaphor and a metaphor which still needs to be shown to be appropriate. A similar comment needs to be made on the use of the expression "performative." However Ramsey may be using this expression, he is not using it as J. L. Austin used it. A little explanation might be in order.

II

My own argument began with some reflections on the impact of Nazism on medical ethics. At first sight, of course, any Christian position will seem in stark contrast with the Nazi view.

Yet it may help to identify a central weakness in Ramsey's argument if, for a moment, I stress the similarities.

Let me summarize what was involved in the doctrine of *Ein Volk, Ein Reich, Ein Führer*. It was that ethics was subordinate to the spirit of the German nation; that the norms of ethical practice should be derived from what the Lord of Germany was believed to have been doing and be doing. The German people were to be conceived as a community of faith. We thus have two rival communities of faith, each invoking the name of a different Lord—the Nazi and the Christian. How are we to decide between these claims? Why are we to prefer Jehovah to Hitler (remembering that the existence of the latter—until 1945—is perhaps more soundly established than that of the former)?

A central part of the answer is surely that Christianity passes a number of ethical tests that Nazism fails. Yet this argument presupposes just what Ramsey denies, namely, that ethics cannot be subordinated to religion, but does indeed provide an independent criterion by which religions are to be judged. Yet one ought to note that in this Ramsey, although he may have Kierkegaard on his side (the most dubious of allies, I should have thought), is at odds with much Christian and even more Jewish theology. Catholic Christianity has classically been commended by apologists because its revelation is congruent with our natural knowledge of the good for men. One strand in Judaism, at once metaphysically daring and historically accurate, goes further; God is held to moral account in the light of the Torah.

The question then is posed to Ramsey: when faith meets faith, how are we to judge between them, if not in the light of an ethics that is not subordinated to the very religion it is required to judge?

III

Ramsey is right in his view that I hold that we do not as yet know how to provide the kind of warrant that ethics needs. But this is not because, as his quotation from Lessing is gratuitously used to suggest, I prefer to be in such a state. I find it painful. The only state I would find more painful would be one in which I claimed to possess a form of justification, but could not in fact make good my claim. But Ramsey apparently has a superior alternative which, at the very least, involves taking the claims of the Christian community seriously. Only—he nowhere tells us what it is. Ramsey regrets that I am still alive to refute him; alas, I cannot, for I still do not know on what rational ground, if any, he stands.

Commentary

Another Response to MacIntyre, Tragedy, Reason, Religion, and Ramsey*

Corinna Delkeskamp

ACCORDING TO ALASDAIR MACINTYRE, there exists historical evidence for the incapacity of moral considerations to outweigh the forces of evil (MacIntyre, p. 25-6). A philosopher may feel obliged, therefore, to search after reasons by which to fortify the claim of morality. (MI, p. 26) One such reason is offered by religion—a reason, however, concerning which Professor MacIntyre exposes a dilemma (MI, p. 35 ff): either the word of God defines what is morally good, or it is acceptable as the word of God only because it agrees with an independently known morality. If the first, no convincing basis can be conceived for deciding which religious (or ideological) pronouncement of morality to choose. Yet it is just such a choice between the pronouncements of Jahweh and those of the Führer (MI, Rejoinder, p. 77) to which the quest for a fortified morality commits one. If the second, an independent standard of morality is acknowledged. Yet, then, religion cannot be the ground of morality.

MacIntyre's refutation of a religious foundation for morality presupposes that the only sensible ground on which one could prefer, say, Christianity to any of the more "neurotic" belief-systems (MI, p. 31) would have to be its agreement with an indepeneent code of behavior. In particular, the first horn of his

79

dilemma implies that these systems—as to their dogmatic content—are all equally closed to rational scrutiny.

In defending religion against this charge of irrationality, and of a consequent irrelevance to morality, Professor Ramsey's feelings are divided. On the one hand, he argues that neither should God be abused for the insurance of secular morals (Ramsey, p. 46) nor should His word be judged by external standards. (R, p. 46) Morality is then no real issue for religion. On the other hand, Ramsey cannot deny that a moral concern is implied in the truly holy life (R, p. 59) and that religion is closely linked with morality. Analogously, an on-the-one-hand oblivion to the question of rationality in religion corresponds to an on-the-other-hand obligation to define a rational basis on which the superiority of the Christian faith and its moral norms can be defended. (R, p. 60).

It is this indecision about how to defend his case, and Ramsey's ensuing double play with two incompatible strategies of attack on MacIntyre's position, which calls for two separate sections in which to evaluate these strategies. My first section will deal with Professor Ramsey's attempt to prove the rationality of religion and thereby to refute MacIntyre's charge of irrationality. The second section will focus on Ramsey's contention that religion need not be rational, because it is sanctioned by God, and on his attempt to prove Professor MacIntyre's morality equally irrational although not so sanctioned. A third section will be devoted to consequences following from MacIntyre's position.

I

The quarrel concerning the rationality of religion belongs to a larger, albeit speculative, history. True to the narrative requirements, (MI, p. 39 ff.) the story exhibits an established genre: *de nuptiis philosophiae et theologiae*;[1] it is properly tragic in character (arising from a fatal misunderstanding among the protagonists) and undoubtedly true, since it is documented by a historian who is noted for critical accuracy, viz., David Hume in his *Dialogues concerning Natural Religion*.[2] We will—though with some hesitation—assign the devilish railleries of Philo to Professor MacIntyre, and the friendly moderation—with equal reservations—to

Professor Ramsey (whose flirtations with the role of Demea will be considered in the next section). The argument, in both cases, revolves around three issues: 1. the rationality of religion; 2. the meaning of religious terms; 3. the role of evil in the world.

1. The rationality of religion. Bishop Butler[3] and Cleanthes and also Professor Hare have argued that religious thought is, after all, no less rational than the ordinarily accepted secular reasoning. All secular knowledge of nature rests on uncertain generalizations derived from fallible experience. Yet we act on a (indefensible) presumption of its certainty. The canons for scientific rationality are grounded on basic decisions, which, although not rationally defensible themselves, define the acceptable standards of belief. Only by an unfounded partiality of reason could we withhold a similarly practical assent from the tenets of religion (in Butler's case natural and revealed, in Cleanthes's case only the former), as they are based on analogous evidence.

The Humean, just as the MacIntyrean Philo, challenges this analogy. Even at a time when knowledge about the world could still (by non-sophisticated Newtonians) be presumed to rest on sensible experience, the similarity between generalizations on the basis of known samples, and generalizations on the basis of unknowable ones, had to be denied.[4] Equally, at a time when scientific knowledge is known to transcend experience, one irrational code of acceptability determines, and is thus confirmed as valid by, daily life, whereas the other, equally unfounded, in a thoroughly secularized world has lost the power to command assent (MI, p. 37)—a difference that again precludes comparison. It seems less rational today to disbelieve in electrons than in God, even though both are equally invisible.

A similar parallel exists for the problem of moral obligation. Professor Ramsey defines the validity of Christian morality by using a contemporary philosophical account of the rationality of such claims. (R, p. 60). Frankena's notion of a metaethical community implies that all ethical reasoning starts with certain "performatives" denoting basic decisions. These are not further rationally grounded, but define the commitments of a community in such a way that ethical discourse subsequently will exhibit an internal consistency which renders it "rational." Yet if such "decoding" is not to reduce Christian morals to just another set of taboos, the specific claim for universal validity (or the overarching recommendation of this set of taboos) can only be worked in by holy cheating: the Christian community is special because it determines that its own particular ethical discourse should include everybody; hence it is valid for everybody (R, pp. 65 ff., 67 ff.).

Against this inference, it must be maintained that this universal claim is still the (hybrid) claim of a particular group. Nothing warrants the move from its description to its acceptance. The required additional premise, that this hybrid claim is somehow justified, cannot be rationally grounded.

A similar transition from the statement of a fact (accessible in *this* world) to the assertion of an imperative (pertaining to the *next*) is employed by Butler in drawing moral conclusions from the design argument: if the laws of nature bespeak an intelligent author, and if it is a law of nature that we seek the good and avoid the evil, then this law must have been intended to inform us of a similar arrangement to continue for the *next* life, and thus to teach us what to seek and to avoid in *this* one.[5] Cleanthes only alludes to this argument,[6] for Philo has already refuted the verifiability of an additional premise that is again required to render the argument valid: God is good, and his goodness means retributive justice.

Thus the issue of rationality in knowledge and morality, as raised between MacIntyre and Ramsey, exhibits the same dilemmas found in the discussion of reason in religion between Philo and Cleanthes.

2. The meaning of religious terms. In a second attempt to rationally defend the validity of Christian morals, Ramsey derives this validity from a primary divine institution of "moral obligation." To acknowledge such an obligation in human affairs constitutes the only proper response to a prototypical behavior on the side of God: his primordial promise to man is the original from which we derive the fundamental notion of moral norms and the respect due to them (R, p. 67).

Against this argument MacIntyre's *Rejoinder* points to the oblique manner in which God's actions function as "premises," and demands a method of "extrapolation." In his view, the assumption that the "obligation" inaugurated by God is of a kind with human commitments, such as to allow inferences from the former to the latter, cannot be defended.

He thus reminds us of the dilemma Philo had exposed in Cleanthes's claim that God is "good." We can, on the one hand, assert his goodness on the grounds of that which in his creation appears to us a "good." But then we have likened the principles of divine estimation to our human standards. Such anthropomorphism leaves us with the inconsistency of simultaneously asserting and denying the essential difference between the human and the divine mind.[7] On the other hand, we can assert his goodness as being different in kind from what fits our judgment—which also makes it easier to account for the manifest imperfections of his world machine (at least from our viewpoint).[8] But then our notion of God is as "mystical" as it is incomprehensible, and empty as any atheist could desire.[9]

Similarly, either God's "obligation" is conceived according to "obligations" defined within the Christian community—but then this "God" is but a projection of tribal self-assertion—or "obligation" is not so conceived—but then it is (humanly) incomprehensible and cannot even function to define prototypically any ethical community whatsoever. Ramsey's attempt to solve the problem of rationality by claiming a privileged access to the divine meaning has failed as well; not only can that claim not be defended, but it cannot even be consistently understood.

3. The role of evil in the world. Professor Ramsey, just as Cleanthes, is more concerned about God and hence preoccupied with doxology. Professor MacIntyre, just as Philo, is filled with compassion for people (hence concerned with the victims of vice) and worried about the evils of life.[10] Considering the "divine nonchalance" with which Professor Ramsey shrugs off the infernal shadows conjured by MacIntyre, it is hard to decide who would have been the better atheist had not Ramsey—like Cleanthes—piously harkened to what religion ideally is, and while MacIntyre—like Philo—mischievously exposed its historical manifestations.

Even if Professor MacIntyre's final tragic vision may count as a narrative enactment of Philo's Manichaean hypothesis, the hero now abandons his prescribed part and improvises tradition as he plays along. Where Philo could only deplore the existence of evil, MacIntyre, by demanding a rigorous understanding of morality and by placing this understanding in a tragic perspective, will endeavor to account for it.

This endeavor is motivated by the contention that the behavior of German physicians in the Nazi euthanasia program arose from an insufficiency in scope and power of the best moral arguments then available. The Aristotelian tradition of ethical thought lacks a notion of "positive evil." (MI, p. 28) Therefore, it cannot account for the necessity of self-sacrifice as the only proper response in cases where evil must be prevented from entering the world. The Christian tradition and its Kantian modification are rigorous enough for an unconditional imperative, but this imperative derives its motivating force from a *summum bonum* to be secured in an afterlife, the believability of which cannot be rationally defended. Hence, there is no reason why we should obey its edicts. (MI, p. 30, 36)

II

The first section of our commentary has in part been addressed to Professor MacIntyre's refutation of a religious foundation for morality. This refutation rested on his refusal to accept the rationality of Christian beliefs. The second section will discuss, first, MacIntyre's own endeavor to fortify morality on rational grounds, and second, the consequences of the "rationality" thus established for a reconsideration of the role of reason in religion.

1. MacIntyre's own solution. Professor MacIntyre's own endeavor to provide both an adequate and a rational foundation for morality must allow for a *summum bonum* which is rationally defendable and also provides an incentive powerful enough to balance the desire for survival. Kant's (adequate) imperative, as it was not directed toward a particular group of believers but to humans in general, was rational in its universality of scope. But this rationality did not by itself make the imperative compelling (MI, p. 30). MacIntyre needs an incentive to render the universally valid imperative an equally universal motivative force.

The "triviality" (MI, p. 38) attending all previous descriptions of a promised "fulfilled life" points to their lack of universal appeal. The suggested *summum bonum* must therefore not be described as a "happy state," but must be thought to disclose itself as humanity changes and develops, or must evolve *in via* (MI, p. 39). Regarding this suggestion, Professor Ramsey points out that the *homo viator* ideal really derives from Christianity (R, p. 51). But where MacIntyre meant a goal that *changes* as we go along, Ramsey describes it as what *accompanies* us as we go along. He thereby wants to prove that Christian "happiness" is not a (trivial) superadded state "crowning virtue," but is realized in every virtuous act itself.

This undertaking is surprising when we consider that Ramsey had wished to prove the Christian belief system rational, and hence as universal in scope as any Kantian imperative. Such a view would have been quite compatible with superadding the divine reward as an additional motivating reason, thereby retaining the (now questionable) cardinal virtue of hope, and still not exposing his account to the charge of triviality: the fate of the blessed remains sufficiently obscure. Of course, Ramsey has already charged MacIntyre with "futuristic obscurity" (R, p. 48), and since his own claim for religious rationality has rested on weak foundations, we must understand Ramsey's argument by reference to his second strategy of embracing the a-rationality (and hence the non-universality in scope) of religion. Yet in this case the religious imperative should oblige simply because God commands, and the *summum bonum* of faithful joy claimed to attend obedience is not even needed.

Quite apart from Professor Ramsey's argument, the compelling force MacIntyre trusts to a goal that is in the process of developing is hard to comprehend. Why should I be moved to sacrifice my life by envisaging different value systems arising out of those I have come to cherish? It seems that the requirements of universality and motivating force in Professor MacIntyre's quest for rationality are hard to reconcile.

Should these requirements have been separated in the first place? Ramsey adduces the identity of justifying and moving reasons in religious morality (R, p. 71), but he can do so only because he has identified "what moves" with "what justifies" (a position not very helpful for those not yet moved) and hence abandons the demand for universality.

One may, however, wonder whether that universality of application, which is meant to distinguish a valid code from a cluster of taboos, should be established on rational grounds at all. For a counterexample, the "Schöne" and "erhabene Seelen"[11] as portrayed in Schiller's dramas, present human beings who, by their very thought and action, are capable of instilling in us love for "Sittlichkeit selbst."[12] They function, thus, as incentives to morality in a non-trivial and more noble way than by simply promising a cheerful future.[13] It was this—pointedly a-rational—quality which made it impossible for the national socialist authorities in the later years to permit the staging of *Wilhelm Tell*. Moreover, while Schiller's art was designed to work on the feelings of his audience, he could—rationally—argue why and how.[14]

In order to remedy his own position, Professor MacIntyre must specify the meaning of the narrative history emerging with the development of his *summum bonum* to such a degree that it can compel our willingness to obey the moral imperative. Since he wants to avoid specifying a goal for the future, and since his enumeration of alternative histories (MI, p. 39-40) is not meant to encourage a random selection (which might in the end justify even Nazi-narratives), MacIntyre places this history into the context of a determinate tradition. Or, the "right" direction of historical change is entrusted to the "narrative" inaugurated by Vico, Herder, and Hegel (MI, p. 42). His stipulation that this is a "true" history (MI, p. 40) betrays a quaint sense of irony, but is also necessary in order to solicit that universal assent which would render such an appeal "rational" and the values expounded in the suggested tradition universally compelling.

Yet, what guarantees that this story is not just another myth? In order to have such an interpretation of history warrant the sacrifice of (my, your, his) life, a universal claim must be established. Why should the context of "oughts" suggested here be granted the dignity of a quasi-theological "super-oughthood"? Professor Ramsey's diagnosis of a hidden "seeing eye" (R, p. 53) seems to expose a principle of validation which cannot be rationally grounded. Hence MacIntyre's solution appears to be just as irrational as the Christian one.

This accusation is, however, not quite just. The fact that ultimately no reasons can be given becomes less relevant when we consider that the scope, not only of the validity of the moral imperative but of reason-giving itself, has been extended. The region where questions meet with silence has shrunk. A Kantian "ought" is reduced to embarrassment when someone asks: "why ought I?" while a Humean "ought" can still be defended: "because we all profit."[15] Similarly, MacIntyre can reason still further that those values determining "our" profit belong to a chosen tradition and, finally, that the choice of this tradition can be corroborated on a yet higher level: this tradition, in that it avoids the pitfalls of individualism, restores human history to its former place in a cosmic order (MI, p. 42). The values it revives do justice, in a more comprehensive manner, to the humanity of the past. By addressing humans on a more fundamental level of self-understanding, this tradition derives its universal appeal from a more complete account of what is humanly desirable. In this sense it has been proven superior to the Nazi—or any similarly tribal—ideology.

2. The rationality of religion reconsidered. Professor MacIntyre has placed the ultimate rational ground for our willingness to obey moral norms in an appeal to the legacy of history. This legacy is meant to provide not only some orientation for that goal toward which history is progressing, but also an incentive to take an active part in promoting that progress. One may then wonder whether Christian morality (even though he discarded it as an impasse) could not be established on a similar basis. Obviously, the kind of declamatory assertions offered by Professor Ramsey for the notion of "faithing" (R, p. 59, 66) are not very helpful. However, if we consider the Hebraic, Greek, and Roman traditions the Christian religions have accommodated, then it becomes increasingly difficult to decide which tradition has done more justice to the humanity of the past.

Yet two considerations stand in the way of Christianity as a possible opponent in a rhetorical contest over tradition-choosing. First, Professor MacIntyre would insist that an "obsolete" opponent, as it is no longer capable of compelling commitment by providing universally desirable goals, does not even qualify for such a contest.[16] Professor Ramsey's refutation of this claim is weak: he argues (R, p. 50) that religion does not have to prove itself credible, because its credibility was never effectively disproven. Yet even scientific hypotheses are often not formally refuted but quietly abandoned when they fail to make a difference for the theory to which they belong. Thus, the only ground for Ramsey's claim that the "obsoleteness" of religion need not be disproven is unconvincing.

The second consideration by which the possibility of such a contest is repudiated concerns the fact that there seems to be something wrong with a faith in one's having been chosen when it is defended as an object of such a "choosy" choice. A detached assessment of various cultural heritages squares poorly with the unconditional claim the Christian God is supposed to have on his creatures. This very fact, however, also provides a reason for refuting the first consideration; it leads us to admit that reason, as it occurs in religion, cannot be foundational. Consequently, religious reasoning, when employed for "legislating" a given culture, does not—as MacIntyre assumes—perform its proper office, but has been misused. Hence, that religion, even once such a legislating function has ceased to be believable (MacIntyre's central argument), or once the goals it advocates are no longer universally accepted as desirable, is not, therefore, liable to obsolescence.

On the analogy of the difference between "looking for" and "looking after," we suggest that one cannot reason "for" but only "after" religion. The function of such a "second digestion" of what is "already known" by faith is determined by a triple purpose: mediation, demarcation, and communication. First, just as the "sacred" object (place, institution) consists of a worldly thing (building, administration) which is "sanctified" such as to render it capable of pointing beyond its mundane existence and mediating between world and God,[17] so reason, when employed to interpret revealed truth, serves as a mediator, by which a mind trained in secular rationality can partake of a truth beyond its grasp.[18] Second, the Christian religion must be rendered "rational" so as to demarcate the dividing line separating it from superstition and enthusiasm within, and from non-Christian beliefs and ideologies outside its domain. Third, the adaptation of theological content to the vernacular of current philosophical and scientific thought is to insure a medium of reasonable (and hence somewhat humane) communication between those believers who have learned not to abuse their reasonings for superfluous proofs (e.g., Ramsey in his rational moods), and those unbelievers (e.g., MacIntyre) who have accepted the skeptical truth that a discourse may be "rational" if one can reason "up to a point," even though not all the way.[19] As a consequence, the tenets of theology (just as sacred objects, churches, and ecclesiastical hierarchies) have a history in the world; or they respond to historical change.[20] Once a given socioeconomic, and hence intellectual, climate has been transformed, the reasoned exposition of a constant revelation (as this exposition is bound to none of its particular manifestations) will have to be transformed accordingly. The demythologization of the New Testament was but one response to the existentialist humor; MacIntyre correctly diagnoses that both are dying out together. The fate of faith is trusted to the inertia of its administration and to the chaos of laymen's divinations, until another Aristotle will lend his thought to pious abuse.[21]

We are, then, left not with conflicting claims to rationality and accusations of irrationality, but with different manners of relating the two. Foundational rationality is concerned with exhibiting reasons. In its application to moral problems we may conceive these reasons as the several lower floors, as constructive elements conceptually reconstructed by those on the top executive level, who wish to secure a base on which to operate. Yet if the inquiry is pushed beyond a certain limit, we discover that the solid building we had hoped to inhabit floats on unstable waters. We are reduced to rigging up some steering facilities so as to keep our houseboat from drifting into the open sea where it might be tossed to pieces.

Mediating rationality, on the other hand, is concerned with offering reasons. It proceeds on the assumption that we are thrown into a dangerous current, that the top floor is like a bridge, and that the structure of the whole derives its stability from a careful parsimony of foundations which, starting with an almost imperceptible line deep down, are only slowly allowed to broaden, until they finally expose their modest upper decks. (From whence it follows that those who have not yet discovered the water in their own basement must marvel, when they descend into the narrow keel, what could hold such a monstrous work in balance.)

But let me, before this simile strands us on some shallow contradiction, debark, and draw the appropriate conclusions regarding Ramsey's argument for, and MacIntyre's argument against, religion. My sketch of reason's role in religion differs from the view reflected in Professor Ramsey's methodical oscillation between rational claims and humble agnosticism. Ramsey's faith is like a universal insurance which releases him from the risk of losing an argument: whenever the matter gets sticky, he can escape imminent refutation by piously "faithing away." In contrast to this inconsistency, I have tried to show the different meanings rationality must acquire in a religious context, and have cited some reasons which make such modification desirable.[22]

Professor MacIntyre's charge that religion has lost its credibility and hence its power to motivate moral behavior rested on the assumption that religion makes sense only as the foundation of a culture, and that modern culture precludes such a foundation. If, on the other hand, religion is conceived as a peculiar kind of addition to secular culture, somewhat like a counterculture with the appropriate parasitical inclinations, then it functions instead as a "standing offer" to exchange one set of problems for another. The public acceptability of such an offer is then not a fact which can be asserted or denied for any given society, but a task to be fulfilled. Considering MacIntyre's threat that we may fail to inherit a worthwhile tradition (MI, p. 41), nothing in his account prevents those who choose to from trying to render *this* tradition more "compellingly rational"—and nothing in that account excuses them for not trying to do so.

III

The first two sections dealt with the issue of rationality, first, with MacIntyre on the offensive (disproving the rationality of religion), then with a defensive position (with regard to the rationality of his own view). This view must now be scrutinized as to its conceivable practical consequences. I shall try to show why, even though it was intended as a superior alternative to, say, Nazism, some safeguards are lacking which would more effectively preclude such undesirable interpretations.

The vulnerability of MacIntyre's position to such a charge follows from some implications of his account: unlike the Aristotelian idea of the *summum bonum*, Professor MacIntyre's vision allows for a tragic conflict of values (MI, p. 28, 39-40). In this conflict the sacrifice of an individual's life can be required for the sake of the welfare of his chosen collective unit. Hence his life must rank lower in value than such envisaged welfare. Moreover, as our moral notions and our perception of that larger good must be expected to evolve as we go along, it is hard not to infer that for the sake of such evolution yet another sacrifice may be required, that of the individual's conscience. It was precisely this order of priorities which made National Socialism so seductive for a people disposed toward the nobility and confusion attending reckless idealism.

Nobody who knows and, hence, admires MacIntyre's work can believe that this is what he means, but the lack of safeguards in his account has deeper roots, and it may be useful to examine them with the help of a comparison.

The occurrence of evil in the world motivated the choice of a moral theory which allowed for unconditional obligations and thus for the possibility that self-sacrifice may be required. This Kantian commitment Professor MacIntyre shares with Friedrich Schiller, and they both agree that something is amiss in Kant's account. Yet where MacIntyre addresses this lack with the question: How do we come to respect the law? (MI, p. 30) or: How do we come to desire what we must? Schiller asks: Is there a better way to elicit such a desire than by subjecting our feelings to the tyranny of reason? or: Can the dignity of man as a unity of both feelings and reason be better accounted for?[23]

It seems that the horrors of the recent past have rendered us less choosy about how to obey the moral law, as long as we do so. This is why MacIntyre does not hesitate to smooth over the tragic presence by offering the hope of a future collective good that will justify the hardships of the voyage. The positive outcome transforms a human tragedy into a no longer divine but societal comedy.

Schiller, on the contrary, is prepared to face a harder truth. No future salvation can console the ones who are caught between conflicting forces, and can thus present an interior motive by which our interest is aroused. Rather, the sacrifice of life is conceived as a celebration of freedom and power—as the exaltation of a deified self.[24]

It would be wrong to charge Schiller's account with individualism (MI, p. 42). The fact that it is essentially an individual who acts, rather than the contingently particular manifestation of a communal spirit, (MI, p. 39) does not imply that he acts for the sake of his individuality. It is exactly such individuality, as defined by a particular body with its natural necessities, and by particular feelings and passions, which, even though it constitutes the necessary condition for our coming to desire what we must, is yet overcome in the act.[25] The power to assert one's freedom, when informed by "Sittlichkeit," raises the individual to the realization of a universal ideal of humanity similar to what MacIntyre has in mind when he thinks of people giving their lives in order that evil may not enter the world.

The difference emphasized here does not concern simply an individualist versus a collectivist account, but, rather, two manners by which one might overcome concern for the merely private self. With MacIntyre, the initial choice commits us ever after to viewing ourselves as safely placed in a larger tradition. Our death will be that of a martyr, asserting our mystical communion with the common cause. With Schiller, on the other hand, the principle of beauty is meant to mediate between our individual self and the general forms of grace and dignity it teaches.[26] The subsumption of the particular under the general, or the decision for a given hierarchy of values with ascending prerogatives (as in MacIntyre), is here replaced by an ever reiterated interplay which can, by its fictional synthesis in the tragic hero, only be suggested to the onlooker for imitation. Individuality itself is transformed into what transcends it.

As a consequence, Schiller's vision allows for controls where MacIntyre's does not. Just as in a Hobbesian state the subjects transfer their individual powers to the sovereign and henceforth submit to his definition of justice, but at the same time retain the right to think, and thus to protest when the sovereign has violated the natural laws, so Schiller's distinction between what we ought and what we want, or between what is morally pleasing and what is esthetically so (as a pure affirmation of power), preserves an awareness of possible conflicts[27] between courses of action which only seem to raise us above ourselves (i.e. the incentives of personal ambition) and courses of action which actuallly do so (i.e. incentives to perform a duty). In opposition to this ever-present ambiguity of human greatness, a happy harmony of both incentives is placed in MacIntyre's hope that his story be true. Once such a hope has motivated our choice we are—if we want to be consistent—no longer free to doubt. The difference between a Wallenstein and a Max Piccolomini becomes incomprehensible.[28]

For Schiller this distinction roots in a further difference between (the beautiful) appearance (or the dramatic work of art) and historical reality.[29] When MacIntyre puts the narrated facts on stage, or admits the company of historical actors simultaneously into the illustrious audience of Juno's birthday party,[30] he claims history to be an edifying fable and morality an esthetic occasion. But Schiller knew that we can trust a moral story only if *we* made it. Only if a clear distinction between appearance and reality is maintained, can the moral inspiration derived from the former be hoped to gradually inform and ennoble the latter—thus raising it to a state which allows for the realization of the (ideally) moral impulse.[31] For the poet, history is the stuff from which dramas are made; for MacIntyre that drama is entrusted to history. Who, then, can restrain Robespierre and St. Just from wishing to *play* the ancient Romans and also claiming that it is for *real*?

Of course the beautiful appearance from which the classic theater derived its dignity as "moral institution" has faded into a cultural product for complacent consumption. The safeguards introduced to preclude its abuse have not precluded its eventual loss of inspirational power. Yet if history is to be conceived as that in terms of which we may define our obligation toward the future, then it implies an equally pressing obligation toward conceptual distinctions which served a purpose in the past and which, when integrated into present thought, may help avoid unnecessary danger. It is the concern for such possible misunderstanding of MacIntyre's endeavor to delineate a foundation for morality acceptable for the nonreligious part of humanity which has inspired Professor Ramsey's criticism. But then, we must not forget, religious morality has suffered from false defenders as well.

NOTES

*My special gratitude goes to Dodie R. Meeks for her imaginative criticism, and to H. Tristram Engelhardt for his unwavering and public-spirited belief in clarity.

1. Martianus M. F. Capella, *De nuptiis philologiae et Mercurii et de septem artibus liberalibus libri novem*, F. Kopp, ed. (Frankfurt/M.: Franciscus Varrentrapp, 1836).
2. David Hume, *Dialogues concerning Natural Religion*, 1st ed., London, 1779 (Indianapolis: Bobbs Merrill Company, 1947).
3. Joseph Butler (Bishop of Durham), *The Analogy of Religion Natural and Revealed*, 1st ed., London, 1736 (London: J. M. Dent, 1906), Author's Introduction.
4. Hume, *Dialogues*. . ., p. 134 ff., p. 144 ff.
5. Butler, *The Analogy of Religion*. . ., p. 24.
6. Hume, *Dialogues*. . ., p. 219, ff.
7. Ibid., p. 156, ff.
8. Ibid., p. 198.
9. Ibid., pp. 199, 203.
10. Ibid., p. 193, ff.
11. Both concepts are defined by Schiller in "Über Anmut und Würde," *Friedrich Schiller, Werke in drei Bänden*, 1st ed., *Neüe Thalia*, 1793 (München: Carl Hanser, 1966) II, 408, 413.
12. "Wenn der gütige August dem Verräter Cinna, der schon den tödlichen Spruch auf seinen Lippen zu lesen meint, gross wie seine Götter, die Hand reicht: 'Lass uns Freunde sein, Cinna!'—Wer unter der Menge wird in *dem* Augenblick nicht gern seinem Todfeind die Hand drücken wollen, dem göttlichen Römer zu gleichen?' etc., Friedrich Schiller, "Was kann eine gute stehende Schaubühne eigentlich wirken?' *ed. cit.*, I, 723 (public lecture, held in 1784; later title: Die Schaübuhne als moralische Anstalt betrachtet).
13. "Rücksicht auf eine belohnende Zukunft schliesst die Liebe aus. Es muss eine Tugend geben, die auch ohne den Glauben an Unsterblichkeit auslangt, die auch auf Gefahr der Vernichtung das

nämliche Opfer wirkt," Friedrich Schiller, "Philosophische Briefe," *ed. cit.*, I, 713 (1st ed., *Thalia*,1786-7).

14. See Schiller, "Was kann eine . . . Schaubühne . . .," *ed. cit.*, p. 722.

15. See Alasdair MacIntyre, *Against the Self-Images of the Age* (New York: Schocken Books, 1971), p. 169 ff.

16. In A. MacIntyre, *The Religious Significance of Atheism* (New York: Columbia University Press, 1969) such "obsolescence" is inferred from the fact that, while in the seventeenth through the nineteenth century the transformation of natural science and of its canons of acceptability directly confronted religious claims about the world, modern society is dominated by a physics and a politics (p. 19) which do not encounter any more resistance from orthodox Christianity. Since atheism is no longer an issue, theism has lost its relevance (p. 24). What content, after all, should we ascribe to a theory that does not even lend itself to refutation? This argument, however, does not address Christian theism as such, but only those endeavors to defend its truth which use the secular scientific knowledge as a universal basis of consent on which to establish the tenets of faith. Once religious writers derive the validity of their claims from a scientific world view, any change in this world view will indeed repudiate that validity. But one may argue that any attempt at apologetics is inappropriate in the first place. (I have tried to argue thus in "La Sécularisation Philosophique—Une Apologie provisoirement Non-sécularisante," in *Herméneutique de la Sécularisation*, E. Castelli, ed. [Paris: Aubier, 1976], pp. 297 ff.) Hence the charge of irrefutability (MacIntyre, ibid., p. 10) misses the point. Even on the level of facts one might quarrel with Professor MacIntyre's contention that there is nothing left worth quarreling about in religion. His own usage of terms such as "guilt" and "evil" is strangely at odds with the contemporary psychological, sociological, and psychiatric inclination to keep the description of human conduct free from value implications and to address moral problems in terms of behavioral maladaptation or of mental disease. Kant very prudently relegated the notion of "evil," as it is incomprehensible in philosophical terms, to religion (see Immanuel Kant, "Der Streit der Fakultäten in drei Abschnitten," *Immanuel Kants Werke,* 1st ed., 1798. E. Cassirer *et al.,* ed. [Berlin: Bruno Cassirer, 1922], VI, 319.) Indeed, the paradox of a being presumed to be fundamentally opposed to what is "good," and yet on equal standing with it as to its existence, can only be accommodated in a

system where the "good" itself encompasses the evil and accounts for its presence. Whether the devil is merely the instrument of a divine justice, or whether a state of sin is a necessary condition for the assertion of divine love through salvation, the Judaeo-Christian tradition offers a meaning for the existence of evil in the world. Professor MacIntyre's discussion of the problem of evil in "The Logical Status of Religious Belief," (*Metaphysical Beliefs, S.* Toulmin *et al.* ed. [London: SCM Press Ltd., 1957], p. 181 ff.), disregards this aspect of occidental theism. His analysis of the relation of morals to religion, moreover, as the final issue with regard to which he proves Christianity to be outmoded, is equally deficient: while religious morality is represented by austere sex rules, the central commandment "love thy neighbour" is not mentioned once in *The Religious Significance . . .*, (*ed. cit.*), where a whole section is devoted to "Atheism and Morals." Nobody will deny the fact that religion, historically speaking, has presupposed a particular antecedent morality, and that, systematically speaking, its practical requirements presuppose some secular morality or other. But it is also hard to deny that some seasoning with such "love of neighbor" may take the "edge" off occasionally disagreeable moralism.

17. My concept of the "sacred" is derived from Henri Bouillard, "La catégorie du sacré dans la science des religions," in *Le Sacré*, E. Castelli, ed. (Paris: Aubier, 1974).

18. This implies a third alternative for religion's self-understanding, over and above the two which MacIntyre has discussed and discarded (see *The Religious Significance . . ., ed. cit.* pp. 11, 26, and also *Against the Self-Images . . ., ed. cit.,* p. 20). Even though there are times when the factual content of religious claims is emphasized, and other times when religion so to speak recoils into its private theological vernacular, both possibilities (of fundamentalism and of proclaiming a "double truth") present only extremes (of identification and separation) on a continuous scale of possible manners, in which the available facts and their transcendent interpretations can be related one to another. It is not necessary, therefore, to put the Christian theism *only* into a defensive position. The adaptation of the mechanistic system to the needs of a theological world view (or the occasionalist hypothesis), for example, provided *also* a gain, i.e. a hitherto unsuspected manner in which God's presence in the world could be conceived and, thus, enriched the store of pious metaphors (cf. the discussion in Samuel Clarke, *The Leibniz-Clarke Correspondence* [New York: Philosophical Library,

1956]). There is no reason conceivable why what is accessible to human comprehension should agree with what is given as a mythical hint at what is beyond comprehension. There is also no reason, however, why those issues, in which our scientific understanding is acknowledged to surpass our comprehension, should not be used also to assess what is known to be principally incomprehensible and serve as yet another "stepping stone."

19. A similar reasoning can be applied to morality, for here as well the moral requirements are added to those of a pious life so as to mediate what is right in the eyes of man with what is so in the eyes of God. Similarly, morality serves as a criterion by which to identify the mere pretenders to holy dignities, and provides a condition for civilized commerce with non-religious humanity.

20. It might, therefore, simply be asking too much if one were to challenge Christians (and Marxists) to "clearly discriminate the truths of which their tradition is a bearer from what are merely defensive or aggressive responses to their social situation." (A. MacIntyre, *Marxism and Christianity* [New York: Schocken Books, 1968], p. ix). The fact that, say, thoughts and imaginations cannot be assessed independently of a language expressing them does not defeat the claim that it makes sense to believe in the existence of thoughts and imaginations over and above their—often incomplete—expressions. The fact, moreover, that different languages permit us to express different facets of what we "had in mind," or that different styles and techniques allow the manifestation of different aspects of an otherwise inaccessible aesthetic inspiration, seems to corroborate the assumption that there exist contents which are distinguishable (and discoverable, as our habit of juxtaposing an original and its skilful copy suggests), but not separable from their formulations.

21. The possibility, of course, of subsequent such mediative undertakings does not imply their desirability. The relevance of a religious interpretation over and above our worldly assessment of the nature of things cannot be proven, but only recommended wherever the secular system is felt to fail. MacIntyre has hard words for those who, while professing atheism, still want divine sanctions for birth, marriage, and death. Maybe, however, it is not just "dumbness" and "self-indulgence" (*The Religious Significance* . . ., *ed. cit.*, p. 19) which makes us plead for a handsome funeral, but rather a shamefaced admission that for the more spectacular aspects of life the more humdrum notions are not quite sufficient.

22. Religious language, therefore, presupposes a secular language in a

similar sense in which the religious transformation of morality presupposes some secular morality upon which to transform. Just as in poetry words are taken from their prosaic employment and yet "mean more," or "differently," and just as each attempt at "decoding" ("The Logical Status. . .", *ed. cit.*, p. 174) will yield a different interpretation—with the history of such interpretations ("Rezeptionsgeschichte") constituting that tradition which explicates the meaning of the original poem—so the Schleiermachian, Barthian, Bultmannian, etc. attempts at "decoding" religious language present us with isolated facets of what we should understand as "the word of God." All this is "misleading" only if we restrict the function of speaking to "saying what is the case." Perhaps we can compare the *decorum* for secular terms in religious contexts to that of a well-bred guest in a properly conducted household: There are quite a number of things which he may do, and a number of manners in which he is expected to assert his presence. But they all are to be tempered by the considerate endeavor not to upset established routines, violate sacred privileges, take off his shoes, and, above all, by the skill to discreetly evanesce when matters get complicated.

23. See Schiller, "Über Anmut und Würde," *ed. cit.*, II, 406 ff.
24. ". . . Gefühl unsrer Übermacht, welche vor keinen Grenzen erschrickt und dasjenige sich geistig unterwirft, dem unsre sinnlichen Kräfte unterliegen." (Schiller, "Über den Grund des Vergnügens an tragischen Gegenständen," *ed. cit.*, II, 344.)
25. "Durch die ästhetische Gemütsstimmung wird also die Selbsttätigkeit der Vernunft schon auf dem Felde der Sinnlichkeit eröffnet, . . . und der physische Mensch so weit veredelt, dass nunmehr der geistige sich nach Gesetzen der Freiheit aus demselben bloss zu entwickeln braucht . . . Soll der Mensch . . . aus jedem beschränkten Dasein den Durchgang zu einem unendlichen finden, . . . so muss dafür gesorgt werden, dass er in keinem Momente bloss Individuum sei und bloss dem Naturgesetz diene." (Schiller, Über die ästhetische Erziehung des Menschen," 23rd letter, *ed. cit.*, II, 500 ff., 1st ed., *Horen*, 1795.)
26. "Der Übergang von dem leidenden Zustande des Empfindens zu dem tätigen des Denkens und Wollens geschieht also . . . durch einen mittleren Zustand ästhetischer Freiheit" (Ibid., p. 499).
27. "Das Interesse der Einbildungskraft aber ist: sich *frei von Gesetzen* im Spiele zu erhalten. Diesem Hange zur Ungebundenheit ist die sittliche Verbindlichkeit des Willens, . . . nichts weniger als

günstig; und da die sittliche Verbindlichkeit des Willens der Gegenstand des moralischen Urteils ist, so sieht man leicht, dass bei dieser Art zu urteilen die Einbildungskraft ihre Rechnung nicht finden könne. . . . denn die Gesetzmässigkeit, welche die Vernunft als moralische Richterin fordert, besteht nicht mit der Ungebundenheit, welche die Einbildungskraft als moralische Richterin verlangt." (Schiller, "Über das Pathetische," *ed. cit.*, II, 439, 441; 1st ed. 1801.)

28. Wallenstein, after all, justifies his decision to lead the Austrian Army into the Swedish camp with a narrative history: "Was tu ich Schlimmres, / Als jener Cäsar tat, des Name noch / Bis heut das Höchste in der Welt benennet? / Er führte wider Rom die Legionen / Die Rom ihm zur Beschützung anvertraut." (Schiller, "Wallensteins Tod," II, 2, *ed. cit.*, III, 149 [staged in Weimar, 1799, 1st ed., 1800]).

29. ". . . wie wenig die poetische Kraft des Eindrucks, den sittliche Charaktere oder Handlungen auf uns machen, von ihrer *historischen Realität* abhängt. . . . Die poetische Wahrheit besteht aber nicht darin, dass etwas wirklich geschehen ist, sondern darin, dass es geschehen konnte, also in der innern Möglichkeit der Sache." (Ibid., p. 442.)

30. See Ludovicus Vives, "A Fable about Man," in *The Renaissance Philosophy of Man,* E. Cassirer *et al.*, eds. (Chicago: The University of Chicago Press, 1948 [after: *J. L. Vivis Valentini* (1492-1540) *Opera omnia,* Valentiae 1783, IV, 3-8]), p. 387 ff.

31. "Sobald der Mensch einmal so weit gekommen ist, den Schein von der Wirklichkeit, die Form von dem Körper zu unterscheiden, so ist er auch imstande, sie von ihm abzusondern; denn das hat er schon getan, indem er sie unterscheidet. . . . je sorgfältiger er die Gestalt von dem Wesen trennt, und je mehr Selbständigkeit er derselben zu geben weiss, desto mehr wird er nicht bloss das Reich der Schönheit erweitern, sondern selbst die Grenzen der Wahrheit bewahren; denn er kann den Schein nicht von der Wirklichkeit reinigen, ohne zugleich die Wirklichkeit von dem Schein frei zu machen." ("Ästhetische Erziehung," 26th letter, *ed. cit.*, II 512.)

32. "Bei welchem einzelnen Menschen oder ganzen Volk man den aufrichtigen und selbständigen Schein findet, da darf man auf Geist und Geschmack und jede damit verwandte Trefflichkeit schliessen— da wird man das Ideal das wirkliche Leben regieren, die Ehre über den Besitz, den Gedanken über den Genuss, den Traum der Unsterblichkeit über die Existenz triumphieren sehen." (Ibid., p. 513.)

Commentary

Morality and Religion

Jack Bemporad

IN THIS ESSAY, I am concerned with delineating the interrelationship between ethics, science, and theology. This is an old and well-worn topic. However, what I shall endeavor to do here is to indicate where moral issues transcend those of ethics proper and constrain us to introduce religious questions. In particular I will be concerned with four issues.

I. The relationship of ethical questions to the development of a concept of an ideal self.
II. The significance of repentance.
III. The relationship between the good and the holy.
IV. The sense in which ethics and science demand a backdrop that more properly can be delineated as religious or theological.

I. Ethics and the Self

When we consider action, we cannot avoid questions of motives, goals, and results. We are immediately aware that reality is not homogeneous in all respects, or one-dimensional. We recognize that some actions or goals are better than others, we distinguish what is from what ought to be, and we recognize that our moral values are conceived independently of their actual concrete instances. They even seem to claim a certain preeminence over what actually is.

We continuously decide what is good or bad, right or wrong. This process is reflexive, for it affects not merely how we influence others (and we can never avoid influencing others by who we are and by what we do) but makes a difference to ourselves. Our acts contribute to our future selves. We, as it were, make ourselves in the sense that what we do will help to determine the self that will be, whether we want to be that self or not.

Every moral act not merely has its own intrinsic value but also directs us beyond the present act toward the horizon of something else, something larger and not fully exhausted in the particular act. This is true even in any plausible hedonistic ethic which must take account of at least short-term consequences of actions. It is not enough just to seek pleasure since the particular experience of pleasure has to be seen in the context of a total life. We are forced to ask how any particular experience fits into the context or nexus of experiences which will determine the kind of self we want to be. There is a context to any act that forms a backdrop to it. Thus one can always ask: With respect to what total or whole self does this act or series of acts contribute?

Social mores and the teachings of our traditions offer guidelines for judging our particular acts through portrayals of what the whole self should be like. Such are the functions of taboos, rules, regulations, and moral codes. Yet there is always sufficient ambiguity in these that the individual must decide for himself what his overall unified self is, and how each act and experience applies to this unity. The less traditions constrain a society, the greater will be the ambiguity and the role of individual responsibility.

Now, for two reasons, I submit that what kind of self I want to be or produce through my actions is not simply a moral or ethical question. First, the search for the whole of the self requires categories that are not reducible to purely moral notions. They involve questions of hope and despair, of the purpose and significance of one's life, of self-realization and self-sacrifice. Second, when these issues are introduced, the ideal around which the self organizes itself becomes universal and all-encompassing. My point is that ethics may claim certain actions to be right or wrong. It may evaluate or order a hierarchy of values or goods. Yet when one asks the more radical questions of hope and faith, of the meaning of it all and the meaning of one's life, then one transcends the strictly ethical and scientific pursuits. That is, one moves to a concept of an ideal in terms of which one judges particular actions.

The more one attempts to take familial and social considerations into account in one's actions, the more one is brought to judge one's actions in terms of an ideal self, and thus in terms of more than immediate satisfactions insofar as one judges in terms of overarching considerations. This ideal self gives a consistency to one's life and one's actions. Which is to say, one internalizes the surrounding mores.

But beyond that, one creates a portrait of oneself as a moral agent that can come into conflict with the moral ambience that inspired it, insofar as the mores one draws upon are not fully self-consistent. Such incompatibilities can culminate or display themselves as conflicts between one's view of oneself as a moral agent and one's generally accepted mores. This engenders what some have seen as the core of the genuine ethical dilemma, in distinction from a moral dilemma. Vivas, for example, claims that a genuine ethical dilemma does not consist of knowing what is right and wrong, but in lacking courage and willpower to choose the right.[1] In a genuine ethical dilemma a person does not know the right thing to do. For if he knew the right thing to do, but did not have the courage to do it, it is not a genuine ethical perplexity; it is rather a matter of failure of courage or will. A genuine ethical perplexity lies in a situation where an individual is undergoing stresses and strains in the organization of his inner values. It is one in which he must reconstitute those values through a radical decision involving a choice favorable not to our idea of our actual moral personality, but to our *ideal* moral personality. My contention is that there are situations in which he does not know what the right choice is, and where he has to refashion his moral decisions through a struggle and a creative act. Through an inward search for our essential moral personality we create an ideal person. We may act toward this ideal person as though he were real. A genuine moral perplexity invites a descent into the depths of our very being, a painful inquiry into our actual, rather than our ostensible, motivations and values. And since the formulation is constitutive of an ideal not yet fully formed, this is an act of self-creation.

The monotheistic vision of one God, one mankind, and one universal history, with a concomitant belief in the intrinsic dignity of every person as made in God's image, is an ideal which has furnished the means of judging and changing more parochial and limited ideals. It has been the corrective to various idolatries, chief among which are nationalism and the excessive use of power.

This insight should be seen in the context of the broadest and most universal ideals, and historically has led us to various religious visions. Isaiah was the first to give us a vision of international morality. It is not enough for Isaiah, for example, to have the sword forbidden to individuals. Isaiah claims it is incredible that murder is a crime but war is not. "Nation shall not lift up sword against nation neither shall they learn war anymore."[2] Isaiah's view of morality transcends nationalism—our class, our clan, our tribe—and is seen to be universal and applicable to all. In this fashion, monotheism provides grounds for universal values and functions as a corrective to narrower visions.

II. The Significance of Repentance

The attempt to fulfill ethical demands inevitably fails. And man's failure, his feelings of guilt and remorse at not having fulfilled his ethical goals, leads to contrition, repentance, and endeavors at self-transcendence and self-transformation. It often leads as well to a search for spiritual cleansing, purification, and forgiveness for one's sins.

This search for forgiveness and spiritual cleansing is not simply an ethical need but has numerous religious overtones. This is clear in the context of the self's awareness that ethically he has done wrong, and that yet there must be room for a new beginning, another chance, and not simply condemnation. Still, the more moral faults involve injury to persons generally, the more it becomes impossible to set aside moral debts within the ethical order. Especially as one comes to judge one's moral actions in terms of an ideal self, and the more that ideal self reflects a commitment to general goals of moral conduct, guilt for moral failure requires repentance and forgiveness in terms of that ideal self.

What comes to the fore is the consciousness of the connection of ethics with the self-transcendent aspect of man, his spiritual generation. It is here, as Hermann Cohen points out, that the correlation with God emerges.[3] The Psalmist phrases, "He restoreth my soul," or "Create in me a clean heart and *restore* a steadfast spirit within me," testify to man's need for spiritual healing and regeneration. One cannot refer to this need simply in ethical terms in the sense that ethics seeks general rules of correct behavior and does not give grounds for the very singular act of forgiveness—especially when the offences involve justice generally, not simply particular individuals who could forgive the offence to them. What ethics does not fully confront, and here the religious element comes to the fore, is, as Hermann Cohen has indicated, the self-recognition of sin and failure and the need for repentance and self-transcendence. Repentance makes it possible to redeem the past. As Max Scheler states, ". . . there is no part of our past life which—while its component natural reality is of course less freely alterable than the future—might not still be genuinely altered in its *meaning* and *worth*, through entering our life's total significance as a constituent of the self-revision which is always possible."[4] Scheler continues,

> Repenting is equivalent to re-appraising part of one's past life and shaping for it a mint-new worth and significance. People tell us that Repentance is a senseless attempt to drive out something 'unalterable'. But nothing in this life is 'unalterable' in the sense of this argument. Even this 'senseless' attempt alters the 'unalterable' and places the regretted conduct or attitude in a new relation within the totality of one's life, setting it to work in a new direction.[5]

Thus Max Scheler sees repentance as the way in which one can "totally kill and extinguish the *reactive* effect of the deed within the human soul, and with it the root of an eternity of renewed guilt and evil." Repentance seeks "forgiveness of sin" and "an infusion of new strength from the center of things."[6]

The need for forgiveness and the recognition that we can be regenerated, start anew as it were, is the heart of repentance. It is an appeal to a transcendent source of power to give us strength, hope, and faith to continue. That is, it is an appeal beyond the ethical order for reinstatement within that order. The possibility for ethical failure, the reality of guilt, the lack of a ground for forgiveness for general moral failures signal beyond the ethical order. Forgiveness, as a general moral category, transcends the ethical in requiring a locus for the giving of forgiveness. One is returned thus to the concept of an ideal self, but now in correlation to the source of forgiveness—God.

III. The Relationship Between the Good and the Holy

There is another aspect of the ethical which, when fully amplified, transcends ethics and makes it enter the domain of the religious: the feeling of reverence and awe that is related to certain ethical acts, such as self-sacrifice. In such acts the individual often feels that his whole life and the meaning of his life are at stake. Here one has intimations of the holy and the sacred. This point has been raised by MacIntyre with regard to the motivations requisite for self-sacrifice. Even if one recognizes that one can only act coherently if one obeys the categorical imperative, still one may choose to act incoherently—especially if one's own life is at stake. How can the ethical order give adequate motivations for ethical action, especially when these are at the cost of self-sacrifice? Self-sacrifice requires an appeal to something of absolute value.

John Oman has argued that we cannot by building up natural, mundane values arrive at anything of absolute worth.[7] He claims that only in the experience of the holy does one stand in the presence of a reality before which one cannot simply seek one's own pleasure. What Oman distinguishes is the natural and supernatural; he indicates that it is in the recognition of absolute worth or of the holy that an intuition of the supernatural appears.

Hans Jonas also reinforces this concept when he states:

> We must, in other words, distinguish between moral obligation and the much larger sphere of moral value. (This, incidentally,

shows up the error in the widely-held view of value theory that the higher a value the stronger its claim and the greater the duty to realize it. The highest are in a region beyond duty and claim.) The ethical dimension far exceeds that of the moral law and reaches into the sublime solitude of dedication and ultimate commitment, away from all reckoning and rule—in short, into the sphere of the holy. From there alone can the offer of self-sacrifice genuinely spring, and this—its source—must be honored religiously.[8]

In short, the search for an ideal focus in terms of which one's particular acts can be judged and given coherence, and the need for a source of forgiveness, coincide with the holy—the adequate ground for ultimate dedication and self-sacrifice. Reflection upon the ethical leads one beyond the ethical in order that coherence in the ethical life, repentance and forgiveness, and ultimate dedication and self-sacrifice can make sense. The argument is clearly not a strict one. It is rather an ascent from lesser to greater coherence of moral vision. The argument turns on an appeal to an interest in a moral life of greater compass and intensity. Thus, as Henry Slonimsky puts it, the religious man is:

> . . . one who is willing to bear the burdens—and on a higher and more difficult plane, the sorrows—and on the highest and most difficult and almost superhuman plane, the sins of the world. A religious person is one who feels responsible for every one else.[9]

This feeling of general responsibility and moral interest is one to which monotheism gives purpose and coherence. If God is one, then there is one moral history—grounded in that God. Moreover, this one God, as the God of all creation, suggests that there is one account or story of the world which is, in principle, a general story. Cosmology and moral history come to coincide in an appeal to universality and generality.

IV. Ethics, Science and Theology

Ethics makes a demand that the universe be such as to enable ethics to succeed. This is similar to the Kantian postulates in the *Critique of Practical Reason*. It is the task of theology to seek to determine the kind of universe wherein the presuppositions and demands of both science and ethics can be realized and fulfilled. That is, religion gives a view in terms of which the kingdom of nature and the kingdom of grace can be reconciled—in terms of which the otherwise senseless suffering of the innocent can have enduring meaning. Which is to say, religion makes a claim that morality at best can only leave as a postulate—that reality is, in fact, susceptible to morality—that being and goodness are not irreconcilable or opposed, but rather that at least in the Divine Being they are united in a supreme form.

Religion thus forwards an ideal of coherence that extends beyond that of giving unity to particular moral actions. It comes to include giving unity to both our descriptive and normative interests, both our interests in science and ethics. While science is primarily concerned with what is (i.e., with an accurate or true description of the state of things as they are), science as such is not concerned with that aspect of reality that needs changing and transformation. In this respect, science is concerned with what is, morality with what ought to be, and theology is concerned with the interrelationship of these two through an attempt to understand the structure of things as making possible both science and morality. As Montague has argued:

> Religion as we shall conceive it is the acceptance neither of a primitive absurdity nor of a sophisticated truism, but of a momentous possibility—the possibility namely that what is highest in spirit is also deepest in nature, that the ideal and the real are at least to some extent identified, not merely evanescently in our own lives but enduringly in the universe itself. If this possibility were an actuality, if there truly were at the heart of nature something akin to us, a conserver and increaser of values, and if we could not only know this and act upon it, but really feel it, life would suddenly become radiant. For no longer should we be alien accidents in an indifferent world, uncharacterized by-products of the blindly whirling atoms; and no longer would the things that matter most be at the mercy of the things that matter least.[10]

Implicit in Montague's characterization of religion are three concepts: meaning, order, and value. Religion is the assurance or reassurance that life and the universe have meaning and that meaning is impossible without order attuned to values.

Religion as the quest for meaning is not an abstract or intellectual pursuit but lies at the very depths of the human self. The quest for religion begins when man searches for the meaning of his existence, when he seeks the purpose and significance of his life, and when he judges himself by terms that transcend his finite self. This religious quest does not begin in wonder or amazement or in the ineffable, but in the self-questioning of the meaning and purpose of one's existence, and from questioning one's own existence to the existence of all that is. The question man ultimately asks himself is: Why is there something rather than nothing? What is the reason and meaning of the being that is? This question of meaning is never a question of fact. It is not raised by asking what is, but rather by asking the why for, the why.

It is necessary to point out that science makes certain presuppositions which are neither intelligible in themselves nor self-contained, but which require a metaphysical and theological context for their intelligibility. All science presupposes being and order. It takes them for granted and does not discuss the more radical question of the ground for the being and order of what is. But we are still inescapably aware of our contingency and of the contingency of all that is. We are still struck with the question: What is the ground of the being that is? Why is there order and not chaos? What is the ground of the order that is? No attempt at juggling theories of chance and randomness can successfully address itself to these questions. Being cannot come from non-being by chance. The laws of chance could intelligibly answer the question as to the probability of coming to be of a certain pattern with respect to a range of actualities. But they could never ask or answer the question about the universe, its coming into being. This question transcends the range and scope of science.

This religious quest for meaning, though, does not contradict science or ethics. After all, it stems from a concern to put science and ethics into a more encompassing framework. Religion in this sense affords a truly interdisciplinary, in fact, trans-disciplinary perspective within which ultimate justifications are sought for both ethics and science, for both honoring obligations and having confidence in predictions. Religion offers a coincidence of the *termini ad quos* of our interests in an ideal vantage point for judging our particular moral actions, in a source of forgiveness, in a justification for moral self-sacrifice, and in grounds for confidence regarding our place as moral agents and knowers. A final authentication of ourselves as doers and knowers is to be found, if anywhere, only in religion. To quote Schubert Ogden:

> Religious questions do not ask either about particular phenomena as do scientific questions, or about particular courses of action as do moral questions; they ask, rather, about the fundamental conditions that everything particular presupposes. Thus what gives rise to religious questions is the common experience of the apparent unreality and final meaninglessness of all that is and is done. . . . religion is a matter of enabling us so to understand our inalienable confidence in the worth of life that it may be reasonably affirmed.[11]

When one looks for foundations of ethics that also underlie science, I believe one finds them in religion. It is only in terms of a transcendent ground, a universal rationale underlying both the world of experience and the world of moral action, that the domains of ethics and science are assured of integration. Again, this is similar to Kant's suggestion—that only by presuming the existence of God does it become possible to be assured that the kingdoms of Grace and of Nature, of autonomous action and scientific investigation, can be reconciled. The religious viewpoint looks beyond particular vantage points, which give fragmentary portrayals of the human condition, to affirm in one God a unity to being, and a unification to the diverse elements of human existence.

NOTES

1. Eliseo Vivas, *The Moral and the Ethical Life* (Chicago: Henry Regnery Co., 1963).
2. *Isaiah* 2:4b.
3. Hermann Cohen, *Religion of Reason* (New York: Unger Pub. Co., 1972), p. 168.
4. Max Sheler, *On the Eternal in Man* (London: SCM Press Ltd., 1960), p. 40.
5. Ibid., p. 41.

6. Ibid., p. 55.
7. John Oman, *The Natural and the Supernatural* (Cambridge: Cambridge University Press, 1931), p. 310.
8. Hans Jonas, *Philosophical Essays* (Englewood Cliffs, New Jersey: Prentice Hall, 1974).
9. Henry Slonimsky, *Essays* (Chicago: Quadrangle Press, 1967), p. 115.
10. W. P. Montague, *Belief Unbound* (New Haven: Yale University Press, 1930), pp. 6-7.
11. Schubert Ogden, personal communication.

From System to Story:
An Alternative Pattern
for Rationality in Ethics

David Burrell
Stanley Hauerwas

I. Narrative, Ethics, and Theology

IN THE INTEREST of securing a rational foundation for morality,
contemporary ethical theory has ignored or rejected the significance of narrative for ethical reflection. It is our contention that
this has been a profound mistake, resulting in a distorted account
of moral experience. Furthermore, the attempt to portray practical
reason as independent of narrative contexts has made it difficult
to assess the value which convictions characteristic of Christians
or Jews might have for moral existence. As a result, we have lost
sight of the ways these traditions might help us deal with the
moral issues raised by modern science and medicine.[1]

To substantiate this thesis we will develop a negative and
positive argument. Negatively, we will characterize the standard
account of ethical rationality and the anomalies that such an
account occasions. This aspect of our argument will hold no
surprises for anyone acquainted with recent ethical theory. Most
of the criticisms we will develop have already been made by
others. However, we hope to show that these criticisms cannot be
met within the standard account and at least suggest why narra-

tive might be significant for an adequate analysis of moral existence. In developing this negative argument we will use
"narrative" and "character" without trying to analyze them fully.

Positively, we will analyze the concept of narrative and show
how it provides a pattern for moral rationality. We will argue that
the standard account of moral rationality has been wrong to
associate the narrative aspects of our experience with the subjective or arbitrary. In contrast we will suggest that narrative constitutes the form that does justice to the kind of objectivity proper
to practical reason. In order to show how it is possible to
discriminate between the truth of stories we will pay particular
attention to the way this was done by a master of narrative, St.
Augustine. Building on his story, we will suggest how the ve-
racity of stories can be tested.

Our argument involves two independent but interrelated theses.
First, we will try to establish the significance of narrative for
ethical reflection. By the phrase, "the significance of narrative,"
we mean to call attention to three points:[2] (1) that character and
moral notions only take on meaning in a narrative; (2) that
narrative and explanation stand in an intimate relationship, and,
therefore, moral disagreements involve rival histories of explanation; (3) that the standard account of moral objectivity is the
obverse of existentialist ethics, since the latter assumes that the
failure to secure moral objectivity implies that all moral judgments must be subjective or arbitrary. By showing the way
narrative can function as a form of rationality, we hope to
demonstrate that these do not represent the only alternatives.

Secondly, we will try to show how the convictions displayed
in the Christian story have moral significance. We will call
particular attention to the manner in which story teaches us to
know and do what is right under finite conditions. For at least
one indication of the moral truthfulness of a particular narrative is
the way it enables us to recognize the limits of our engagements
and yet continue to pursue them.

II. The Standard Account of Moral Rationality

At least partly under the inspiration of the scientific ideal of
objectivity,[3] contemporary ethical theory has tried to secure for

moral judgments an objectivity that would free such judgments from the subjective beliefs, wants, and stories of the agents who make them. Just as science tries to insure objectivity by adhering to an explicitly disinterested method, so ethical theory tries to show that moral judgments, insofar as they can be considered true, must be the result of an impersonal rationality. Thus moral judgments, whatever else they may involve, must at least be non-egoistic in the sense that they involve no special pleading colored by the agent's own history, community identification, or other particular point of view in order to establish their truthfulness.

Thus the hallmark of contemporary ethical theory, whether in a Kantian or utilitarian mode, has been to free moral behavior from the arbitrary and contingent nature of the agent's beliefs, dispositions, and character. Just as science strives to free the experiment from the experimenter, so, ethically, if we are to avoid unchecked subjectivism or relativism, it is thought that the moral life must be freed from the peculiarities of agents caught in the limits of their particular histories. Ethical rationality assumes it must take the form of science if it is to have any claim to being objective.[4]

There is an interesting parallel to this development in modern medical theory. Eric Cassell has located a tension between the explanation of a disease proper to science and the diagnosis a clinician makes for a particular patient.[5] The latter is well described by Tolstoy in *War and Peace*,

> Doctors came to see Natasha, both separately and in consultation. They said a great deal in French, in German, and in Latin. They criticised one another, and prescribed the most diverse remedies for all the diseases they were familiar with. But it never occurred to one of them to make the simple reflection that they could not understand the disease from which Natasha was suffering, as no single disease can be fully understood in a living person; for every living person has his complaints unknown to medicine—not a disease of the lungs, of the kidneys, of the skin, of the heart, and so on, as described in medical books, but a disease that consists of one out of the innumerable combinations of ailments of those organs.[6]

The scientific form of rationality is represented by B. F. Skinner's commentary on this quote. Skinner suggests that

Tolstoy was justified, during his day, in calling every sickness a unique event, but uniqueness no longer stands in the way of the development of the science of medicine since we can now supply the necessary general principles of explanation. Thus happily, according to Skinner, "the intuitive wisdom of the old-style diagnostician has been largely replaced by the analytic procedures of the clinic, just as a scientific analysis of behavior will eventually replace the personal interpretation of unique instances."[7]

Even if we were competent to do so, it would not be relevant to our argument to try to determine whether Tolstoy or Skinner, or some combination of their theories, describes the kind of explanation most appropriate to medical diagnosis (though our hunch lies with Tolstoy). Rather, it is our contention that the tendency of modern ethical theory to find a functional equivalent to Skinner's "scientific analysis" has distorted the nature of practical reason. Ethical objectivity cannot be secured by retreating from narrative, but only by being anchored in those narratives that best direct us toward the good.

Many thinkers have tried to free the objectivity of moral reason from narrative by arguing that there are basic moral principles, procedures, or points of view to which a person is logically or conceptually committed when engaged in moral action or judgment. This logical feature has been associated with such titles as the categorical imperative, the ideal observer, universalizability, or, more recently, the original position. Each of these in its own way assumes that reasons, if they are to be morally justified, must take the form of judgments that can and must be made from anyone's point of view.[8] All of the views assume that "objectivity" will be attained in the moral life only by freeing moral judgments from the "subjective" story of the agent.

This tradition has been criticized for the formal nature of its account of moral rationality, i.e., it seems to secure the objectivity of moral judgment exactly by emptying the moral life of all substantive content. Such criticism fails to appreciate, however, that these accounts of moral rationality are attempts to secure a "thin" theory of the moral life in order to provide an account of moral duty that is not subject to any community or tradition. Such theories are not meant to tell us how to be good in relation to some ideal, but rather to insure that what we owe to others as strangers, not as friends or sharers in a tradition, is non-arbitrary. What I am morally obligated to do is not what derives from being a father, or a son, or an American, or a teacher, or a doctor, or a Christian, but what follows from my being a person constituted by reason. To be sure all these other roles or relations may involve behavior that is morally good, but such behavior cannot be required except as it can be based upon or construed as appropriate to rationality itself. This is usually done by translating such role-dependent obligations as relations of promise-keeping that can be universalized. (Of course, what cannot be given are any moral reasons why I should become a husband, father, teacher, doctor, or Christian in the first place.)

It is our contention, however, that the standard account of moral rationality distorts the nature of the moral life by: (1) placing an unwarranted emphasis on particular decisions or quandaries; (2) by failing to account for the significance of moral notions and how they work to provide us with skills of perception; (3) by separating the agent from his interests. We will briefly spell out each of these criticisms and suggest how each stems in part from the way standard accounts avoid acknowledging the narrative character of moral existence.

II:1. Decisions, Character, and Narrative

In his article, "Quandary Ethics," Edmund Pincoffs has called attention to the way contemporary ethics concentrates on problems—situations in which it is hard to know what to do—as paradigmatic concerns for moral analysis.[9] On such a model, ethics becomes a decision procedure for resolving conflict-of-choice situations. This model assumes that no one faces an ethical issue until they find themselves in a quandary—should I or should I not have an abortion, etc. Thus the moral life appears to be concerned primarily with "hard decisions."

This picture of the moral life is not accidental, given the standard account of moral rationality. For the assumption that most of our moral concerns are "problems" suggests that ethics can be construed as a rational science that evaluates alternative "solutions." Moral decisions should be based on rationally derived principles that are not relative to any one set of convictions.

Ethics becomes a branch of decision theory. Like many of the so-called policy sciences, ethics becomes committed to those descriptions of the moral life that will prove relevant to its mode of analysis, that is, one which sees the moral life consisting of dilemmas open to rational "solutions."

By concentrating on "decisions" about "problems," this kind of ethical analysis gives the impression that judgments can be justified apart from the agent who finds himself or herself in the situation. What matters is not that David Burrell or Stanley Hauerwas confronts a certain quandary, but that anyone may or can confront X or Y. The intentions or reasons proper to a particular agent tend to become irrelevant. Thus, in considering the question of abortion, questions like: Why did the pregnancy occur? What kind of community do you live in? What do you believe about the place of children?—may be psychologically interesting but cannot be allowed to enter into the justification of the decision. For such matters are bound to vary from one agent to another. The "personal" can only be morally significant to the extent that it can be translated into the "impersonal."

(Although it is not central to our case, one of the implications of the standard account of rationality is its conservative force. Ethical choice is always making do within the societal framework we inherit, because it is only within such a framework that we are able to have a problem at all. But often the precise problem at issue cannot arise or be articulated given the limits of our society or culture. We suspect that this ineptness betrays a commitment of contemporary ethical theory to political liberalism: one can concentrate on the justification of moral decisions because one accepts the surrounding social order with its moral categories. In this sense modern ethical theory is functionally like modern pluralist democratic theory—it can afford to be concerned with incremental social change, to celebrate "issue" politics, because it assumes the underlying social structures are just.)[10]

By restricting rationality to choices between alternative courses of action, moreover, the various normative theories formed in accordance with the standard account have difficulty explaining the moral necessity to choose between lesser evils.[11] Since rational choice is also our moral duty, it must also be a good duty.

Otherwise one would be obliged rationally to do what is morally a lesser evil. There is no place for moral tragedy; whatever is morally obligatory must be good, even though the consequences may be less than happy. We may subjectively regret what we had to do, but it cannot be a moral regret. The fact that modern deontological and teleological theories assume that the lesser evil cannot be a moral duty witnesses to their common commitment to the standard view of moral rationality.

The problem of the lesser evil usually refers to tragic choices externally imposed, e.g., the necessity of killing civilians in order to destroy an arms factory. Yet the language of "necessity" is often misleading, for part of the "necessity" is the character of the actors, whether they be individuals or nations. Because moral philosophy, under the influence of the standard account, has thought it impossible to discuss what kind of character we should have—that, after all, is the result of the accident of birth and psychological conditioning—it has been assumed that moral deliberation must accept the limits of the decision required by his or her character. At best, "character" can be discussed in terms of "moral education"; but since the "moral" in education is determined by the standard account, it does not get us very far in addressing what kind of people we ought to be.

As a result, the standard account simply ignores the fact that most of the convictions that charge us morally are like the air we breathe—we never notice them, and do not do so precisely because they form us not to describe the world in certain ways and not to make certain matters subject to decision. Thus we assume that it is wrong to kill children without good reason. Or, even more strongly, we assume that it is our duty to provide children (and others who cannot protect themselves) with care that we do not need to give to the adult. These are not matters that we need to articulate or decide upon; their force lies rather in their not being subject to decision. And morally we must have the kind of character that keeps us from subjecting them to decision.

(What makes "medical ethics" so difficult is the penchant of medical care to force decisions that seem to call into question aspects of our life that we assumed not to be matters of decision, e.g., should we provide medical care for children who are born with major disabilities such as meningomyelocele.[12] In this respect the current interest in "medical ethics" does not simply represent a response to issues arising in modern medicine, but also reflects the penchant of the standard account to respond to dilemmas.)

Another way to make this point is to indicate that the standard account, by concentrating on decision, fails to deal adequately with the formation of a moral self, i.e., the virtues and character we think it important for moral agents to acquire. But the kind of decisions we confront, indeed the very way we describe a situation, is a function of the kind of character we have. And character is not acquired through decisions, though it may be confirmed and qualified there, but rather through the beliefs and dispositions we have acquired.

From the perspective of the standard account, beliefs and dispositions cannot be subject to rational deliberation and formation.[13] Positions based on the standard account do not claim that our dispositions, or our character, are irrelevant to how we act morally. But these aspects of our self are rational only as they enter into a moral decision. It is our contention, however, that it is rather character, inasmuch as it is displayed by a narrative, that provides the context necessary to pose the terms of a decision, or to determine whether a decision should be made at all.[14]

We cannot account for our moral life solely by the decisions we make; we also need the narratives that form us to have one kind of character rather than another. These narratives are not arbitrarily acquired, although they will embody many factors we might consider "contingent." As our stories, however, they will determine what kind of moral considerations—that is, what reasons—will count at all. Hence these narratives must be included in any account of moral rationality that does not unwarrantedly exclude large aspects of our moral existence—i.e., moral character.[15]

The standard account cannot help but view a narrative account as a retreat from moral objectivity. For if the individual agent's intentions and motives—in short, the narrative embodied in his or her character—are to have systematic significance for moral judgment, then it seems that we will have to give preference to the agent's interpretation of what he has done. So the dreaded first person singular, which the standard account was meant to purge from moral argument, would be reintroduced. To recall the force of "I," however, does not imply that we would propose "because I want to" as a moral reason. The fact is that the first person singular is seldom the assertion of the solitary "I," but rather the narrative of that "I." It is exactly the category of narrative that helps us to see that we are not forced to choose between some universal standpoint and the subjectivistic appeals to our own experience. For our experiences always come in the form of narratives that can be checked against themselves as well as others' experiences. I cannot make my behavior mean anything I want it to mean, for I have learned to understand my life from the stories I have learned from others.

The language the agent uses to describe his behavior, to himself and to others, is not uniquely his—it is *ours*, just as the notions we use have meanings that can be checked for appropriate or inappropriate use. But what allows us to check the truthfulness of these accounts of our behavior are the narratives from which our moral notions derive their paradigms. An agent cannot make his behavior mean anything he wants, since at the very least it must make sense within his own story, as well as be compatible with the narrative embodied in the language he uses. All our notions are narrative-dependent, including the notion of rationality.

II:2. Moral Notions, Language, and Narrative

We can show how our very notion of rationality depends on narrative by noting how the standard account tends to ignore the significance and meaning of moral notions. The standard account pictures our world as a *given* about which we need to make decisions. So terms like "murder," "stealing," "abortion," although admitted to be evaluative, are nonetheless regarded as descriptive. However, as Julius Kovesi has persuasively argued, our moral notions are not descriptive in the sense that yellow is, but rather describe only as we have purposes for such descriptions.[16] Moral notions, in other words, like many of our non-moral notions (though we are not nearly so sure as is the standard account how this distinction should be made), do not merely describe our activity; they also form it. Marx's claim, that the point of philosophy should be not to analyze the world but to change it, is not only a directive to ethicists but also an astute observation about the way our grammar displays the moral direction of our lives. The notions that form our moral perceptions involve skills that require narratives, that is, accounts of their institutional contexts and purposes, which we must know if we are to know how to employ them correctly. In other words, these notions resemble skills of perception which we must learn how to use properly.

The standard account's attempt to separate our moral notions from their narrative context by trying to ground them in, or derive their meaning from, rationality in itself has made it difficult to account for two reasons why moral controversies are so irresolvable. The standard account, for example, encourages us to assume that the pro- and anti-abortion advocates mean the same thing by the word "abortion." It is assumed, therefore, that the moral disagreement between these two sides must involve a basic moral principle, such as "all life is sacred," or be a matter of fact, such as whether the fetus is considered a human life. But this kind of analysis fails to see that the issue is not one of principle or fact, but one of perception determined by a history of interpretation.

Pro- and anti-abortion advocates do not communicate on the notion "abortion," since each group holds a different story about the purpose of the notion. At least as far as "abortion" is concerned, they live in conceptually different worlds. This fact does not prohibit discussion, but if abortion takes place, it cannot begin with the simple question of whether it is right or wrong. It is rather more like an argument between a member of the PLO and an Israeli about whether an attack on a village is unjustified terrorism. They both know the same "facts" but the issue turns on the story each holds, and within which those "facts" are known.

The advocates of the standard account try to train us to ignore the dependence of the meaning and use of notions on their narrative contexts, by providing a normative theory for the derivation and justification of basic moral notions. But to be narrative-dependent is not the same as being theory-dependent, at least in the way that a utilitarian or deontological position would have us think. What makes abortion right or wrong is not its capacity to work for or against the greatest good of the greatest number in a certain subclass. What sets the context for one's moral judgment is rather the stories we hold about the place of children in our lives, or the connection one deems ought or ought not to hold between sexuality and procreation, or some other such account. Deontological or utilitarian theories that try to free moral notions from their dependence on examples and the narratives that display them, prove to be too monochromatic to account for the variety of our notions and the histories on which they are dependent.

There can be no normative theory of the moral life that is sufficient to capture the rich texture of the many moral notions we inherit. What we actually possess are various and sometimes conflicting stories that provide us with the skills to use certain moral notions. What we need to develop is the reflective capacity to analyze those stories, so that we better understand how they function. It is not theory-building that develops such a capacity so much as close attention to the ways our distinctive communities tell their stories. Furthermore, an analysis of this sort carries us to the point of assessing the worth these moral notions have for directing our life-projects and shaping our stories.

The standard account's project to supply a theory of basic moral principles from which all other principles and actions can be justified or derived represents an attempt to make the moral life take on the characteristics of a system. But it is profoundly misleading to think that a rational explanation needs to be given for holding rational beliefs,[17] for to attempt to provide such an account assumes that rationality itself does not depend on narrative. What must be faced, however, is that our lives are not and cannot be subject to such an account, for the consistency necessary for governing our lives is more a matter of integrity than one of principle. The narratives that provide the pattern of integrity cannot be based on principle, nor are they engaging ways of talking about principles. Rather such narratives are the ones that allow us to determine how our behavior "fits" within our ongoing pattern.[18] To be sure, fittingness cannot have the necessitating form desired by those who want the moral life to have the "firmness" of some sciences, but it can exhibit the rationality of a good story.

II:3. Rationality, Alienation, and the Self

The standard account also has the distressing effect of making alienation the central moral virtue. We are moral exactly to the extent that we learn to view our desires, interests, and passions as if they could belong to anyone. The moral point of view, whether it is construed in a deontological or teleological manner, requires that we view our own projects and life as if we were outside observers. This can perhaps be seen most vividly in utilitarianism (and interestingly in Rawls's account of the original position) since the utilitarian invites us to assume that perspective toward our projects which will produce the best consequences for anyone's life plan. Thus, the standard account obligates us to regard our life as would an observer.

Paradoxically, what makes our projects valuable to us (as Bernard Williams has argued) is that they are ours. As soon as we take the perspective of the standard account, we accept the odd position of viewing our stories as if they were anyone's, or at least capable of being lived out by anyone. Thus, we are required to alienate ourselves from the projects that interest us in being anything at all.

The alienation involved in the standard account manifests itself in the different ways the self is understood by modern ethical theory. The self is often pictured as consisting of reason and desire, with the primary function of reason being to control desire. It is further assumed that desire or passion can give no clues to the nature of the good, for the good can only be determined in accordance with "reason." Thus, the standard account places us in the odd position of excluding pleasure as an integral aspect of doing the good. The good cannot be the satisfaction of desire, since the morality of reason requires a sharp distinction between universal rules of conduct and the "contingent" appetites of individuals.

Not only are we taught to view our desires in contrast to our reason, but the standard account also separates our present from our past. Morally, the self represents a collection of discontinuous decisions bound together only in the measure they approximate the moral point of view. Our moral capacity thus depends exactly on our ability to view our past in discontinuity with our present. The past is a limitation, since it can only prevent us from embodying more fully the new opportunities always guaranteed by the moral point of view. Thus, our moral potentiality depends on our being able to alienate ourselves from our past in order to grasp the timelessness of the rationality offered by the standard account.[19]

(In theological terms the alienation of the self is a necessary consequence of sinful pretensions. When the self tries to be more than it was meant to be, it becomes alienated from itself and all its relations are disordered. The view of rationality offered by the standard account is pretentious exactly as it encourages us to try to free ourselves from history. In effect it offers us the possibility of being like God. Ironically enough, however, this is not the God of the Jews and the Christians since, as we shall see, that God does not will himself to be free from history.)

In fairness, the alienation recommended by the standard account is motivated by the interest of securing moral truthfulness. But it mistakenly assumes that truthfulness is possible only if we judge ourselves and others from the position of complete (or as complete as possible) disinterest. Even if it were possible to assume such a stance, however, it would not provide us with the conditions for truthfulness. For morally there is no neutral story that insures the truthfulness of our particular stories. Moreover, any ethical theory that is sufficiently abstract and universal to claim neutrality would not be able to form character. For it would have deprived itself of the notions and convictions that are the necessary conditions for character. Far from assuring truthfulness, a species of rationality that prizes objectivity to the neglect of particular stories distorts moral reasoning by the way it omits the stories of character formation. If truthfulness (and the selflessness characteristic of moral behavior) is to be found, it will have to occur in and through the stories that we find tie the contingencies of our life together.

It is not our intention to call into question the significance of disinterestedness for the moral life, but rather to deny that recent accounts of "universality" or the "moral point of view" provide adequate basis for such disinterest. For genuine disinterest reflects a non-interest in the self occasioned by the lure of a greater good or a more beautiful object than we can create or will into existence.[20] In this sense we are not able to choose to conform to the moral point of view, for it is a gift. But as a gift it depends on our self being formed by a narrative that provides the conditions for developing the disinterest required for moral behavior.

II:4. The Standard Account's Story

None of the criticisms above constitute a decisive objection to the standard account, but taken together they indicate that the standard account is seriously inadequate as a description of our moral existence. How then are we to account for the continued dominance of the standard account for contemporary ethical theory? If our analysis has been right, the explanation should be found in the narrative that provides an apparent cogency for the standard account in spite of its internal and external difficulties.[21]

It is difficult, however, to identify any one narrative that sets the context for the standard account, for it is not one but many narratives that sustain its plausibility. The form of some of these stories is of recent origin, but we suspect that the basic story underlying the standard account is of more ancient lineage— namely, humankind's quest for certainty in a world of contingency.

It seems inappropriate to attribute such a grand story to the standard account, since one of its attractions is its humility: it does not pretend to address matters of the human condition, for it is only a method. As a method it does not promise truth, only clarity. .

Yet the process of acculturating ourselves and others in the use of this method requires a systematic disparaging of narrative. By teaching us to prefer a "principle" or "rational" description (just as science prefers a statistical description) to a narrative description, the standard account not only fails to account for the significance of narrative but also sets obstacles to any therapy designed to bring that tendency to light. It thus fails to provide us with the critical skills to know the limits of the narrative which currently has us in its grasp.

The reason for this lack of critical perspective lies in the narrative that was born during the Enlightenment. The plot was given in capsule by Auguste Comte: first came religion in the form of stories, then philosophy in the form of metaphysical analysis, and then science with its exact methods.[22] The story he tells in outline is set within another elaborated by Hegel, to show us how each of these ages supplanted the other as a refinement in the progressive development of reason. Therefore, stories are pre-scientific, according to the story legitimizing the age that calls itself scientific. Yet if one overlooks that budding contradiction, or fails to spell it out because everyone knows that stories are out of favor anyway, then the subterfuge has worked and the way out been blocked off.

Henceforth, any careful or respectable analysis, especially if it is moral in intent, will strike directly for the problem, leaving the rest for journalists who titillate or novelists who entertain. Serious folk, intent on improving the human condition, will have no time for that (except, maybe, after hours) for they must focus all available talent and resources on solving the problems in front of them. We all recognize the crude polarities acting here, and know how effectively they function as blinders. It is sufficient for our interests to call attention only to the capacity stories hold for eliciting critical awareness, and how an awareness of story enhances that approach known as scientific by awakening it to its presuppositions. Hence, we have argued for a renewed awareness of stories as an analytic tool, and one especially adopted to our moral existence, since stories are designed to effect critical awareness as well as describe a state of affairs.

By calling attention to the narrative context of the standard account, we are not proposing a wholesale rejection of that account or of the theories formed under its inspiration. In fact, the efforts expended on developing contrasting ethical theories (like utilitarianism or formalism) have become part of our legacy, and offer a useful way to introduce one to ethical reasoning. Furthermore, the manner of proceeding that we associate with the standard account embodies concerns that any substantive moral narrative must respect: a high regard for public discourse, the demand that we be able to offer reasons for acting, at once cogent and appropriate, and a way to develop critical skills of discrimination and judgment. Finally, any morality depends on a capacity to generate and to articulate moral principles which can set boundaries for proper behavior and guide our conduct.

Our emphasis on narrative need not militate against any of these distinctive concerns. Our difficulty rather lies with the way the standard account attempts to express and to ground these concerns in a narrative-free manner of accounting. We are given the impression that moral principles offer actual grounds for conduct, while in fact they present abstractions whose significance continues to depend on original narrative contexts. Abstractions play useful roles in reasoning, but a continual failure to identify them as abstractions becomes systematically misleading: a concern for rationality thereby degenerates into a form of rationalism.

Our criticism of the standard account has focused on the anomalies that result from that rationalism. We have tried to show how the hegemony of the standard account in ethics has in fact ignored or distorted significant aspects of moral experience. We do not wish to gainsay the importance of rationality for ethics; only expose a pretentious form of rationalism. Though the point can be made in different ways, it is no accident that the stories that form the lives of Jews and of Christians make them peculiarly sensitive to any account that demands that human existence fit a rational framework. The legitimate human concern for rationality is framed by a range of powers of quite another order. It is this larger contingent context which narrative is designed to order in the only manner available to us.

In this way, we offer a substantive explication of narrative as a constructive alternative to the standard account. Our penchant has been to rely upon the standard account as though it were the only lifeboat in a sea of subjective reactions and reductive explanations. To question it would be tantamount to exposing the leaks in the only bark remaining to us. In harkening to the narrative context for action, we are trying to direct attention to an alternative boat available to us. This one cannot provide the security promised by the other, but in return it contains instructions designed to equip us with the skills required to negotiate the dangers of the open sea.

III. Stories and Reasons for Acting

Ethics deals explicitly with reasons for acting. The trick lies in turning reasons into a form proper to acting. The normal form for reasoning requires propositions to be linked so as to display how the conclusion follows quite naturally. The very skills that allow us to form statements lead us to draw other statements from them as conclusions. The same Aristotle who perfected this art, however, also reminded us that practical syllogisms must conclude in an action rather than another proposition.[23] As syllogisms, they will display the form proper to reasoning, yet they must do so in a way that issues in action.

This difference reflects the fact that practical wisdom cannot claim to be a science, since it must deal with particular courses of action (rather than recurrent patterns); nor can it call itself an art, since "action and making are different kinds of thing." The alternative Aristotle settles for is "a true and reasoned . . . capacity to act with regard to the things that are good or bad for man" (*N. Ethics* 6.4, 1140b5). We have suggested that stories in fact help us all to develop that capacity as a reasoned capacity. This section will focus on the narrative form as a form of rationality; the following section will show how discriminating among stories develops skills for judging truly what is "good or bad for man." Using Aristotle's discriminations as a point of reference is meant to indicate that our thesis could be regarded as a development of his—in fact, we would be pleased to find it judged to be so.

III:1. Narrative Form as Rational Discourse

There are many kinds of stories, and little agreement on how to separate them into kinds. We distinguish short stories from novels, while acknowledging the short novel as well. We recognize that some stories offer with a particular lucidity patterns or plots that recur in countless other stories. We call these more archetypal stories myths, and often use them as a shorthand for referring to a typical tangle or dilemma that persons find themselves facing—whether in a story or in real life. That feature common to all stories, which gives them their peculiar aptitude for illuminating real life situations, is their narrative structure.

Experts will want to anatomize narrative as well, of course, but for our purposes let it be the connected description of action and of suffering which moves to a point. The point need not be detachable from the narrative itself; in fact, we think a story better that does not issue in a determinate *moral*. The "point" we call attention to here has to do with that form of connectedness that characterizes a novel. It is not the mere material connection of happenings to one individual, but the connected unfolding that we call *plot*. Difficult as this is to characterize—independently of displaying it in a good story!—we can nonetheless identify it as a connection among elements (actions, events, situations) which is neither one of logical consequence nor one of mere sequence. The connection seems rather designed to move our understanding of a situation forward by developing or unfolding it. We have described this movement as gathering to a point. Like implication, it seeks to make explicit what would otherwise remain implicit; unlike implication, the rules of development are not those of logic but stem from some more mysterious source.

The rules of development are not logical rules because narrative connects contingent events. The intelligibility which plot affords is not a necessary one, because the events connected do not exhibit recurrent patterns. Narrative is not required to be explanatory, then, in the sense in which a scientific theory must show necessary connections among occurrences. What we demand of a narrative is that it display how occurrences are actions. Intentional behavior is purposeful but not necessary. We are not possessed of the theoretical capacities to predict what will happen on the basis of what has occurred. Thus, a narrative moves us on to answer the question that dogs us: what happened next? It cannot answer that question by arbitrary statement, for our inquiring minds are already involved in the process. Yet the question is a genuine one precisely because we lack the capacity for sure prediction.

It is the intentional nature of human action that evokes a narrative account. We act for an end, yet our actions affect a field of forces in ways that may be characteristic yet remain unpredictable. So we can ask: What would follow from our hiring Jones?—as though certain events might be deduced from his coming on board. Yet we also know that whatever follows will not do so deductively, but rather as a plot unfolds. Nevertheless, we are right in inquiring into what might *follow from* our hiring him, since we must act responsibly. By structuring a plausible response to the question—and what happened next?—narrative offers just the intelligibility we need for acting properly.

III:2. What the Narrative Unfolds

But what makes a narrative plausible? The field of a story is actions (either deeds or dreams) or their opposite, sufferings. In either case, whatever action or passion is seen to unfold is something we call "character." *Character*, of course, is not a theoretical notion, but merely the name we give to the cumulative source of human actions. Stories themselves attempt to probe that source and discover its inner structure by trying to display how human actions and passions connect with one another to develop a character. As we follow the story, we gain some insight into recurrent connecting patterns, and also some ability to assess them. We learn to recognize different configurations and to rank some characters better than others.

Gradually, then, the characters (or ways of unifying actions) that we can recognize offer patterns for predicting recurring ways of acting. Expectations are set up, and the way an individual or others deal with those expectations shows us some of the capacities of the human spirit. In this way, character can assume the role of an analytic tool even though it is not itself an explanatory notion. Character is neither explanatory in origin nor in use, for it cannot be formulated prior to nor independently of the narrative that develops it. Yet it can play an illuminating or analytic role by calling attention to what is going on in a narrative as the plot unfolds: a character is being developed. Moreover, this character, as it develops, serves as a relative baseline for further developing itself or other characters, as we measure subsequent actions and responses against those anticipated by the character already developed. In this way, character plays an analytic role by offering a baseline for further development. That the baseline itself will shift represents one more way of distinguishing narrative development from logical implication.

We may consider the set of expectations associated with a developing character as a "language"—a systematic set of connections between actions that offers a setting or syntax for subsequent responses. Since character cannot be presented independently of the story or stories that develop it, however, the connection between a syntactical system and use, or the way in which a language embodies a form of life, becomes crystal clear. By attending to character, stories will display this fact to us without any need for philosophical reminders.

Similarly, we will see how actions, like expressions, accomplish what they do as part of a traditional repertoire. What a narrative must do is to set out the antecedent actions in such a way as to clarify how the resulting pattern becomes a tradition. In this way, we will see why certain actions prove effective and others fail, much as some expressions succeed in saying what they mean while others cannot. Some forms of story, like the three-generational Victorian novel, are expressly designed to display how a grammar for actions develops, by adopting a deliberately historical, even explicitly generational, structure. Lawrence's *Rainbow*, for example, shows how the shaping habits of speech and personal interaction are altered over three generations in response to industrial development. As he skillfully displays this alteration in grammar over against a traditional syntax, we can grasp something of the capacities latent in us as human beings. In articulating the characters, Lawrence succeeds in making explicit some reaches of the human spirit as yet unexplored.

Stories, then, certainly offer more than entertainment. What they do offer, however, cannot be formulated independently of our appreciating the story, so seeking entertainment is less distracting than looking for a moral. The reason lies with the narrative structure, whose plot cannot be abstracted without banality, yet whose unity does depend on its having a point. Hence it is appropriate to speak of a plot, to call attention to the ordering peculiar to narrative. It is that ordering, that capacity to unfold or develop character, and thus offer insight into the human condition, which recommends narrative as a form of rationality especially appropriate to ethics.

III:3. How a Narrative Unfolds

If a narrative becomes plausible as it succeeds in displaying a believable character, we may still ask how *that* achievement offers us an intelligibility appropriate to discriminating among courses of action. Using Aristotle's language, how can stories assist in the formation of a practical wisdom? How can stories themselves develop a capacity for judging among alternatives, and further: how does discriminating among stories make that capacity even keener? Since reading stories for more than mere entertainment is usually described as "appreciating" them, some skills for assessing among them are already implied in one's appreciating any single story.

We often find ourselves quite unable, however, to specify the grounds for preferring one story to another. Critics, of course, develop a language for doing this, trying to formulate our normally inchoate criteria. Yet these criteria themselves are notoriously ambiguous. They must be rendered in utterly analogous terms, like "unity," "wholeness," "consistency," "integrity," etc. We cannot hope to grasp the criteria without a paradigmatic instance, yet how present an exemplary instance without telling a story?[24] Criticism thus can only conceive itself as disciplining our native capacity to appreciate a good story.

A complete account of the way narrative functions, then, would be a narrative recounting how one came to judge certain stories as better than others. Since this narrative would have to be autobiographical, in the perceived character of its author we would have a vantage for judgment beyond the intrinsic merit of the narrative itself. If stories are designed to display how one might create and relate to a world and so offer us a paradigm for adopting a similar posture, this autobiographical story would have to show how a person's current manner of relating himself to the world itself represents a posture towards alternative stances. The narrative will have to recount why, and do so in the fashion proper to narrative: that one stance comes after another, preferably by improving upon its predecessor.[25]

Augustine's *Confessions* offer just such an account by showing how Augustine's many relationships, all patterned on available stories, were gradually relativized to one overriding and ordering relationship with the God revealing himself in Jesus. Augustine's life story is the story of that process of ordering.

III:4. Augustine's *Confessions*: A Narrative Assessment of Life Stories

Writing ten years after the decisive moment in the garden, Augustine sees that event as culminating a quest shaped by two questions: How to account for evil, and how to conceive of God? That quest was also dogged by demands much more immediate than questions, of course. These needs were symbolically ordered in the experience recounted in Book 9, and monitored sense by sense, passion by passion, in Book 10. What interests us here, however, is the step-like manner in which Augustine describes himself relating to the shaping questions: How explain evil? How conceive divinity?

The pear-tree story allows him to telegraph to the reader how he was able to discriminate one question from the other early on, even though the skills developed to respond to one would help him meet the other. For his own action, reflected upon, allowed him to glimpse an evil deed as wanton or pointless (2.4-10). From the perspective displayed by the *Confessions*, he formulates clearly an intimation that guided his earlier quest: what makes an action evil is not so much a reason as the lack of one. So we would be misled to attribute evil to the creator who orders all things, since ordering and giving reasons belong together.

By separating in this way the query into the source of evil from the attempt to conceive divinity, Augustine took a categorial step. That is, he was learning how to slip from the grip in which Manichean teaching held him, as he came to realize that nothing could properly explain the presence of evil in the world. Nothing, that is, short of a quality of human freedom that allowed us to act for no reason at all. Since explanations offer reasons, and evil turns on the lack of reasons, some form other than a causal explanation must be called for. The only form that can exhibit an action without pretending to explain it is the very one he adopted for the book itself: narrative. So Augustine took his first decisive step toward responding to the shaping questions by eschewing the pretense of explanation in favor of a reflective story.

Categorial discriminations are not usually made all at once, of course. If we are set to turn up an explanation, we will ordinarily keep trying to find a satisfactory one. We cannot give up the enterprise of looking for an explanation unless our very horizon shifts. (It is just such a horizon-shift or paradigmatic change that we identify as a categorial discrimination.) Yet horizons form the stable background for inquiry, so normally we cannot allow them to shift. In Augustine's case, as in many, it only occurred to him to seek elsewhere after repeated attempts at explaining proved fruitless. Furthermore, the specific way in which the Manichean scheme failed to explain the presence of evil also suggested why seeking an explanation was itself a fruitless tack.

To be sure, the Manichean accounts to which Augustine alludes strike us as altogether too crude to qualify as explanations. In fact, it sounds odd to identify his rejection of Manichean teachings with the explicit adoption of a story form, since it is their schemes which sound to us like "stories." The confusion is understandable enough, of course; it is the very one this essay addresses: stories are fanciful, while explanations are what offer intelligibility. Yet fanciful as they appear to us, the Manichean schemes are explanatory in form. They postulate causes for behavior in the form of diverse combinations of "particles" of light or darkness. The nature of the particles is less relevant, of course, than the explanatory pretense.

What first struck Augustine was the scheme's inability to explain diverse kinds of behavior coherently (5.10, 7.1-6). What he came to realize, however, was that *any* explanatory scheme would, in principle, undermine a person's ability to repent because it would remove whatever capacity we might have for assuming responsibility for our own actions (6.5, 7.12-13, 8.10). This capacity to assume responsibility would not always suffice to accomplish what we (or at least a part of us) desire (8.8-9); but such a capacity is logically necessary if we are to claim our actions as our own—and so receive praise or blame for them. If our contrary actions could be explained by contrary substances within us, then we would not be able to own them. And if we cannot own our actions, then we have no self to speak of. So the incoherence of the explanations offered led Augustine to see how the very quest for explanation itself failed to cohere with the larger life project belonging to every person.

As the narrative of Augustine's own life project displays, this deliberate shift away from the explanatory modes of the Manichees or the astrologers led to adopting a form which would also help him better to conceive divinity. If evil is senseless, we cannot attribute it to the one who creates with order and reason. If we commit evil deeds, we must be able to own up to them—to confess them—if we want to open ourselves to a change of heart. And the more we examine that self who can act responsibly—in accomplishing deeds or in judging among opinions—the more we come into possession of a language for articulating divinity. It was a language of inwardness, as practiced by the Platonists of his day (7.10). It assumed a scheme of powers of the soul, but made its point by transcendental argument: if we are to make the discriminations we do, we must do so by virtue of an innate light or power (7.17). This way of articulating the power by which we act responsibly, then, becomes the model for expressing divinity. The path which led away from seeking an explanation for evil offers some promise for responding to the second question as well.

Augustine must take one more step, however, lest he forfeit the larger lesson of his struggle with the Manichees, and simply substitute a Platonist explanatory scheme for theirs.[26] They appeal to formal facts by way of transcendental argument. His life, however, was framed by facts of another kind: of rights and wrongs dealt to others (6.15); of an order to which he now aspired to conform, but which he found himself unable to accomplish (8.11). What he misses in the Platonists' books is "the mien of the true love of God. They make no mention of the tears of confession" (7.21). He can read there "of the Word, God . . ., but not read in them that 'the Word was made flesh and came to dwell among us' (John 1:14)" (7.9). While they speak persuasively of the conditions for acting and judging aright, they do not tell us how to do what we find ourselves unable to do: to set our hearts aright.

The key to that feat Augustine finds not in the books of the Platonists, but in the gospels. Or better, he finds it in allowing the stories of the gospels to shape his story. The moment of permission, as he records it, is preceded by stories of others allowing the same to happen to them—recounting how they did it and what allowing it to happen did to them. The effect of these stories is to insinuate a shift in grammar tantamount to the shift from explanation to narrative, although quite in line with that earlier shift. Since we think of stories as relating accomplishments, Augustine must use these stories together with his own to show us another way of conceiving them.

It is not a new way, for it consciously imitates the biblical manner of displaying God's great deeds in behalf of his people. Without ceasing to be the story of Israel, the tales of the Bible present the story of God. Similarly, without ceasing to be autobiography, Augustine's *Confessions* offer an account of God's way with him. The language of will and of struggle is replaced by that of the heart: "as I came to the end of the sentence, it was as though the light of confidence flooded into my heart and all the darkness of doubt was dispelled" (8.12). Yet the transformation is not a piece of magic; the narrative testifies to that. And his narrative will give final testimony to the transformation of that moment in the measure that it conforms to the life story of the "Word made flesh." So the answer to his shaping questions is finally received rather than formulated, and that reception is displayed in the narrative we have analyzed.

IV. Truthfulness as Veracity and Faithfulness

The second step which Augustine relates is not a categorial one. It no longer has to do with finding the proper form for rendering a life project intelligible. The narrative Augustine tells shows us how he was moved to accept the gospel story by allowing it to shape his own. In more conventional terms, this second step moves beyond philosophical therapy to a judgment of truth. That is why recognizable arguments surround the first step, but not this one. Assent involves more subtle movements than clarification does, notably, assent of this sort, which is not assent *to* evidence but an assent *of* faith. Yet we will grasp its peculiar warrants better if we see how it moves along the same lines as the categorial discrimination.

Accepting a story as normative, by allowing it to shape one's own story, in effect reinforces the categorial preference for story over explanation as a vehicle of understanding. Augustine adumbrates the way one step leads into the other towards the beginning of Book 6:

> From now on I began to prefer the Catholic teaching. The Church demanded that certain things should be believed even though they could not be proved. . . . I thought that the Church was entirely honest in this and far less pretentious than the Manichees, who laughed at people who took things on faith, made rash promises of scientific knowledge, and then put forward a whole system of preposterous inventions which they expected their followers to believe on trust because they could not be proved (6.5).

The chapter continues in a similar vein, echoing many contemporary critiques of modern rationalist pretensions.

IV:1. Criteria for Judging among Stories

The studied preference for story over explanation, then, moves one into a neighborhood more amenable to what thirteenth-century theologians called an "assent of faith," and in doing so, helps us develop a set of criteria for judging among stories. Books 8-9-10 of the *Confessions* record the ways in which this capacity for discriminating among stories is developed. It is less a matter of weighing arguments than of displaying how adopting different stories will lead us to become different sorts of persons. The test of each story is the sort of person it shapes. When examples of diverse types are offered to us for our acceptance, the choices we make display, in turn, our own grasp of the *humanum*. Aristotle presumed we could not fail to recognize a just man, but also knew he would come in different guises (*N. Ethics* I, 1-7).

The criteria for judging among stories, then, will most probably not pass an impartial inspection. For the powers of recognition cannot be divorced from one's own capacity to recognize the good for humankind. This observation need not amount to a counsel of despair, however. It is simply a reminder that on matters of judgment we consult more readily with some persons than others, because we recognize them to be in a better position to weigh matters sensibly. Any account of that "position" would have to be autobiographical, of course. But it is not an account we count on; it is simply our recognition of the person's integrity.

Should we want to characterize the story that gives such coherence to a person's life, however, it would doubtless prove helpful to contrast it with alternatives. The task is a difficult one, either for oneself or for another, for we cannot always identify the paths we have taken; Augustine continued to be engaged in mapping out the paths he was actually traversing at the very time of composing the *Confessions—vide* Book 10. Yet we can certainly formulate a list of working criteria, provided we realize that any such list cannot pretend to completeness or achieve unambiguous expression.

Any story which we adopt, or allow to adopt us, will have to display:

(1) power to release us from destructive alternatives
(2) ways of seeing through current distortions
(3) room to keep us from having to resort to violence
(4) a sense for the tragic: how meaning transcends power.

It is inaccurate, of course, to list these criteria as features that a story must display. They envisage rather the effect that stories might be expected to have on those who allow them to shape their lives. The fact that stories are meant to be read, however, forces one to speak of them as relational facts. So we cannot help regarding a story as something that (when well constructed) will help us develop certain skills of perception and understanding. This perspective corresponds exactly to the primary function of narratives by contrast with explanatory schemes: to relate us to the world, including our plans for modifying it. Those plans have consequences of their own, but their shape as well as their execution depends on the expectations we entertain for planning.

Such expectations become a part of the plans themselves, but they can be articulated independently and when they are, they take the form of stories, notably of heros. Thus the process of industrialization becomes the story of tycoons, as the technology we know embodies a myth of man's dominating and transforming the earth. Not that industrial processes are themselves stories, or technological expertise a myth. In fact, we are witnessing today many attempts to turn those processes and that expertise to different ends by yoking them to a different outlook. Stories of these experiments suggest new ways of using some of the skills we have developed, and illustrate the role of narrative in helping us formulate and practice new perspectives.[27]

Stories, then, help us, as we hold them, to relate to our world and our destiny: the origins and goal of our lives, as they embody in narrative form specific ways of acting out that relatedness. In allowing ourselves to adopt and be adopted by a particular story, we are, in fact, assuming a set of practices that will shape the ways we relate to our world and destiny. Lest this sound too instrumental, we should remind ourselves that the world is not simply waiting to be seen, but that language and institutions train us to regard it in certain ways.[28] The criteria listed above assume this fact; let us consider them in greater detail.

IV:2. Testing the Criteria

Stories that (1) empower us to free ourselves from destructive alternatives can also (2) offer ways to see through current distortions. To judge an alternative course to be destructive, of course, requires some experience of its effects on those who practice the skills it embodies. It is the precise role of narrative to offer us a way of experiencing those effects without experimenting with our own lives as well. The verisimilitude of the story, along with its assessable literary structure, will allow us to ascertain whether we can trust it as a vehicle of insight, or whether we are being misled. In the absence of narratives, recommendations for adopting a set of practices can only present themselves as a form of propaganda and be judged accordingly.[29] Only narrative can allow us to take the measure of a scheme for human improvement—granting that we possess the usual skills for discriminating among narratives as well.

For we can learn how to see a current ideology as a distortion by watching what it can do to people who let it shape their story. The seduction of Manichean doctrine for Augustine and his contemporaries lay precisely in its offering itself as a *story* for humankind—much as current problem-solving techniques will invariably also be packaged as a set of practices leading to personal fulfillment. Therefore, Augustine's subsequent discrimination between explanation and story first required an accurate identification of Manichean teaching as explanatory pretense in the guise of a story.

The last two criteria also go together: (3) providing room to keep us from having to resort to violence, and (4) offering a sense for the tragic: how meaning transcends power. We can watch these criteria operate if we contrast the story characteristic to Christians and Jews with one of the prevailing presumptions of contemporary culture: that we can count on technique to offer eventual relief from the human condition. This conviction is reflected in the penchant of consequential ethical theories not only to equate doing one's duty with the greatest good for all, but also to presume that meeting our obligations will provide the satisfaction we seek. Surely, current medical practice is confirmed by the conviction that harnessing more human energies into preventing and curing disease will increasingly free our lives from tragic dilemmas.[30] Indeed, science as a moral enterprise has provided what Ernest Becker has called an anthropodicy, as it holds out the possibility that our increased knowledge serves human progress toward the creation of a new human ideal—namely, to create a mankind free of suffering.[31]

But this particular ethos has belied the fact that medicine, at least as characterized by its moral commitment to the individual patient, is a tragic profession. To attend to one in distress often means many others cannot be helped. To save a child born retarded may well destroy the child's family and cause unnecessary burdens on society. But the doctor is pledged to care for each patient because medicine does not aim at some ideal moral good, but to care for the needs of the patient whom the doctor finds before him. Because we do not know how to regard medicine as a tragic profession, we tend of course to confuse caring with curing. The story that accompanies technology—of setting nature aright—results in the clinical anomalies to which we are subjecting others and ourselves in order to avoid the limits of our existence.[32]

The practice of medicine under the conditions of finitude offers an intense paradigm of the moral life. The moral task is to learn to continue to do the right, to care for this immediate patient, even when we have no assurance that it will be the successful thing to do. To live morally, in other words, we need a substantive story that will sustain moral activity in a finite and limited world. Classically, the name we give to such stories is tragedy. When a culture loses touch with the tragic, as ours clearly has done, we must describe our failures in acceptable terms. Yet to do so *ipso facto* traps us in self-deceiving accounts of what we have done.[33] Thus, our stories quickly acquire the characteristics of a policy, especially as they are reinforced by our need to find self-justifying reasons for our new-found necessities.

This tactic becomes especially troublesome as the policy itself assumes the form of a central story that gives our individual and collective lives coherence. This story then becomes indispensable to us, as it provides us with a place to be. Phrases like "current medical practice," "standard hospital policy," or even "professional ethics," embody exemplary stories that guide the way we use the means at hand to care for patients. Since we fail to regard them as stories, however, but must see them as a set of principles, the establishment must set itself to secure them against competing views. If the disadvantaged regard this as a form of institutional violence, they are certainly correct.

Such violence need not take the form of physical coercion, of course. But we can detect it in descriptions that countenance coercion. For example, an abortion at times may be a morally necessary, but sorrowful, occurrence. But our desire for righteousness quickly invites us to turn what is morally unavoidable into a self-deceiving policy, e.g., the fetus, after all, is just another piece of flesh. It takes no mean skill, certainly, to know how to hold onto a description that acknowledges significant life, while remaining open to judging that it may have to be destroyed. Yet medical practice and human integrity cannot settle for less. Situations like these suggest, however, that we do not lie because we are evil, but because we wish to be good or preserve what good we already embody.[34]

We do not wish to claim that the stories with which Christians and Jews identify are the only stories that offer skills for truthfulness in the moral life. We only want to identify them as ways to countenance a posture of locating and doing the good which must be done, even if it does not lead to human progress. Rather than encourage us to assume that the moral life can be freed from the tragedies that come from living in a limited and sinful world, these stories demand that we be faithful to God as we believe he has been faithful to us through his covenant with Israel and (for Christians) in the cross of Christ.[35]

IV:3. A Canonical Story

Religious faith, on this account, comes to accepting a certain set of stories as canonical. We come to regard them not only as meeting the criteria sketched above (along with others we may develop) but find them offering ways of clarifying and expanding our sense of the criteria themselves. In short, we discover our human self more effectively through these stories, and so use them in judging the adequacy of alternative schemes for humankind.

In this formal sense, one is tempted to wonder whether everyone does not accept a set of stories as canonical. To identify those stories would be to discover the shape one's basic convictions take. To be unable to do so would either mark a factual incapacity or an utterly fragmented self. Current discussion of "polytheism" leads one to ask whether indiscriminate pluralism represents a real psychic possibility for a contemporary person.[36] In our terms, arguing against the need for a canonical story amounts to questioning, "Why be good?" Just as we do not require ethics to answer that question, so we need not demand a perspicuously canonical story. But we can point to the endemic tendency of men and women to allow certain stories to assume that role, just as ethicists remind us of the assessments we do, in fact, count on to live our lives.[37]

NOTES

1. For example, James Gustafson ends his recent Marquette Lecture, "The Contributions of Theology to Medical Ethics," by saying: "For most persons involved in medical care and practice, the contribution of theology is likely to be of minimal importance, for the moral principles and values needed can be justified without reference to God, and the attitudes that religious beliefs ground can be grounded in other ways. From the standpoint of immediate practicality, the contribution of theology is not great, either in its extent

or in its importance." (p. 94) While we have no wish to challenge this as a descriptive statement of what pertains today, we think we can show that even though "moral principles can be justified without reference to God," how they are accounted for still makes a difference for the meaning of the principle and how it works to form institutions and ways of life that may have practical importance. To be sure, Christians may have common moral convictions with non-Christians, but it seems unwise to separate a moral conviction from the story that forms its context of interpretation. Moreover, a stance such as Gustafson's would seem to assume that medicine as it is currently formed is the way it ought to be. In this respect, we at least want to leave open the possibility of a more reformist, if not radical, stance.

2. We wish to thank Professor MacIntyre for helping us clarify these issues. As will be obvious to anyone acquainted with his work we are deeply influenced by his argument that the "conflict over how morality is to be defined is itself a moral conflict. Different and rival definitions cannot be defended apart from defending different and rival sets of moral principles." ("How to Identify Ethical Principles," unpublished paper prepared for the National Commission for the Protection of Human Subjects of Biomedical and Behavioral Research, p. 8.)

3. The search for ethical objectivity, of course, is also a response to the social and political diversity of our day. Thus the search for a "foundation" for ethics involves the attempt to secure rational agreement short of violence. The attraction of the ideal of science for ethicists may be partly because science appears to be the last form of universal culture we have left. Of course this strategy comes to grief on the diversity of activity and disciplines that constitute what we generally call science. For example see Ernest Becker's reflection on this in his *The Structure of Evil* (New York: Braziller, 1968).

4. We do not mean to claim the actual practice of science involves this sense of objectivity. Indeed we are very sympathetic with Toulmin's analysis of science not as a tight and coherent logical system, but "as a conceptual aggregate, or 'population,' within which there are—at most—localized pockets of logical systematicity." *Human Understanding* (Princeton: Princeton University Press, 1972), p. 128. It is exactly his stress on necessity of understanding the history of the development of a discipline in order to understand its sense of "rationality" that we feel must be recovered in science as well as, though with different significance,

in ethics. As he suggests, "In science as much as in ethics the historical and cultural diversity of our concepts gives rise to intractable problems, only so long as we continue to think of 'rationality' as a character of particular systems of propositions or concepts, rather than in terms of the procedures by which men change from one set of concepts and beliefs to another" (p. 478). Rather what must be seen is that rationality "is an attribute, not of logical or conceptual systems as such, but of the human activities or enterprises of which particular sets of concepts are the temporary cross-sections" (p. 133).

5. Eric Cassell, "Preliminary Exploration of Thinking in Medicine," *Ethics in Science and Medicine*, 2, 1 (1975), pp. 1-12. MacIntyre and Gorovitz's "Toward a Theory of Medical Error" also obviously bears on this issue. See *Science, Ethics and Medicine*, ed. by H. Tristram Engelhardt, Jr. and Daniel Callahan (Hastings-on-Hudson: The Hastings Center, 1976).

6. Quoted by B. F. Skinner in *Science and Human Behavior* (New York: MacMillan, 1953), pp. 18-19. Eric Cassell's, "Illness and Disease," *Hastings Center Report*, 6, 2 (April, 1976), pp. 27-37 is extremely interesting in this respect. It is his contention that we as yet have failed to appreciate the obvious fact that doctors do not treat diseases but patients who have diseases.

7. Ibid., p. 19. In the light of Skinner's claim it is interesting to reflect on John Wisdom's observation in *Paradox and Discovery* (New York: Philosophical Library, 1965). "It is, I believe, extremely difficult to breed lions. But there was at one time at the Dublin zoo a keeper by the name of Mr. Flood who bred many lion cubs without losing one. Asked the secret of his success, Mr. Flood replied, 'Understanding lions'. Asked in what consists the understanding of lions, he replied, 'Every lion is different'. It is not to be thought that Mr. Flood, in seeking to understand an individual lion, did not bring to bear his great experience with other lions. Only he remained free to see each lion for itself." (p. 138.) We are indebted to Professor Ed Erde for the Tolstoy and Wisdom quotes.

8. We are aware that this judgment would need to be qualified if each of these positions were considered in detail. Yet we think that this does characterize a tendency that these positions share. For each position is attempting to establish what Frankena calls the "institution of morality,"—that is to show that morality is an institution that stands on its own, separate from other human activities such as politics, religion, etiquette. (We suspect that connected with this attempt to establish the independence of ethics is the desire to give

ethics a disciplinary character like that of the sciences. For an excellent discussion of ethics as a "quasi-discipline" see Toulmin, *Human Understanding*, pp. 406-411.) The language of obligation tends to become central for these interpretations of the moral life as they trade on our feeling that we ought to do our duty irrespective of how it effects or relates to our other interests and activities. Obligation and rationality are thus interpreted in interdependent terms as it is assumed that an ethics of obligation can provide the standpoint needed to establish the independence of moral discourse from all the relativities of interests, institutions, and commitments save one—the interests of being rational. Thus the moral life, at least as it involves only those obligations that we owe one another apart from any special relationships, needs no further grounding apart from our common rationality. It should be obvious that our criticisms of this approach have much in common with such thinkers as Foot, MacIntyre, Toulmin, and Hampshire. For a critique of the emphasis on obligation to the exclusion of virtue in contemporary accounts of the moral life, see Hauerwas, "Obligation and Virtue Once More," *Journal of Religious Ethics* 3, 1 (Spring, 1975), 27-44, and the following response and critique by Frankena.

9. *Mind*, 80 (1971), 552-71. For similar criticism see Hauerwas, *Vision and Virtue: Essays in Christian Ethical Reflection* (Notre Dame: Fides, 1974).

10. To our mind one of the most disastrous aspects of the standard account of rationality is the resulting divorce of ethical reflection from political theory. It may be objected that the work of Rawls and Nozick are impressive counters to such a claim. However, it is interesting to note that the political theory they generate exists on a high level of abstraction from the actual workings of the modern state. It is only when ethicists turn their attention to C. B. MacPherson's challenge to the liberal democratic assumptions that Rawls and Nozick presuppose that they will address questions that are basic, for liberal political theory and the objectivist's account of moral rationality share the assumption that morally and politically we are strangers to one another. Thus, any common life can only be built on our willingness to qualify our self-interest in order to increase our long-term satisfaction. From this perspective the standard account can be viewed as an attempt to secure a basis for rational politics for a society that shares no interests beyond each individual increasing his chance for survival. It is our hunch that historically the disputes and disagreements in ethical theory, such as that between Rawls and Hare, will appear as scholastic debates

within a liberal framework. For the disputants agree far more than they disagree. For MacPherson's critique of these assumptions see his *Democratic Theory* (Oxford: Clarendon Press, 1973). For a radical critique of liberal democracy, both in terms of the liberal understanding of rationality and the self similar to our own, see Roberto Unger's *Knowledge and Politics* (New York: Free Press, 1975).

11. For a critique of this assumption see Michael Walzer, "Political Action: The Problem of Dirty Hands," *Philosophy and Public Affairs*, 2, 2 (Winter, 1973), 160-80. He is responding to Hare's "Rules of War and Moral Reasoning," *Philosophy and Public Affairs*, 1, 2 (Winter, 1972), 161-81. Hare argued that though one might wrongly think he was faced with a moral dilemma this could not be the case if a course of action suggested itself that was moral. See also John Ladd's very useful discussion of this issue in his "Are Science and Ethics Compatible?" *Science, Ethics and Medicine*, edited by Engelhardt and Callahan (Hastings-on-Hudson: Hastings Center Publication, 1976). This is also the issue that lies behind the theory of double effect in Roman Catholic moral theology although it is seldom explicitly discussed in these terms. For example, see Richard McCormick's *Ambiguity in Moral Choice* (Marquette Theology Lectures: Marquette University, 1973). (See Hauerwas, "Natural Law, Tragedy, and Theological Ethics," *American Journal of Jurisprudence* 20 (1975), 1-19 for a different perspective.)

For a fascinating study of the problem of moral evil in terms of the economic category of scarcity see Vivian Walsh, *Scarcity and Evil* (Englewood Cliffs: Prentice-Hall, 1961). Ms. Walsh argues that we are often mistaken to try to ascribe responsibility for actions that are the result of scarcity even when the scarcity is not the result of the "external" limits but in the person doing the action. What we often must do is the lesser good because of our own limits, but we must learn to know it is a lesser good without implying that we are morally blameworthy. Even though we are sympathetic with Ms. Walsh's analysis we think the concept of character provides a way to suggest what is an inappropriate "scarcity" for anyone to lack in their character given the form of their engagements. Albert Speer lacked political sense that became morally blameworthy because of his political involvement, but that does not mean that morally there is no way to indicate that his character should have provided him with the skills to know what kind of politics he was involved with. In classical terms the concept of character gives the means to assess in what ways we are blameworthy or praiseworthy for that which we have omitted as well as for what we have "done."

12. For a discussion of these issues see Hauerwas, "The Demands and Limits of Care: Ethical Reflections on the Moral Dilemma of Neonatal Intensive Care," *American Journal of the Medical Sciences*, 269, 2 (March-April, 1975), 222-36; and Hauerwas, "Meningomyelocele: To Treat or Not to Treat: An Ethical Analysis of the Dispute between Drs. Freeman and Lorber" (forthcoming).

13. It is not just Prichard that argues in this way but, as Henry Veatch suggests, Kant is the primary inspiration behind those that would make interest, desires, and beliefs in principle unjustifiable. This, of course, relates to the matter discussed in footnote 4 as Kant wanted to provide a basis for morality not dependent on any theological or anthropological assumption—except that of man's rational capacity. That is why Kant's principle of universalizability, which has so often been misinterpreted, applies only to men as rational beings and not just to all human beings. As Veatch points out in this latter case, "the maxim of one's action would be based on a regard simply for certain desires and likings characteristic of human nature—albeit desires that all human beings happen to share in. But any mere desire or inclination or liking or sentiment of approbation, even if it be shared by the entire human race, would still not be universalizable in the relevant sense, simply because it was something characteristic of and peculiar to human kind, and hence not truly universal." "Justification of Moral Principles," *Review of Metaphysics*, XXIX, 2 (December, 1975) p. 225.

14. For example witness this exchange between Lucy and Linus as Lucy walks by while Linus is preparing a snowball for launching.
Lucy: "Life is full of Choices.
    You may choose, if you so wish, to throw that snowball at me.
    You may also choose, if you so wish, not to throw that snowball at me.
    Now, if you choose to throw that snowball at me I will pound you right into the ground.
    If you choose not to throw that snowball at me, your head will be spared."
Linus: (Throwing the snowball to the ground) "Life is full of choices, but you never get any."

15. For a more extended analysis of the concept of character see

Hauerwas, *Character and the Christian Life: A Study in Theological Ethics* (San Antonio: Trinity University Press, 1975).

16. Julius Kovesi, *Moral Notions* (New York: Humanities Press, 1967); and Hauerwas, *Vision and Virtue*, pp. 11-29. For a detailed account of the historical development of meaning of words, see Raymond Williams, *Keywords* (New York: Oxford, 1976).

17. For example R. S. Downie and Elizabeth Telfer attempt to argue that "the ordinary rules and judgments of social morality presuppose respect for persons as their ultimate ground . . . (and) that the area of private or self-referring morality also presupposes respect for persons as its ultimate ground." *Respect for Persons* (New York: Schocken, 1970), p. 9. They interpret respect for persons in a Kantian fashion of respecting the claim another rational capacity— that is, capable of self-determining and rule-governing behavior— can demand. It never seems to occur to them that the "ordinary rules of social morality" or "self-referring morality" may not need an "ultimate ground." Moreover, they have a good deal of trouble explaining why we owe respect to children or "idiots" on such grounds. They simply assert that there "are sufficient resemblances between them and persons" to justify extending respect to them. (p. 35.) (For a different perspective on this issue see Hauerwas, "The Retarded and the Criteria for the Human," *Linacre Quarterly*, 40 (November, 1973), 217-22.) It is Downie and Telfer's contention that "respect for persons" is the basis of such Christian notions as agape. It is certainly true that much of what a "respect for persons" ethic represents has been assumed by Christian morality, but we think that it is misleading to assume that the story that informs the latter can be translated into the former. One of the places to see this is where each construes the relationship between obligation and supererogation. The Christian ethic of charity necessarily makes obligatory what a follower of "respect for persons" can see only as supererogation. For an analysis of agape in terms of equal regard see Gene Outka, *Agape: An Ethical Analysis* (New Haven: Yale University Press, 1972).

18. For an account of the moral life that makes "fittingness" central see H. R. Niebuhr, *The Responsible Self* (New York: Harper and Row, 1963).

19. It would take us too far afield to explore this point further, but surely it is Kant that stands behind this understanding of the self. It is impossible to document this, but it is at least worthwhile calling attention to two passages from *Religion Within the Limits of Reason*

Alone, translated by Theodore Green (New York: Harper, 1960). "In the search for the rational origins of evil action, every such action must be regarded as though the individual had fallen into it directly from a state of innocence. For whatever his previous deportment may have been, whatever natural causes may have been influencing him, and whatever these causes were to be found within or outside him, his action is yet free and determined by none of these causes; hence it can and must always be judged as an original use of his will. . . . Hence we cannot inquire into the temporal origins of this deed, but solely into its rational origin, if we are thereby to determine and, whereby possible, to elucidate the propensity, if it exists, i.e., the general subjective ground of the adoption of transgression into our maxim." (p. 36.) In case it is objected that Kant is only dealing with moral evil, consider "To reconcile the concept of freedom with the idea of God as a *necessary* Being raises no difficulty at all: for freedom consists not in the contingency of the act, i.e., not in indeterminism, but rather in absolute spontaneity. Such spontaneity is endangered only by predeterminism, where the determining ground of the act is in *antecedent time*, with the result that, the act being now no longer in my power but in the hands of nature, I am irresistibly determined; but since in God no temporal sequence is thinkable, this difficulty vanishes." (p. 45.) It is, of course, the possibility of the moral law that Kant thinks gives men the possibility to be like God—timeless. It is not a far distance from Kant to the existentialist in this respect.

20. For this point and much else that is involved in this paper see Iris Murdoch, *The Sovereignty of the Good Over Other Concepts* (Cambridge: Cambridge University Press, 1967).

21. We have not based our criticism of the standard account on the debates between those that share its presuppositions. It is, of course, true that as yet no single theory of the standard account has proved to be persuasive to those that share its presuppositions. We still find Kant's theory the single most satisfying statement of the program implied by the standard account.

22. Ernest Becker, however, argues that Comte has been misunderstood, as his purpose was not to free science from morality but to call attention to what kind of moral activity science involved. Thus, Becker suggests, "Comte's Positivism, in sum, solved the problem of science and morals by using science to support a man-based morality. With all the force at his command he showed that life is a moral problem, and science only a tool whose unity would serve the larger unity of life. Like de Maistre and de Bonald, and

like Carlyle in England, he looked approvingly on the Middle Ages. But he did not pine nostalgically for their institutions; he saw the Middle Ages as possessing what man needed most, and has since lost: a critical, unitary world view by which to judge right and wrong, good and bad, by which to subordinate personal desire to social interest. But instead of basing this knowledge on theological fiat, man could now settle it firmly on science. In this way, the Enlightenment could achieve what the Middle Ages almost possessed; but it could do this on a much sounder footing than could ever have been possible during the earlier time, namely, it could achieve the subordination of politics to morality on a scientific rather than on a theological basis. Social order and social harmony would be a call of the new day, and human progress could then be progress in social feeling, community, and love—all of it based on the superordinate science of man in society, serving man, elevating humanity." (*The Structure of Evil*, p. 50.)

In this respect consider Simone Weil's observation that "The criticism of religion is always, as Marx said, the condition for all progress; but what Marx and the Marxists have not clearly seen is that, in our day, everything that is most retrograde in the spirit of religion has taken refuge, above all, in science itself. A science like ours, essentially closed to the layman, and therefore to scientists themselves, because each is a layman outside his narrow specialism, is the proper theology of an ever increasingly bureaucratic society."

23. Cf. G. E. M. Anscombe, "Thought and Action in Aristotle," in R. Bambrough (ed.), *New Essays on Plato and Aristotle* (New York: Humanities Press, 1965), pp. 151-52. See also Hauerwas, *Character and the Christian Life*, Ch. 2.

24. For an account of the way analogous terms can be used once they are effectively linked to a paradigmatic instance, cf. Burrell, *Analogy and Philosophical Language* (New Haven and London: Yale University Press, 1973).

25. It may, of course, happen that one cannot sustain a particular relationship and "fails." Again, the way he deals with that becomes a story. Stories often seem better the more they overturn conventional assessments and challenge settled attitudes.

26. Peter Brown shows how this choice represented an existential decision as well. The *Platonici* formed an identifiable group of noble humanists, and as such offered a viable alternative to Christianity. While they were not formed into a church, their common aspirations could well be imagined to constitute a community of like-

minded persons—*Augustine of Hippo* (Berkeley: University of California Press, 1967).

27. This is the point of Peter Winch's oft-cited analysis: "Understanding a Primitive Society," reprinted in Bryan R. Wilson (ed.), *Rationality* (New York: Oxford University Press, 1970). More constructively, it forms the focus of alternative endeavors like *Creative Simplicity* (Minneapolis, Minn. 55410).

28. For further elaboration of this, see Iris Murdoch, *The Sovereignty of the Good Over Other Concepts*.

29. Cf. James Cameron's efforts to offer perspective to current writing on the "sexual revolution," in *The New York Review of Books*, 23 (May 13, 1976), 19-28.

30. MacIntyre's argument in "Towards a Theory of Medical Error," that medicine must necessarily deal with explanations of individuals, only makes this claim more poignant. For the attempt to claim that the only errors in medicine were those characteristic of a science of universals was necessary if medicine was to make good its claim to be the means to free mankind of the limits of disease. To recognize that medical explanation and prediction are subject to the same limits as explanation and prediction of individuals will require a radical reorientation of the story that morally supports and directs medical care.

31. Becker, *The Structure of Evil*, p. 18. "The central problem posed by the Newtonian revolution was not long in making itself felt. This was the momentous new problem; it is still ours today—I mean of course the problem of a new theodicy. If the new nature was so regular and beautiful, then why was there evil in the human world? Man needs a new theodicy, but this time he could not put the burden on God. Man had to settle for a new limited explanation, an anthropodicy which would cover only those evils that allow for human remedy." Science naturally presented itself as the "remedy."

32. It is tempting to try to make, as many have, the ethic of "respect for persons" sufficient as a moral basis for medical care. (Cf. Paul Ramsey's *The Patient as Person*.) But if, as we suggest, medicine is necessarily involved in tragic choices, a more substantive story than that is needed to sustain and give direction to medical care. Without such a story we will be tempted to make technology serve as a substitute, since it allows us to delay further decisions of life and death that we must make in one or another arena. For a critique of the way "person" is being used as a regulative moral notion in medical ethics see Hauerwas, "Must a Patient Be a 'Person' To Be

a Patient, or My Uncle Charlie is Not Much of a Person But He Is Still my Uncle Charlie," *Connecticut Medicine*, 39, 12 (December, 1975), 815-17.

33. For an analysis of the concept of self-deception see Burrell and Hauerwas, "Self-Deception and Autobiography: Theological and Ethical Reflections on Speer's *Inside the Third Reich*," *Journal of Religious Ethics*, 2, 1 (1974), 99-117.

34. Jules Henry's analysis of the phenomenon of "sham" is perhaps the most graphic depiction of this. He says, "Children in our culture cannot avoid sham, for adults cannot escape depression, hostility and so on. Since sham consists in one person's withholding information, while implying that the other person should act as if he had it all; since sham consists also in giving false information while expecting the other person to act as if the information were true; since sham consists in deriving advantage from withholding or giving information—and since, on the whole, our culture is sham-wise, it might seem that the main problem for the mental health of children is to familiarize them with the edges of sham. Yet, if we were to do that, they would be 'shot' for Albee is right. Our main problem then is to tell them the world lies but they should act as if it told the truth. But this too is impossible, for if one acted as if all sham were truth he might not be shot, but he certainly would lose all his money and marry the wrong person though he would have lots of friends. What then is the main problem; or rather, what does mankind do? People do not like children who lack innocence, for they hold the mirror up to adults. If children could not be deceived they would threaten adults beyond toleration, they would never be orderly in elementary school and they clearly could not be taught the rot-gut dished out to them as truth. Personally I do not know what to do; and I anticipate a geometric increase in madness, for sham is at the basis of schizophrenia and murder itself." *On Sham, Vulnerability, and Other Forms of Self-Destruction* (New York: Vintage Books, 1973), pp. 123-4. See also his *Pathways to Madness* (New York: Vintage Books, 1971), pp. 99-187.

35. For a fuller development of the issues in this last section see Hauerwas, "Natural Law, Tragedy, and Theological Ethics," *American Journal of Jurisprudence*, 20 (1975), 1-19. Moreover for a perspective similar to this see Ernest Becker, *The Denial of Death* (New York: Free Press, 1975). In a broad sense Becker suggests man's situation is tragic because, "Man has a symbolic identity that brings him sharply out of nature. He is a symbolic self, a creature with a name, a life history. He is a creator with a mind that soars

to speculate about atoms and infinity, who can place himself imaginatively at a point in space and contemplate bemusedly his own planet . . . . Yet at the same time man is a worm and food for worms. This is the paradox: He is out of nature and hopeless in it; he is dual, up in the stars and yet housed in a heart-pumping, breath-grasping body that once belonged to a fish. Man literally is split in two: he has awareness of his own splendid uniqueness in that he sticks out of nature with a towering majesty, and yet he goes back into the ground a few feet in order blindly to rot and disappear forever. It is a terrifying dilemma to be in and to have to live with." (p. 26.)

36. In his *Revisioning Psychology* (New York, 1975), Ch. 1, James Hillman questions whether psychic integration has not been conceived in too "monotheistic" a manner. His discussion is flawed by failing to see how an analogical "reference to one" offers a feasible way of mediating between an ideal which is too confining and a *laissez faire* program which jettisons ideals altogether.

37. A special note of gratitude to Larry McCullough of Texas A & M Medical School for his careful reading of our argument. Many of his suggestions would have clarified our argument had we been able to incorporate them more organically into our text.

Commentary

Rationality, the Normative and the Narrative in the Philosophy of Morals

E. D. Pellegrino

A CONSUMING TASK of the modern philosophy of morals is to locate precisely the contributions to ethical judgment of reason and normative principles, on the one hand, and human experience and the particular case, on the other. Kant exposed the issues in the most radical way when he inquired into what reason can know apart from experience, and then elaborated a metaphysic of morals purged of all empiric elements. Modern ethical theorists have ever since been forced to reexamine the possibility of normative ethics, and the utility of reason in its pursuit. The resultant congeries of ethical objectivism, subjectivism, skepticism, and metaethics speaks eloquently of the unsettled state of the question.

Burrell and Hauerwas plunge boldly into this turbulent stream with a radical criticism of classical and modern assumptions about rationality in ethics. They assert that the neglect of narrative in ethical reflection constitutes a serious flaw in all contemporary theories. They propose an alternative form of rationality that employs narrative and "character" as a primary instrument for apprehending ethical—and even theological—truths.

Their argument is of genuine significance for the philosophy of morals and for theology, and, by implication, for moral decision in medicine as well. In my examination of the line of their argument, I shall attempt the following:

1. locate the precise foci of the critique within the framework of the "standard" account;
2. examine the validity of narrative as a source of rationality in ethics;
3. examine the validity of narrative as a source of the normative;
4. offer a possible reconciliation which preserves the value of narrative as well as certain elements of the "standard" account.

I. The "Standard" Account or Accounts: Foci of the Critique

The nosography of modern ethical theories is a prickly thicket, not to be entered even by the professional ethicist without good reason. Yet, we must enter this thicket at the outset, since Burrell and Hauerwas level their criticisms at what they call the standard account. Our first task must be to discern more precisely what constitutes the standard account, and then locate within its framework the points of the attack. Only then can we respond to the suggestions of an alternative pattern for rationality in ethics.

There are at least two "standard" accounts, each containing elements under criticism by the authors, a classical and a modern account.

The classical account of normative ethics makes two claims: that moral philosophy begins in human nature and experience, and that reason reflecting on these realities can derive general principles which will guide men to good actions. The classical account assumed a synergy of reason and experience, and this was the leitmotiv of ethical discourse from Socrates and Aristotle to Aquinas.

This synergy was first seriously impaired by being over-stretched in opposing directions in post-medieval thinking. The metaphysical rationalists, especially Spinoza, made ethical judgments almost exclusively the domain of a deductive logical system. The empiricists moved in just the opposite direction and denied that reason can arrive at ethical distinctions. Hume, for example, located ethical judgments not in reason, but in the personal experience and sentiments of the subject.

It was Kant's powerful metaphysic of morals which most radically questioned the twin assumptions of the classical account and spun off the host of theories that comprise the modern account. Having grounded all philosophy on a priori forms in the knowing subject, Kant insisted that ethics too must be based in pure reason: ". . . the ground of obligation must be looked for not in the nature of man, nor in the circumstances of the world in which he is placed, but solely in the concepts of pure reason . . . ."[1] The concepts of pure duty, and the categorical imperative thus derived, became the absolute foundations of morals. In a very special sense, these concepts were "objective," in that their validity was independent of the subject and the details of his moral situation.

Kant's critique of the classical synergism of reason and reality in ethics had an effect similar to the Cartesian assault on the unity of mind and body. His successors were forced to build their accounts out of the fragments of a former unity whose probity could never be fully restored. Some followed the Humean lead into a variety of forms of subjectivism, while others took the objectivist turn.

The standard account, against which Hauerwas and Burrell argue, is not easily identifiable. I take it to consist largely of some combination of Kantian ethical absolutism and the scientific and logical forms of ethical objectivism. They share an "objective" quality in that they seek for the validity of ethical judgments independently of who utters them, and under what circumstances.

Burrell and Hauerwas, though they express some sympathy for the more traditional uses of reason, have in actuality leveled serious criticisms against both the modern and the classical accounts of rationality in ethics.

Against the modern objectivist account, they argue that ethics is not a rational science dealing with judgments apart from the agent, and that only the narrative context of moral choices can give those choices meaning or rationality. Kantian a priorism and the modern forms of ethical objectivity err in trying to derive meaning from rationality separated from narrative.

Against the classical account, Burrell and Hauerwas deny the validity of general normative principles on which judgments about moral decisions can be made. They also question any attempt to ground ethics in "human nature," abstractly defined. They insist that the central significance of personal experience is not simply to serve as the ground for deriving moral principles. In place of deductive reasoning, they would put narrative and "character" as new tools of rationality.

What is the basis for the authors' renunciation of the validity and utility of general moral principles? The difficulty, they say, is that such principles must, by definition, be abstracted from the particulars of personal narrative: what we are in life, how our moral notions are formed by our life story, how our beliefs and dispositions shape what count for us. The ordinary use of rationality, it is held, forces us to see ethics primarily as problem solving; it undermines our sense of the tragic elements in moral choice, and it enfeebles our capacity to define our moral selves.

Moral differences cannot be resolved by logical or dialectical discourse. They are not clashes of principles, but of individual perceptions, meanings, and language, and these can only emerge from the framework of narrative. Stories are not mere descriptions, however, for even the notion of rationality is dependent upon narrative. Rationality itself and moral justifications, therefore, are meaningless apart from narrative.

A more serious critique of both the classical and the modern accounts of ethics can hardly be devised. Deprived of normative principles, we are left with the individual narrative as the norm; and deprived of the use of explicit reason, we are left with narrative as the only tool of rationality. Paradoxically, even while firing these salvos, the authors express their belief that the alternative is not ethical subjectivism and not a total disregard of traditional concerns for reason.

The major vector in the authors' critique is located in its two counter-claims: that narrative is the instrument of rationality in ethics, and that narrative has normative force. We can now examine each of these claims.

II. Is Narrative a Source of Rationality in Ethics?

The authors formulate a notion of rationality founded not in the logical sequence of necessary events, but in the contingent sequences of a person's story. Words like "meaning," "fitting-ness," "consistency," and "intentionality" are used variously to define this form of rationality that is narrative dependent. The center of this rationality lies in the plot of the story whose rules of development ". . . stem from some mysterious source" (p. 128).

The difficulties of such a vaguely described form of rationality are both logical and epistemological. To begin with, the authors at the outset state clearly that they will not attempt to analyze the concepts of narrative or character fully. It is a peculiar form of rationality which must be derived from "mysterious sources," and which leaves its major analytic instruments undefined, except to refer them back to their origins in narrative. Narrative, by some light—intuitive or otherwise—is then expected to define and justify itself.

Some of the difficulty is evident if, for example, we examine the notion of "plausibility." Plausibility in a narrative is defined as the way human actions connect with each other to form character. Character then gives us the pattern for predicting the further development of a story. But this pattern must be built out of contingent events, since logical necessity has been ruled out as having no meaning in the unfolding of a story. With contingency built into the predictive instrument, how can we know that the next step in the narrative is "plausible"? The authors face a serious paradox: they recommend a form of rationality "especially appropriate to ethics," which is based on an ordering principle itself unpredictable in its operations.

On the authors' view, plausibility seems to rest in a post facto judgment of the internal consistency of a given moral judgment with what precedes it in a particular narrative. Since the essence of the unfolding of stories is their non-predictiveness, everything within a narrative is plausible simply because it is in the narrative. We must not seek plausibility outside the narrative. That would be to adduce some critical principle which, by definition, would be invalid. We could seek the criterion in some other story—a canonical story—which would keep the rationality bound to narrative. But then, how can we distinguish between the competing claims of stories?

What, then, is the specific nature of this special form of rationality which is the preeminent contribution of narrative to ethical discourse? Deductive logic seems to be ruled out by the emphasis on the contingency of the events unfolding in a story. Inductive logic would be of little use, since the generation of general principles must, of necessity, eschew the richness of particulars that constitute a narrative. Scientific reasoning is especially interdicted, since it is the paradigm of the objectivity so roundly condemned. Finally, "explanation" is excluded, since explanations are said to be incoherent and the search for them pointless.

The authors appreciate the difficulties of this "strong" version of their proposals. On pages 125 and 126, they give us a "weaker" version. They say they do not intend to reject "wholesale" that part of our legacy contained in the standard account. Being able to offer reasons for our actions, to engage in public discourse, to use critical skills, and even to generate moral principles to guide our conduct—all must be respected in any "substantive moral narrative." They protest that all they wish to do is offer a criticism of the neglect of narrative and the overemphasis on principles, as well as the confusion of principles which are abstractions with actual grounds for conduct. They want to offer an alternative to the standard account as the only safeguard against subjectivism and reductionism; narrative is such a viable alternative.

This section of the paper is quite unconvincing. If we take it on face value, it contradicts the bulk of what the authors say elsewhere about the powers of narrative. They cannot have it both ways. The strong version of their argument leads to subjectivism and relativism; the weak version reasserts the value of all those things they criticize in objectivism. If they hold to the weaker version, then why not make the major case for that version, emphasizing the neglect of narrative and not the emergence of a new form of rationality?

An equally serious set of difficulties of an epistemological kind arises when we look more closely at the story they use to illustrate how narrative can work as an alternative form of rationality. The powerful story of St. Augustine's *Confessions* is the paradigm which, the authors say, sustains their proposition that narrative is a form of rationality. What we have in St. Augustine is the exquisitely described spiritual odyssey of a man who spent years examining and reexamining the notions or "stories" of Manicheanism and Platonism. He could find no satisfying answers to his twin desires for understanding evil and God until, in one moment of searing truth in the garden, "the darkness of doubt was dispersed." The search of many years suddenly came to an end in Augustine's acceptance of the Gospel story, and, thereafter, that story shaped every moment of his life.

How does this story justify the function of narrative as an analytic tool? Is it because it reveals a process whereby one may order one's life (p. 131); or because narrative is the only way we can exhibit an action without attempting to explain it (p. 132); or because the "incoherence" of the explanations offered shows how futile all explanations really are (p. 133); or does rationality consist in the change from "the language of will and struggle to the language of the heart" (p. 135); or is it when questions are "received rather than formulated" (p. 135)?

Such variations in phraseology, and the consequent shifting nuances and meanings, make it almost impossible to assign a clear and specific character to the way narrative can provide the skills for rationality in ethics. There is more than a little irony in the lengthy explanations and appeals to reason required to prove that explanation and ordinary rationality have little place in Augustine's story. The point must be labored simply because the narrative is clearly not sufficient to speak directly to us of its own rationality.

Stories do have an extraordinary power to sensitize us, to provide a whole set of particulars out of which the meaning of our lives may suddenly emerge. Therein lies their singular strength. They can work on reader and author as well. Huysmans, who created Des Esseintes, one of the most bizarre characters in literature, describes the effect of the story he created on his own beliefs years later. "Only little by little, I was shaking myself loose from my shell of impurity; I was beginning to have a disgust of myself, but at the same time I kicked against the articles of faith. The objections I raised in my own mind sounded irresistible; and lo! one fine morning when I woke they were solved—I never knew how. I prayed for the first time and the catastrophe was over."[2]

One of Huysman's readers summarizes his reaction to the same book, as follows: "After such a book, it only remains for the author to choose between the muzzle of a pistol or the foot of the cross."[3]

These are secular parallels of the way the Gospel narrative affected St. Augustine. The experiences are in many ways identical; they cannot be argued by explicit reason. These need not be called a special form of rationality. They are inconsistent with rationality in any current construal of that term. Burrell and Hauerwas blunt the opportunity to make the strongest case for narrative. They dissipate their energies and induce unnecessary opposition by leveling their critique at the rationality of the standard accounts. Story apprehends unerringly a part of reality we have yet to understand well. But to understand it, we must not weaken the value of ordinary rationality or general moral principles. No theory of logic or epistemology can yet explain the full power of stories to affect our interior lives.

What the authors are struggling to express in their search for the special rationality of Augustine's narrative is some way to understand his leap from non-acceptance of the Gospel story to acceptance. That leap is often described in literature, just as it is in St. Augustine, as a sudden and inexplicable movement of the mind and heart. What was once just a story, suddenly, in a flash of recognition, becomes a canonical story—one which we allow to shape our lives thereafter. Having made the leap of acceptance, the story we accept does indeed sharpen our skills for judging all other stories. But those skills are, still, only the usual skills of reason and use of evidence. They do not differ radically from ordinary reason, except that reason operates in a new and clearer context of presuppositions, now an integral part of our interior life following the act of acceptance. This is especially true when we try to justify our choice of stories to others.

The seminal act is the act of acceptance, and the subsequent internalization of a story or some part of it. There is little to be gained from positing this as a special form of rationality, superior to the explicit forms of reasoning characteristic of the standard accounts. A long time ago, Anselm said it succinctly and well (borrowing from St. Augustine's use of a phrase in the Septuagint translation of *Isaiah* 7:9): *"Credo ut intelligam."* We still have no theory of logic or epistemology which will adequately explain the transformation of unbelief into belief.

There might be some potentials for an explanation of this phenomenon in some of the more recent theories of knowledge. One possibility might be the logic of tacit understanding proposed by Polanyi.[4] He has posited an extension of the Gestalt notion from psychology to epistemology, based on the fact that we know "more than we can tell." On this view, we accept moral teachings not by explicit logic, but by interiorization. "To interiorize is to identify ourselves with the teachings in question by making them function as the proximal term of a tacit framework for our moral actions and judgments."[5] ". . . we cannot choose explicitly a new set of values, but must submit to them by the very act of creating or adopting them."[6]

We can resort to other possible explanations, like the theories of superficial and deep structures discussed in the paper by Stent in this same volume, or even to the Jungian archetypes, or to Freudian metapsychology—all, like Kant, seek some overall unifying principle which gives meaning to all our ideas and experiences.

There are too many unresolved difficulties with all recent theories of knowledge, Polanyi's included. They are no more satisfying than traditional theories, though they may embody in their formulations the novelty of recent psychological and neurophysiological language. We still need to clarify and justify the nature and the sources of the knowledge and logic subsumed under such vague notions as "tacit understanding." Burrell and Hauerwas, too, fail to enlighten us on the nature of their ordering principles like "plot" and "character." All of these theories imply some form of intuitionism and internal illumination, by which ordinary reason is enhanced and shaped to "see" the truth. They are not much different from Bonaventure's notion of the knowledge of God preceding all other knowledge and ordering it. Modern theories leave God out, and substitute archetypes, tacit understanding, deep structures, and the like.

III. Can Narrative be Normative?

All of this only illuminates the *process* whereby a story convinces, teaches, or converts the subject, the teller, or the reader. It still does not deal with the issue of *why* the story does all of this, and why *this* story should be believed rather than dozens of other competing stories that unfold in a myriad of other ways. Even if we grant a special, non-formal rationality based in tacit logic or the special illumination of faith, how do we judge between stories? How can any narrative become normative?

Burrell and Hauerwas offer us two sets of criteria by which we might distinguish between stories and through which narratives can carry normative force—one implicit and the other explicit. The implicit criteria are intermingled throughout their argument and inhere in such notions as coherence, faithfulness, truth, or meaning. The four explicit criteria are set forth on page 137.

As to the implicit criteria, coherence, faithfulness, truth, or meaning are qualities inherent in the unfolding of any narrative. A narrative can show whether the protagonist's decisions are faithful to the flow of his story, whether the events are honestly recorded, what their meaning may be, and whether they relate coherently to each other. Seen from the subject's viewpoint, every narrative can be argued to have these qualities, and is neither inferior nor superior to other narratives.

These criteria are all internal to the narrative and inextricably rooted in what *is*, or what *was*, or what *might be*. The moment we face the question of what *ought to be*—that is to say, when we begin ethical discourse proper—we must choose between narratives. Internal criteria are of little use in trying to decide which story should shape our lives. Stories adumbrate the process, but not the product—the "good" or "bad" person who is formed by a particular narrative. We must step outside the narratives we are comparing and resort to more explicit reason and more general principles to justify the assumptions about what is "good" and "bad." This does violence to the splendid uniqueness and integrity of the narrative.

The same limitations apply to the more explicitly stated criteria on page 137. A preferred story is said to be one which releases from destructive alternatives, helps us to see through distortions; avoids violence, and imparts a sense of the tragic. These criteria help us judge the kind of person we would become, were we to allow a particular story to shape our lives. As with the implicit criteria, these explicit ones can only derive validity from prior, extra-narrative assumptions about what is a good and what a bad person. If we require non-story justifications to judge between stories, how can the story itself carry normative force?

The fundamental dilemma is inescapable. The greatest strength of the narrative—its particularity and uniqueness—is also its greatest weakness as a normative instrument. The narrative is indeed a powerful and indispensable medium without which we cannot fully comprehend what we will become if we permit a particular story to shape our lives. But the gap between that kind of understanding and a commitment to some story as what we *ought to be* seems unbridgeable if we are restricted solely to the narrative. Yet ethical discourse genuinely begins only when we grapple with what *ought to be*, and with the conflicts between different claims on what we ought to be.

St. Augustine clearly understood that even the truth of his story would not convince men by itself:

> And how can they tell, when they hear from me of myself, whether I speak the truth, seeing that no man knoweth what is in man "save the spirit of man which is in him?" . . . But because charity believeth all things . . . I too, O Lord, also so confess the truth, yet do they believe me whose ears charity openeth to me.[7]

To attain normative force, even Augustine's singularly moving story had to be read by a mind prepared to see its plausibility. Ivan in *The Brothers Karamazov* wrestled with the same problem of evil as did St. Augustine; he read the same Gospel story as Augustine. But he ended up rejecting the Gospel story, because it required that we accept the suffering of children.

All stories, since they narrate the moral choices of humans, have some degree of plausibility for other humans in the same situation, and sharing the same moral notions. Nonetheless, all stories are not equally compelling. Nor are the persons they shape equally worthy of emulation. Rational choice among stories requires criteria that transcend the stories judged. Metaphysical presuppositions, the light of faith, intuition, reason, or scientific evidence are "in" our stories in the sense that they become part of our choices, but "outside" in the sense that they can be applied to all stories.

Modern man, especially, has need for some way to judge among merely plausible stories. Rejecting the need for theological, philosophical, or even rational insights, modern men are especially susceptible to the seductive stories of the "picaresque saints," as Lewis calls them, of the modern novel.[8] The confessions—for that is what they are—of Gide's Marcel, Sartre's Mathieu, or Camus's Meursault have greater coherence than Augustine's. Those who share their sense of the absurd, and of the alienation in contemporary existence, easily find "coherence" in these stories.

Neither the strong nor the weak versions of the Burrell and Hauerwas proposal successfully guards against ethical subjectivism or relativism. Every narrative has its own justification simply because it reveals a unique set of moral events. Without insistence on some elements of objectivism, we easily confuse coherence and plausibility with something very different, namely, moral truth.

There are practical dangers in reinforcing the already prevalent tendency to depreciate the possibility of rational discourse about moral decisions. Medical professionals, whose philosophical stance is often positivistic, are particularly prone to treat ethical matters as acts of personal faith, immune to critical inquiry, or too bound to concrete situations to admit of normative generalizations.

Conflicts in moral beliefs between physicians, patients, and society are, however, a growing reality. Each of us has a story that justifies our position. But if society is to function, and the values of both physicians and patients are to be respected, points of resolution and agreement must be sought between opposing positions.

We urgently need a refurbishment of the philosophical bases of professional ethics in medicine and the other health professions. Any ethical code presupposes common assent to some set of principles which sets limits on the actions of all who undertake to serve society. It also places the opposing values and obligations of patients and physicians into some order with reference to each other. In a democratic society, we should permit each person to subscribe to his own narrative to as large an extent as possible. But, as with all freedoms in a complex society, even this freedom must have reasonable limits. Failure to understand these limits easily leads to the imposition of the beliefs of the professional or the institution on those of patients.

IV. Where Narrative Fits—An Attempt at Reconciliation

As Burrell and Hauerwas point out (fn. 12), it is the Kantian inspiration behind the standard accounts with which they take the greatest issue. Their assertions of the personal and the particular in moral experience are most telling against the Kantian rejection of the empirical. Narrative stands somewhere between the Kantian ethics of pure reason and the overzealous attention to personal experience of ethical subjectivism.

Against these extremes, narrative has an incontestible value for narrator and reader. It helps us to see, understand, empathize, and share the moral experience of another human being as manifest in the moral choices and tragedies of his life. For the reader or listener, the effect is twofold. He is moved to compassion, and to a less self-righteous and more humane spirit, as he immerses himself in the moral dispositions, beliefs and language of a fellow human. The reader can begin to glimpse the mystery of character *in statu nascendi* as it is molded by successive moral choices. The reader is, in effect, a privileged observer, able to behold the likely outcome of some of the very choices he himself may have contemplated—without having to experience those outcomes in his own life.

Narrative is of central importance in ethics, medicine, or any human relationship, for that matter, simply because there is no other way we can penetrate, even partially, the mystery of the other. The opening to another person's life, in his own language, with his own nuances and meanings, is only possible if we hear his story, as we must also tell him ours. It is in this entry into the mystery of being—another's and our own—that narrative transcends problem solving. The distinction Gabriel Marcel makes so well between mystery and problem seems especially pertinent here. "A problem is something met with, which bars my passage. It is before me in its entirety. A mystery, on the other hand, is something in which I find myself caught up, and whose essence, therefore, is not to be before me in its entirety. It is as though in this province, the distinction before me and in me loses its meaning."[9]

The great and undeniable power of narrative is its capacity to enable us to see, in Marcel's sense, the mystery of the moral life, as well as the problem. As Marcel goes on to show, mystery is a problem which has intruded itself into the being of the inquirer. Narrative is essential if moral problems are really to engage our selves, rather than simply standing before us as objects of study. The Kantian metaphysics of morals, so strenuously and consciously denuded of the empiric, is also denuded of being and the mystery of being. Burrell and Hauerwas are right to insist on the irreconcilability of narrative with the Kantian groundwork for ethics.

But the mystery of the moral life is not totally unknowable. Nor is it unsusceptible to the philosophical reflection, rational criticism, and analysis intrinsic to the classical account. Only by narrative can we penetrate the mystery, and even understand it better; but that does not mean we must capitulate before it. Narrative provides the particulars that outline the mystery of moral choices. While we can never plumb the full depths of mystery in any personal narrative, we must not surrender our attempts to see the "problem" as well as the "mystery." Marcel warned against the danger of reducing mystery to problem. The only safeguard against that is to place the particulars of the personal narrative in the center of our ethical deliberations, and then to reflect upon them critically in the light of more general principles.

The moral life and the ethics which reflects upon it deal with both problems and mysteries, with principles, and with unique cases that defy comprehension under any normative principle. This is the radical challenge to all ethical theories—whether they follow classical or modern accounts, or the proposal of story in place of system. To understand human actions, we need the fullness of detail the narrative affords; to judge these actions and choose among them, we need to prescind from these particularities. We are compelled, therefore, to cultivate both accounts—the standard and the narrative—at least in part, for each grasps some part of the unbelievably complex fabric of moral reality. Each falls short of ever encompassing all of human moral life.

The fundamental issue is, of course, metaphysical: how does the particular reside in the general, and the general in the particular? How do the singular and the typical, the perfect and the imperfect, the actual and the possible, relate to each other, inasmuch as they reside simultaneously in all of us? How can we extend our understanding beyond given experiences—or can we? The metaphysics of morals, despite Kant's confidence in his resolution of the antinomies, is still a lively problem and will always remain so. It will always be subject to the "opacification" to which Camus alluded and which descends upon us at the junction between our desires for conceptual clarity and our immersion in human experiences which defy clarification.[10]

Narrative, as the authors construe it, is a revelation of the feelings, language, and perceptions of a human making moral—often tragic—choices in a continually unfolding set of circumstances. It is an essential grounding, and perhaps even a meeting ground, for ethics, theology, and medicine. Ethics is called upon to reflect critically on these revelations; medicine to heal the physical and emotional wounds inflicted by them; theology to give them meaning by illumination with a transcendental revelation.

We must not try to "prove" anything with our story. Indeed, the more we consciously try to make it a form of rationality, the less convincing it becomes. Gide had good advice for all of us—ethicists, theologians, physicians—who deal professionally with stories: "I have tried to prove nothing, but to paint my picture well and light it properly."[11]

Burrell and Hauerwas have given us a potent antidote to the excesses which can infect all ethical theories. Narrative, discriminantly used, can temper the overpurified ethics of Kant, the overrationalized and overobjectivized and oversubjectivized ethics of the moderns. Like any antidote, it too can be lethal if taken exclusively and in excessive quantities.

NOTES

1. Immanuel Kant, *Groundwork of the Metaphysics of Morals*. Trans. and analyzed by H. J. Paton (New York: Harper & Row, Harper Torchbook, The Academy Library 1964), p. 57.
2. J.K. Huysmans, *Against The Grain* (New York: Dover Publications, Inc. 1969), p. XLVII.
3. Ibid., p. XLVI.
4. Michael Polanyi, "The Logic of Tacit Inference." In *Knowing and Being*, ed. Marjorie Grene (Chicago: University of Chicago Press, 1969), pp. 138-59.
5. Michael Polanyi, *The Tacit Dimension* (Garden City: Doubleday, Anchor Books, 1967), p. 17.
6. Ibid., p. xi.
7. St. Augustine: *The Confessions*, trans. and annotated by J.G. Pilkington (New York: Liveright, 1943) (X,III,3), pp. 219-20.
8. R.W.B. Lewis, *The Picaresque Saint* (Philadelphia and New York: J.P. Lippincott Company, Keystone edition, 1961).
9. Gabriel Marcel, *Being and Having*, trans. Katherine Farrer (New York: Harper & Row, Harper Torchbooks, 1965), p. 100.
10. Albert Camus, *The Myth of Sisyphus*, trans. Justin O'Brien (New York: Vintage Books, 1959).
11. Andre Gide, *The Immoralist*, Preface (New York: Vintage Books, 1970).

The Concept of Responsibility: An Inquiry into the Foundations of an Ethics for Our Age

Hans Jonas

THE FRAGMENTARY REFLECTIONS presented here are extracted from a much larger body of work in progress, viz., an *Essay on Ethics in the Age of Technology*. Just a few words on this by way of background to what follows. The major premise of the work is: that, with the wielding of contemporary (and foreseeably still rising) technological *power*, the nature and scope of human action has decisively changed; the minor premise: that a relevant ethics must match the types and powers of action for which it is to provide the norms; the conclusion follows: that we must review, and if necessary revise, ethical theory so as to bring it into line with what it has to deal with now and for some time to come. Thus, one has to look at the actions on the one hand, and at the theory of ethics on the other hand. A first obvious finding then is: that the actions that ethics has to deal with now have an unprecedented causal reach into the future. This, together with the sheer magnitude of the effects, moves "responsibility" into the center of ethics, where it has never stood before. And that, in turn, demands an examination of this new arrival on the stage of ethical theory, i.e., an investigation into the nature of responsibility. It should not be surprising that such a task compels the philosopher to probe into the foundations of morals. In what follows, I cannot entirely avoid the inhospitable terrain of first principles and general ethical theory and even metaphysics; but most of my attention will dwell on the more concrete, and more or less familiar, phenomenon of responsibility itself, which seems to me somewhat neglected in traditional ethical discourse.

I. The Objective and the Subjective in Ethics

A theory of responsibility, as any ethical theory, must deal both with the rational ground of obligation, that is, the validating principle behind the claim to a binding "ought," and with the psychological ground of its moving the will, that is, of an agent's letting it determine his course of action. This is to say that ethics has an objective side and a subjective side, the one having to do with reason, the other with emotion. Sometimes the one, sometimes the other has been more in the center of ethical theory, and traditionally the problem of validation, i.e., the objective side, has posed the greater challenge to philosophers. But the two sides are mutually complementary and both are integral to ethics itself. Without our being, at least by disposition, responsive to the call of duty in terms of feeling, the most cogent demonstration of its right, even when compelling theoretical assent, would be powerless to make it a motivating force. Conversely, without some credentials of its right, our de facto responsiveness to appeals of this kind would remain at the mercy of fortuitous predilections (variously preconditioned themselves), and the options made by it would lack justification. This, to be sure, would still leave room for moral behavior from a naively good will whose direct self-certainty asks for no further validation—and, indeed, may not need it in those favored cases where the promptings of the heart are "naturally" in unison with the biddings of the law. A subjectivity so graced (and who will exclude the possibility of it?) could act all by itself. No similar sufficiency can ever be enjoyed by the objective side: its imperative, evident as its truth may be, cannot become operative at all unless it meets with a sensitivity to the like of it. This sheer fact of feeling, presumably a universal potential of human experience, is thus the cardinal datum of the moral life and, as such, implied in the "ought" itself. It is indeed of the very meaning of the normative principle that its call is addressed to recipients so constituted that they are by nature receptive to it (which does not, of course, already insure its being heeded). One may well say that there would be no "thou shalt" if there were no one to hear it and on his own attuned to its message, even straining toward its voice. This is the same as saying that men already *are* potentially "moral beings" by possessing that affectibility, and only thereby can also be immoral. But it is equally true that the moral sentiment itself demands its authorization from beyond itself, and this not merely in defense against challenges from without (including those from rival motives in oneself), but from an inner need of that very sentiment to be in its own eyes more than a mere impulse. Not the validity, to be sure, only the efficacy of the moral command depends on the subjective condition, which is its premise and its object at the same time, solicited, appealed to, claimed with success or in vain. In any case, the gap between abstract validation and concrete motivation must be bridged by the arc of sentiment, which alone can sway the will. The phenomenon of morality rests a priori on this correlation, even though one of its members is only a posteriori given as a fact of our existence: the subjective presence of our moral interest.

In the order of logic, the validity of obligation would have to come first and the responding sentiment second. But in the order of approach, there is advantage in beginning with the subjective side, as not only the immanent given but also as implied in the transcendent summons directed at it. We can take only the briefest of looks at the emotional aspect of morality in past ethical theory.

II. The Role of Sentiment in Past Ethical Theory

Moral philosophers have always recognized that feeling must supplement reason so that the objectively good can exert a force on our will; in other words, that morality, which is meant to have command over the emotions, requires an emotion of its own to do so. Among the great ones, it was probably Kant alone who had to wring this from his rigorism as a concession to our sensuous nature, instead of seeing it as an integral aspect of the ethical as such. Explicitly or implicitly, the insight lives in every doctrine of virtue, however differently the feeling in question may have been determined. Jewish "fear of the Lord," Platonic "eros," Aristotelian "eudaimonia," Christian "charity," Spinoza's "amor dei intellectualis," Hutcheson's "benevolence," Kant's "reverence," Kierkegaard's "interest," Nietzsche's "lust of the will" (and so on), are modes of defining this affective element in ethics. We cannot discuss them here, but we observe that the feeling of responsibility is not among them. This absence must later be explained in defense of our choice. We also observe that most, though not all, of the feelings named were of the kind inspired by and directed at an *object* of supreme worth, a "highest good," which often carried the ontological connotation (a corollary to the idea of perfection) that this must be something timeless, confronting our mortality with the lure of eternity. The aim of ethical striving is, then, to emulate this object in our own condition and also help its approximation in the state of things: the imperishable invites participation by the perishable and elicits in it the desire thereto. By contrast, the object of responsibility is emphatically the perishable qua perishable, yet, in spite of this shared condition, more unsharably an "other" to the agent than any of the transcendent objects of classical ethics; "other" not as the surpassing better but as nothing-but-itself in its own right, with no bridging of *this* otherness by a qualitative assimilation on the part of the subject. Still, this far-from-supreme object, perceived in its perishability and insecurity, must be able to move the subject to a supreme commitment, without any appetite of appropriation, or there could be no "feeling responsible" for it. But there is the fact of such a feeling, given in experience and no less real than the appetitive feelings of the *summum bonum* aspiration. Of this, we have to speak later. Here we note what is nonetheless common between the two contrasting types: that the committing force issues from the claim of an object, and the commitment is to that object, whether eternal or temporal. In both cases, something is to be brought about in the order of things.

Over against these object-inspired and object-committed ethical stances, in which the content of the aim reigns supreme, stand the objectless kinds, in which the form or spirit of the action itself is the theme of the norm, and the external object, provided by the situation, is more the occasion than the aim for the deed. Not the "what" but the "how" of acting really matters. Existentialism is the modern extreme of this ethics of subjective intention (cf. Nietzsche's "will to will," Sartre's "authentic decision," Heidegger's "resoluteness," etc.), where the worldly issue is not by itself endowed with a claim on us but receives its significance from the choice of our passionate concern. Here the self-committing freedom of the self reigns supreme. Whether this position is tenable and does not hide a surreptitious recognition of a value in the object itself for which the decision opts (for which it therefore *ought* to opt), and whether this is not the true ground for the allegedly groundless choice, need not be discussed here. What matters for ethical theory is the conceptual denial of any immanent order of rank or right among objects and, therefore, of the very idea of objectively valid obligations toward them of which they themselves could be the source.

Unique (as in so many other respects) is Kant's position in this quarrel between "material" and "formal," "objective" and "subjective," principles of moral action. While not denying that objects can affect us by their worth, he denies (for the sake of the "autonomy" of reason) that this emotive affection supplies the true motive for moral action; and while stressing the rational objectivity of a universal moral law, he concedes the necessary role of feeling in conforming to it. It was indeed among the profound insights of Kant, the more telling for coming from the champion of unadulterated autonomy of reason in moral matters, that besides reason there must also be sentiment at work so that the moral law can gain the force to affect our will. According to him, this was a sentiment evoked in us not by an object (which would make the morality heteronomous) but by the *idea* of duty, i.e., of the moral law itself; and this sentiment was "reverence"

(*Ehrfurcht*). Kant thought: reverence for the law, for the sublimity of the unconditional "thou shalt" that issues from reason. In other words, reason itself becomes the source of an affect and its ultimate object. Not, of course, reason as a cognitive faculty, but reason as a principle of universality, to which the will is enjoined to conform; and this not through the choice of its objects, but through the form of choosing them, i.e., through the mode of determining itself with a view to possible universalization. This internal form of willing alone is the content of the "categorical imperative," whose sublime right is said to inspire us with reverence. Here is not the place to explain why this thought (which cannot be denied a sublimity of its own) must be rejected. The vacuity into which the purely formal categorical imperative leads with its criterion of noncontradictory "universalizability" of the maxim of the will has been often noted;[1] and we may add that every attempt to conceive the moral law as its own end must similarly fail.[2] We simply state the counterposition that underlies our own reflections on responsibility throughout this paper: What matters are things rather than states of my will. By engaging the latter, the former become ends. Ends may sometimes be sublime—by *what* they are, and even certain acts or lives may be so; but not the formal rule of the will whose observance is for any chosen end, or act, the *condition* of being a moral one, or, more precisely, of not being an immoral one. The law as such can be neither the cause nor the object of reverence; but Being (or instances of it), disclosed to a sight not blocked by selfishness or dimmed by dullness, can be both—and can with this affection of our feeling come to the aid of the, otherwise powerless, moral law which bids us to honor the intrinsic claim of Being. To be "heteronomous" in this way, i.e., to let oneself be moved by the just appeal of entities, need not be feared or disclaimed in the cause of pure principle. Yet not even "reverence" is enough, for this feeling affirmation of the perceived dignity of the object, however vivid, can remain entirely passive. Only the added *feeling of responsibility*, which binds *this* subject to this object, will make us act on its behalf. We contend that it is this feeling, more than any other, which may generate a willingness to sustain the object's claim to existence by our action. Let us then turn to this phenomenon, "responsibility," about which ethical theory has been so silent.

III. Theory of Responsibility

The first and most general condition of responsibility is causal power, i.e., that acting makes an impact on the world; the second, that such acting is under the agent's control; and third, that he can foresee its consequences to some extent. Under these necessary conditions, there can be "responsibility," but in two widely differing senses: (a) responsibility as being *accountable* "for" one's deeds, whatever they are; and (b) responsibility "for" particular objects that commits an agent to particular deeds concerning them. (Note the different referent of "for"!) The one is a formal, the other a substantive concept, and we really speak of two different things when we say that someone is responsible for what happened (which is neither praise nor blame), and that someone is a responsible person, i.e., honors his responsibilities (which is praise). Some further articulation will make the distinction clearer.

a. *Formal responsibility*. "He is responsible, because he did it." That means: the doer must answer for his deed: he is held responsible for its consequences and, where the case warrants it, can be made liable for them. So understood, "responsibility" does not itself set ends or disallow ends but is the mere formal burden on all causal acting among men, viz., that they can be called to account for it. As the mere fact of accountability independent of the agent's consent, it is thus the precondition of morality but not yet itself morality. Consenting to it, i.e., acknowledging one's accountability, is already more than the choiceless fact. To identify with one's deed, e.g., by readiness to take the consequences, has indeed some moral quality which may adorn even utter immorality. That is, owning the deed is better than dissembling it. An example is Mozart's Don Giovanni, whose defiant avowal at the end, paying the extreme price rather than repent, lends a certain grandeur to his misdeeds. But the example also shows that the affirmation of formal responsibility is not a sufficient principle of morality.

b. *Substantive responsibility*. There is, however, the vastly different concept of responsibility that concerns not the ex-post-facto account for what has been done, but the forward determination of what is to do; by whose command, therefore, I feel responsible, not in the first place for my conduct and its consequences, but for the *matter* that has a claim on my acting. For example, responsibility for the welfare of others does not merely "screen" intended actions with respect to their moral acceptability but obligates to actions not otherwise contemplated at all. Here, the "for" of being responsible is obviously distinct from that in the purely self-related sense. The "what for" lies outside me, but in the effective range of my power, in need of it or threatened by it. It confronts this power of mine with its right-to-be and, through the moral will, enlists it for itself. The matter becomes mine because the power is mine and has a causative relation to just this matter. The dependent in its immanent right becomes commanding, the power in its transcendent causality becomes committed, and committed in the double sense of being objectively responsible for what is thus entrusted to it, *and* affectively engaged through the feeling that sides with it, viz., "feeling responsible." In this feeling the abstractly binding finds its concrete tie to the subjective will. This siding of sentiment with the object originates not from the idea of responsibility in general but from the perceived right-plus-need of the object, as it affects the sensibility and puts the selfishness of power to shame. First comes the "ought-to-be" of the object, second the ought-to-do of the subject who, in virtue of his power, is called to its care. The demand of the object in the unassuredness of its existence, on the one hand, and the conscience of power in the guilt of its causality, on the other hand, conjoin in the affirmative feeling of responsibility on the part of a self that anyway and always must actively encroach on the being of things. If love is also present, then responsibility is inspirited beyond duty by the devotion of the person who learns to tremble for the fate of that which is both worthy of being loved and beloved.

This kind of "responsibility" and "feeling responsible" we have in mind, not the empty, formal one of every agent's being responsible for his acts,[3] when speaking of "responsibility for the future" as the mark of an ethics needed today. We come empirically closer to this substantive, goal-committed concept of responsibility by asking what is meant by "*ir*responsible action."

The gambler who puts his whole fortune at stake acts recklessly; when it is not his but another's, then criminally; but when a family depends on him, then irresponsibly, even with ownership indisputable, and no matter whether he loses or wins. The example tells: Only one who *has* responsibilities can act *ir*responsibly. Whether the responsibility violated is of the pervasive and enduring kind as in the example of the pater-familias, or more circumscribed, as that of a physician, a ship's captain, even as casual and passing as that of the driver giving someone a ride, there always obtains a definable, *non*reciprocal *relation* of responsibility. The well-being, the interest, the fate of others has, by circumstance or agreement, come under my care, which means that my control *over* it involves at the same time my obligation *for* it. The exercise of the power with disregard of the obligation is, then, "irresponsible," i.e., a breach of the trust-relation of responsibility. A distinct disparity of power or competence belongs to this relationship. Within its terms and while it lasts, the responsible one is superior: he is responsible *because* of that superiority, whether it anteceded or only originated with the relation of responsibility.

IV. Natural and Contractual Responsibility

In the parental example just used, we have a case of responsibility instituted by nature, which is independent of prior assent or choice, irrevocable, and not given to alteration of its terms by the participants; and, in that prime example, it encompasses its object totally. Not so a responsibility instituted "artificially" by bestowal and acceptance of a task, e.g., appointment to an office (but also that coming about by tacit agreement or the mere fact of competence): This is circumscribed in content and time by the particular task; its acceptance has in it an element of choice, from which one may later resign or be released. Also, in its inception at least, if not in its existence, there is some degree of mutuality involved. Most important is the difference that here the responsibility draws its binding force from the agreement whose creature it is, and not from the intrinsic validity of the cause. (The tax official's responsibility for collecting taxes is not predicated on the merits of the tax system but on his undertaking the office.) We have thus to distinguish between natural responsibility, where the immanent "ought-to-be" of the object claims its agent a priori and quite unilaterally, and contracted or appointed responsibility, which is conditional a posteriori upon the fact and the terms of the relationship actually entered into. In the latter case, even the requisite power, without which there can be no responsibility, is typically generated by the contract itself together with the duty; in the natural case, it is there to begin with and underlies the object's sovereign claim on it. Evidently, in moral (as distinct from legal) status, the natural is the stronger, if less defined, sort of responsibility. What is more, it is the original from which any other responsibility ultimately derives its more or less contingent validity. This is to say that if there were no responsibility "by nature" there could be none "by contract."

V. Self-chosen Responsibility of the Politician

There remains, however, a third possibility which, in a manner eminently distinctive of human freedom, transcends the difference of natural and contractual responsibility. So far we have found that a good of the first, self-validating order, if and insofar as it lies in the effective range of our power, and all the more, if in any case already impinged on by our activity, engages our responsibility without our choosing and knows no discharge from it. The (at least partly) chosen responsibility of the appointed task has, per se, no such commanding good for its immediate object and permits abdication in appropriate ways. But it also occurs that a good of the first order and dignity, that is, one endowed with a "natural" claim, but which of itself lies quite *beyond* one's present range of power, which he thus *cannot* as yet be responsible for at all and may well leave alone—that such a good is *made* the object of a freely chosen responsibility, so that the choice comes first, from the gratuitous and, as it were, presumptuous wish for just that responsibility, and only then procures for itself the power necessary for implementing it; and with it then, indeed, also the duty. This is clearly an *opus supererogationis*, but familiar enough. What is outwardly visible is the reach for power. The paradigm case is the politician, who seeks power in order to gain responsibility, and supreme power for the sake of supreme responsibility. Power, to be sure, has its own lures and rewards—prestige, glamour, the enjoyment of authority, of commanding and initiating, the inscribing of one's trace in the world, even the enjoyment of the mere consciousness of it (not to speak of the vulgar gains). The motives of the ambitious in striving for it are probably always mixed, and some vanity at least will have played its part already in the self-confidence of the initial choice. But leaving aside the most blatantly selfish tyranny, for which the "political" is merely a pretext, it will be the rule that the responsibility going with the power and made *possible* by it is co-intended in the striving for it, and by the genuine *homo politicus* intended in the first place. The real statesman will see his fame (which he may have quite at heart) precisely in that it can be said of him that he has acted for the good of those over whom he had power, i.e., *for* whom he had it. This, that "over" becomes "for," sums up the essence of responsibility.

Here we have a unique privilege of human spontaneity. Unasked, needlessly, without a prior mandate or agreement (which may later add their legitimation) does the aspirant vie for power so as to burden himself with responsibility. The object of the responsibility is the *res publica*, the common cause, which in a republic is latently everybody's cause, but actually only in the limits of the general civic duties. These do not comprise the assumption of leadership in public affairs; nobody is formally bound to compete for public office, usually not even to accept an unsought call to it. But he who feels the calling for it in himself, seeks the call and demands it as his right. Public peril in particular, meeting with the conviction to *know* the way to salvation and to be fit to *lead* it, becomes a powerful incentive for the courageous to offer himself and force his way to responsibility. Thus came Churchill's hour in May, 1940, when in a nearly hopeless situation he assumed the direction of affairs that no fainthearted one could covet. Having made the first necessary arrangements, so he tells us, he went to bed in the serene confidence that the right task had found the right man, and slept a restful sleep.

And yet he could have been wrong. If not his estimate of the situation, that of himself might have been in error. If this had later turned out to be the case, history would pronounce him guilty together with his erroneous conviction. But as little as this conviction, in all its sincerity, could serve him as an excuse, as little can the wagering on its truth in the reach for power, which might eliminate better claimants to the task, be made a straightforward moral duty. For no general rule of ethics can make it a duty, on the mere criterion of subjective certainty, to risk committing possibly fatal mistakes at others' expense. Rather must he who wagers on his own certainty take the never excludable possibility of being in error upon his own conscience. For this, there exists no general law, only the free deed, which in the unassuredness of its eventual justification (even in the mere presumption of its self-confidence, which surely cannot be part of any moral prescription) is entirely its own venture. After this moment of supreme arbitrariness, the law takes over again. Having appropriated the ownerless responsibility, its holder is henceforth owned by it and no longer by himself. The highest and most presumptuous freedom of the self leads into the most imperious and unrelenting bondage.

VI. The Object of Responsibility: Human Existence

Now, it is of the utmost theoretical interest to see how *this* responsibility from freest choice and the one most under the dictate of nature, that of the statesman and that of the parent, have, nonetheless, across the whole spectrum at whose opposite ends they lie, most in common and *together* can teach most about the nature of responsibility. The differences are many and obvious, and we must here forego their elaboration, instructive as they are. What is common to them can be summed up in the three concepts of "totality," "continuity," and "future," referring to the existence and welfare of human beings. Let us first take a look at this fundamental relatum, "human existence." It has the precarious, vulnerable and revocable character, the peculiar mode of transience, of all *life*, which makes it alone a proper object of "caring"; and, moreover, it shares with the agent subject the *humanum*, which has the first, if not the sole, claim on him. Responsibility is first and foremost of men for men. This subject-object kinship in the relation of responsibility implies that the relation, though unilateral in itself and in every single case, is yet, on principle, reversible and includes possible reciprocity. Generically, indeed, the reciprocity is always there, insofar as I, who am responsible for someone, am always, by living among men, also someone's responsibility. This follows from the non-autarky of man; and in any case, at least the primal responsibility of parental care *everybody* has first experienced on himself. In this archetypal paradigm, the reference of responsibility to the animate and to the kindred is most convincingly displayed. Thus, to repeat, only what is alive, in its constitutive indigence and fragility, *can* be an object of responsibility. But this is only the necessary, not the sufficient condition for it. Man's distinction that he alone can *have* responsibility means also that he *must* have it for others of his like—i.e., for such that are themselves potential bearers of responsibility—and that in one or another respect he, in fact, always has it. Here the mere capacity is the sufficient condition for the actuality. To be de facto responsible in some respect for someone at some time (whether acknowledging it or not) belongs so inseparably to the being of man as his a priori capacity for it—as inseparably indeed as his being a speaking creature—and is therefore to be included in his definition if one is interested in this dubious pursuit. In this sense an "ought" is concretely given with the very existence of man; the mere attribute of being a causative subject involves of itself *objective* obligation in the form of external responsibility. With this, he is not yet moral, but a member of the moral order, i.e., one who can be moral or immoral.

VII. Mankind's Existence—the First Commandment

Of man's prerogative among the claimants on human responsibility there is this to say: that it has nothing to do with a balance sheet of mankind's performance on earth, i.e., whether it has so far made itself deserving of the preference. The Socratic life or the Beethoven symphony, which one might cite for the justification of the whole, can always be countered with such a catalogue of incessant atrocities that, depending on the appraiser's disposition, the balance can turn out to be very negative indeed. Pity and outrage of the pessimist are not really refutable here; the price of the human enterprise is, in any case, enormous; man's wretchedness has at least the measure of his greatness; and on the whole, I believe, the defender of mankind, in spite of the great atoners like Saint Francis on his side, has the harder case. But such value assessments have no bearing on the ontological issue, as little as the hedonistic balance of happiness and unhappiness (which also tends to turn out negative when—and because— attempted). The dignity of man per se can only be spoken of as potential, or it is the speech of unpardonable vanity. Against all this, the *existence* of mankind comes first, whether deserved on its past record *and* its likely continuation or not. It is the ever-transcendent *possibility*, obligatory in itself, which must be kept open by the continued existence. To preserve this possibility is a cosmic responsibility—hence the duty for mankind to exist. Put epigrammatically: The possibility of there being responsibility in the world, which is bound to the existence of men, is of all objects of responsibility the first.

"Existence of a mankind" means simply: that there live men on earth; that they live well is the second commandment. The naked ontic fact of their existing at all, in which they had no say, becomes for them the ontological command: that there continue to be such.[4] The immediate execution of this command is entrusted to the instinct of procreation, and so it can normally remain hidden behind the particular commands of human virtue, which work out its wider meaning. Only very exceptional circumstances (as today's) may necessitate its becoming explicit as such. But tacitly, it always stands behind the others as their common sanctioning ground. Groundless itself (for there could be no commandment to invent such creatures in the first place), brought about with all the opaque contingency of brute fact, the ontological imperative institutes on its own authority the primordial "cause in the world" to which a mankind once in existence, even if initially by blind chance, is henceforth committed. It is the prior cause of all causes that can ever become the object of collective and even individual human responsibility.

VIII. Parental and Political Responsibility: Both Are "Total"

Of such causes we have singled out the two eminent ones of parental and political responsibility, and we named "totality," "continuity," and "future" as the distinctive traits by which they most fully exemplify the nature of responsibility as such. Let us run through them briefly, taking "totality" first. By this we mean that these responsibilities encompass the total being of their objects, i.e., all the aspects of them, from naked existence to highest interests. This is obvious for parental responsibility, which really, in time and in essence, is the archetype of all responsibility (and also genetically, I believe, the origin of every disposition for it, certainly its elementary school). The child as a whole and in all its possibilities, not only in its immediate needs, is its object. The bodily aspect comes first, of course, in the beginning perhaps solely; but then more and more is added, all that which falls under "education" in the broadest sense: faculties, conduct, relation, character, knowledge, which have to be stimulated and guided in their development; and together with these also, if possible, happiness. In brief: the pure being as such, and then the best being of the child is what parental care is about. But isn't this precisely what Aristotle said of the *raison d'être* of the state: that it came into being so that human life be possible, and continues in being so that the good life be possible? This then is also the object of the true statesman.

No wonder, then, that the two so divergent responsibilities interpenetrate in remarkable ways from the opposite ends of greatest singularity and greatest generality. First, in their object. Education, for instance, is private *and* public. Even in the closest sphere of the home it includes socialization toward the wider community; and this, in turn, takes a hand in the molding of its future members, the would-be citizens. Thus all developed states have a public school system and an educational policy. This is just one telling example of how parental and political responsibilities, the most private and the most public, the most intimate and the most general, overlap in virtue of the totality of their respective object.

Not only from the side of the object, but also from that of their condition in the subject do the two "total" responsibilities meet. Everybody knows what the subjective conditions are in the parental case: the consciousness of one's total authorship; the immediate appeal of the child's total need for care; and spontaneous love, first as the post-partural, "blindly" compulsive feeling of the mammal mother for the newborn as such, then increasingly, with the emergence of the person, the seeing, personal love for this subject of unique identity. In such choiceless force of immediacy, the subjective condition is as little as the objective replicable in other, less original relations, and the reproductive bond retains a status of primacy that no analogue can equal in evidence of responsibility. The statesman is not the originator of the community for which he assumes responsibility unto himself; rather is its prior existence the ground for his doing so, and from it he also derives whatever power he may concentrate in his hands. Nor is he, parent-like, the source of sustenance for the collective, but at best the guardian of its continued capacity to sustain itself. More generally, the ruler's responsibility concerns independent beings who at a pinch might manage for themselves. And "love," finally, in the genuine sense cannot be felt for a non-individual, collective, largely abstract entity. Nonetheless, to take the last point first, there does exist an emotional relation comparable to love on the part of the political individual toward the community whose destinies he wishes to guide to the best, for it is "his" in a much deeper sense than that of a mere community of interests: he is (in the normal case) descended from it and through it has become what he is; he is thus, indeed, not the father, but a "son" of his people and country (also class, etc.) and thereby in a kind of sibling-relation to all the others—present, future, even past—with whom he shares this bond. This fact engenders, as in the family, from which the symbolism is borrowed, something more than merely a recognition of duty, namely, that emotional identification with the whole, the felt "solidarity," which is analogous to the love for the individual. Even solidarity of fate can in terms of sentiment take the place of common descent. If both coincide (a radical contingency the one as much as the other), their combination is overpowering. The fact of feeling then makes the heart receptive to the duty which of itself does not ask about it, and ensouls the affirmed responsibility with its impulse. It is difficult, though not impossible, to carry responsibility for something one doesn't love, and one rather generates the love for it than do one's duty "free from inclination."

The spectacle of the total dependency of the infant, too, has a somewhat more abstract analogue in the political sphere: the general but always perceptually particularized knowledge that the issues of common welfare do not simply look after themselves but require conscious direction and decision, nearly always improvement, and sometimes salvation from disaster. It is, in brief, the insistent knowledge that the *res publica* too exists precariously. Thus, we have here again the fact of vulnerability and peril in that with which sentiment identifies and of which "one" must take care. This "one," meaning abstractly everybody, turns into the self-chosen concrete "I" of the politician who believes that he at this moment knows best what is best for "all," or is best fitted to carry out an existing consensus about it. Whether the belief is right remains forever objectively moot (for his occupying the role prevents the trying out of others), but subjectively this belief belongs inalienably to the total nature of political responsibility as it responds to the call of public necessity. But he who thus responds to public necessity is himself subject to it and rises to the challenge out of the condition of an equal among equals; in the public cause he promotes his very own cause as included in the former. This clearly sets his role off from that of parents who do not share the child's needs, but must have outgrown them to be able to minister to them. Beyond this automatically fulfilled condition (as concomitant with procreative maturity), no qualification of special ability is required, whereas the political pretender needs that distinction to legitimate his chosen role.

What, therefore, has no equivalent at all in the political sphere is the unilateral and absolute causation of existence, wherein alone, without further supplements, the obligation as well as the qualification for the parental role is grounded, and no analogous feeling unites political responsibility with the parental one. The statesman, however much of a "founder," is himself already a creature of the community whose cause he takes into his hands. Indebted he is, therefore, not to what he has made but to what has made him, to the forebears who transmitted the commonwealth down to the present, to the contemporary joint-heirs as the immediate source of his mandate, and to the continuation of the received into an indefinite future. Something of this applies also to the parental role, in qualification of the purely originative relation toward a *de novo* beginning life. But here we are already touching upon the two other characteristics of our two models of responsibility, "continuity" and "future," which almost automatically follow from the characteristic of "totality."

IX. The Dimension of Future in Total Responsibility

Of these, "continuity" means simply that responsibilities of that kind (unlike limited ones) have no pause as long as they last and permit of no "vacation" from their duties. More interesting is the dimension of "future" in responsibility of the total sort. In its indefinite scope, it presents something of a paradox. Children outgrow parental care, communities outlive statesmen. And yet, the pertinent responsibilities, in all of their particular, timebound tasks, somehow extend into the whole future of their charge, even though that future lies beyond their ken and control. Can the unknowable be included in my duty? Here lies the paradox. For it is the future of the whole existence, beyond the direct efficacy of the responsible agent and thus beyond his concrete calculation, which is the invisible co-object of such a responsibility in each of its single, defined occasions. These occasions, and the interventions they provoke, are each time about the proximate particular, and this lies more or less within the range of informed prescience. The totality that will absorb the long-range effect of the particular decision is beyond such prescience, not only because of the unknown number of unknowns in the equation of objective circumstances, but ultimately because of the *spontaneity* or freedom of the life in question—the greatest of all unknowns, which yet must be included in the total responsibility. Indeed, precisely that in the object for whose eventual self-assertion the original agent can no longer be held responsible himself, viz., the own, autonomous causality of the life under his care, is yet an ultimate object of his commitment. It can be so in one way only: respecting this transcendent horizon, the intent of the responsibility must be not so much to determine as to enable, i.e., to prepare and keep the capacity for itself in those to come intact, never foreclosing the future exercise of responsibility by them. The object's self-owned futurity is the truest futural aspect of the responsibility, which thus makes itself the guardian of the very source of that irksome unpredictability in the fruits of its labors. Its highest fulfillment, which it must be able to dare, is its abdication before the right of the never-anticipated which emerges as the outcome of its care. Its highest duty, therefore, is to see that responsibility itself is not stifled, be it from its source within, be it from constraints without. In the light of such self-transcending width, it becomes apparent that responsibility as such is nothing else but the moral complement to the ontological constitution of our *temporality*.

Where does that leave us practically? For mere mortals, the incalculability of the long-term outcome of any action might seem either to place an impossible strain on responsibility, which could paralyze action, or to provide a facile shelter in the immunity of ignorance, which could excuse recklessness. But the above considerations tell otherwise: in explaining the unknowability and deferring to its cause, they allow us to extract a practical knowledge from ignorance itself. First of all—to say the obvious—as there is no complete knowledge about the future, neither is there complete ignorance, and an agent's *concrete* moral responsibility at the time of action does extend farther than to its proximate effects. How far ahead, that depends on the nature of the "object" and on our power and prescience. In the case of the child, a definite terminus is set by the object itself: parental responsibility has maturity for its goal and terminates with it. Adulthood, if its self-assertive powers have not been impaired in advance (a vital "if" indeed), is trusted to make its own new start of coping with the—generally recurrent—conditions of individual life. Each generation stands on itself, repeating the parental precedent in its own way. The aged onlooker may have occasion to doubt if his educative record was blameless, but he has at least nurtured the chance of autonomous life to make up for his sins. "Maturity" just implies this chance, which takes over where parental responsibility ceases. That preordained threshold defines the latter's terminal goal.

No such intrinsic terminus is set to political responsibility or that for mankind as a whole by the nature of its object. The continuous life of communities has no true analogy to the ages of man, and major deeds in this field are apt to create facts never to be undone, constraining the options of all posterity. Abstractly, therefore, responsibility is here endless: power and prescience of the agent alone limit its concrete span. If the two were coextensive, there were no ethical problem in wielding the one informed by the other. But that preestablished harmony between the power actually wielded and the predictability of its long-term effects does not exist.[5] Political responsibility is plagued by the excess of the causal reach over that of prescience. The consequences of the single action enmesh with the immensity of strands in the causal fabric of the whole, which defies analysis even for the now, and exponentially so into the future. Dispatched into that interplay, the original intent may become immoderately magnified or—just as well—obliterated, and almost surely distorted; in any case, it is set adrift. This amounts to no more than saying that the course of history is unpredictable—and with it the afterlife of political decisions of the moment. Any long-range prognosis is at best an informed guess (usually proved wrong by events: almost every purpose is destined to become estranged from itself in the long run). The spectator, according to his temperament, may be thrilled or chastised by the perennial surprises of the historical drama; the actor must still wager on his guess and live with its uncertainty.

Nonetheless—remembering what we said before—even the most skeptical estimate of historical prognosis leaves at least one basic certainty, itself a prognosis: that political spontaneity will remain necessary at all times, precisely because the excessively intricate web of events will, on principle, never conform to plan. From this there follows a highly general, but by no means empty, *imperative* precisely for the statesman whose action consciously has this enormous causal thrust into the distant unknown, namely, to do nothing that will prevent the further appearance of his like; that is, not to plug up the indispensable though not calculable wellspring of spontaneity in the body politic from which future statesmen can arise—therefore, neither in the goal *nor on the road to it* to create a condition in which the potential candidates for a repetition of his own role have become lackeys or robots. In brief, *one* responsibility of the art of politics is to see that the art of politics remains possible in the future. Nobody can say that this principle, a knowledge wrested from ignorance, is trivial and not capable of intentional violation (which is one of the criteria of the non-triviality of a principle). The general principle here is that any total responsibility, with all its particular tasks and in all its single actions, is always responsible also for preserving, beyond its own termination, the *possibility* of responsible action in the future.

Contemporary civilization has lent a new edge to these considerations. If political action has always been beset by the excess of causal reach over that of prediction and so was never free of an element of gambling, today's global technology has raised the stakes immeasurably and, at the same time, has only widened the gap between the power actually wielded and the predictability of its long-range effects. To be sure, the time span of informed planning has lengthened greatly with the aid of science and its analytical tools, but the span of objective responsibility even more so with the runaway momentum of the novel things set afoot with that same aid. Novelty itself, this greatest boon, has the cost of denying to prediction the benefit of past precedent. Yet no pleading of ignorance will avail the daring innovators. Possibilities discerned by scientifically schooled imagination take the place of familiar experience in distant anticipation, which has become a moral duty. And among them is for the first time, as a realistic danger of progress, the quenching of future spontaneity in a world of behavioral automata. The point is that the changed scale and content of human action have put the whole human enterprise at its mercy.[6]

Reflecting on all this—on the magnitude of our novel powers and the novelty of their products, their impact on the human condition everywhere, and the dynamism they let loose into an indefinite future—we see that *responsibility* with a never known burden has moved into the center of political morality. This is why we make the present effort to clarify the phenomenon of responsibility as such. Here we also have an answer to the question, raised at the beginning, why "responsibility," for which we claim this central place, lacks that prominence and has largely been ignored in traditional ethical theory. Both the fact and the explanation are interesting.

X. Why "Responsibility" Was Not Central in Former Ethical Theory

The fact is that the *concept* of responsibility nowhere plays a conspicuous role in the moral systems of the past nor in the philosophical theories of ethics. Accordingly, the *feeling* of responsibility appears nowhere as the affective moment in the formation of the moral will: quite different feelings, as I have indicated, like love, reverence, etc., have been assigned this office. What is the explanation? Responsibility, so we learned, is a function of power and knowledge, with their mutual relation not a simple one. Both were formerly so limited that, of the future, most had to be left to fate and the constancy of the natural order, and all attention focused on doing right what had to be done now. But right action is best assured by right being: therefore, ethics concerned itself mainly with "virtue," which just represents the best possible being of man and little looks beyond its performance to the thereafter. To be sure, rulers looked to the permanence of the dynasty, and republics to that of the common-wealth. But what was to be done to this end consisted essentially in strengthening the institutional and social orderings (including their ideological supports) that would assure such permanence, and moreover in the right education of the heir (in a monarchy) or of the coming citizens (in a republic). What is being prepared is always the next generation, and later ones are seen as its repetition—generations that can live in the same house with the same furnishings. The house must be well built to begin with, and to its preservation is also directed the concept of virtue. Wherever the classical philosophers, to whom we owe the sci-ence of the state, reflected on the relative goodness of constitu-tions, a decisive criterion was durability, i.e., stability, and to this end, a right balance of freedom and discipline seemed the proper means. The best constitution is that which is most apt to last, and virtue, in addition to good laws, is the best guarantee of lasting. Therefore, the good constitution must through itself promote the virtue of the citizens. Justice, in particular, belongs to the conditions of stability and is accordingly emphasized, but equally for its being a form of personal excellence. (Never is the shaking of the whole edifice recommended for the sake of absolute justice: it is a virtue, that is, a form of conduct, not an ideal of the objective order of things.) The generally held rule is: what is good for man as a personal and public being now will be so in the future; therefore, the best pre-shaping of the future lies in the goodness of the present state which, by its internal properties, promises to continue itself. For the rest, one was conscious of the uncertainty of human affairs, of the role of chance and luck, which one could not anticipate, but against which one could arm with a good constitution of the souls and a sound constitution of the political body.

The premise for this reckoning with the essentially same that is threatened only by inscrutable fate is, of course, the *absence of that dynamism* which dominates all of modern existence and consciousness. Things human were seen not otherwise in flux than those of nature, i.e., like everything in the world of becoming; this flux has no special definite direction, unless toward decay, and against that the existing order must be secured by good laws (just as the cosmos secures its existence by the preservative laws of its cyclical order). It is understandable, therefore, that for those before us, whose present did not throw such a long shadow ahead into the future as does ours, but mainly counted for itself, "responsibility for the coming" was not a natural norm of action: it would have had no object comparable to ours and be considered hubris rather than virtue.

XI. Eternity versus Time

But the explanation can go deeper than to lack of power (control of fate and nature), limited precognition, and absent dynamism, all of them negative traits. If the human condition, compounded of the nature of man and the nature of the environment, is essentially always the same, and if, on the other hand, the flux of becoming wherein it is immersed is essentially irrational and not a creative or directional or otherwise transcending process, then the true goal toward which man should live cannot be seen in the "horizontal," in the prolongation of the temporal, but must be seen in the "vertical," i.e., in the eternal, which overarches temporality and is equally "there" for every now. This is best exemplified by Plato, still the mightiest countervoice to the ontology and ethic of modernity. The object of eros is the good-in-itself, which is not of this world, i.e., the world of becoming and time. The eros is striving relatively for the better, absolutely for perfect being. A measure of perfection is "to be forever." Toward this goal, eros already labors blindly in animal procreation, obtaining a token of eternity in the survival of the species. The "ever again," "always the same," is the first approximation to true being. The seeing eros of man surpasses this in more direct approximations; the eros of the wise aims at it most directly. The drive is upward, not forward, toward being, not into becoming. This direction of the ethical quest is based on a definite ontology. So is ours, but the ontology has changed. Ours is not that of eternity, but of time. No longer is immutability the measure of perfection; almost the opposite is true. Abandoned to "sovereign becoming" (Nietzsche), condemned to it after abrogating transcendent being, we must seek the essential in transience itself. It is in this context that responsibility can become dominant in morality. The Platonic eros, directed at eternity, at the non-temporal, is not responsible for its object. For this "is" and never "becomes." What time cannot affect and to which nothing can happen is an object not of responsibility, but of emulation. Only for the changeable and perishable can one be responsible, for what is threatened by corruption, for the mortal in its mortality. If this alone is left and at the same time our power over it has grown so enormous, then the consequences for morality are immeasurable but still unclear, and this is what occupies us. The Platonic position was clear: he wanted not that the eternal turn temporal, but that by means of the eros the temporal turn eternal ("as far as is possible for it"). This thirst for eternity is ultimately the meaning of eros, much as it is aroused by temporal images. Our concern about the preservation of the species, to the contrary, is thirst for temporality in its ever new, always unprecedented productions, which no knowledge of essence can predict. Such a thirst imposes its own novel duties; the striving for ultimate perfection, for the intrinsically definitive, is not among them.

The turning-around of the millenial "platonic" position is tellingly exhibited in the quasi-eschatological philosophies of history from the eighteenth century on, precisely because they still retain, in the idea of progress, a residue of the ideal of perfection. Kant, Hegel, and Marx, for example, with all their profound differences, have this in common: that the axis of approximation to the absolute has been pivoted from the vertical down to the horizontal, the ordinate has become the abscissa, the goal, e.g., the highest good, the absolute spirit, the classless society, lies in the time-series that stretches before the subject indefinitely into the future, and is to be progressively approximated through the cumulative activity of many subjects along the series.

We today are beyond even that stage. Threatened by catastrophe from the very progress of history itself, we surely can no longer trust in an immanent "reason in history"; and to speak of a self-realizing "meaning" of the drift of events would be sheer frivolity. This relegates all former conceptions to obsolescence and charges responsibility with tasks by whose measure even the great question which has agitated minds for so long—whether a socialist or individualist society, an authoritarian or free one, would be better for man—changes to the second-grade question of which would be better suited to deal with the coming situations—a question of expediency, perhaps even of survival, but no longer of "Weltanschauung."

XII. Parent-Child Relation: the Archetype of Responsibility

To conclude these very incomplete reflections on a theory of responsibility we return once more to the timeless archetype of all responsibility, the parental for the child. Archetype it is in the genetic and typological respect, but also in the epistemological, because of its immediate evidence. What has it to tell us?

1. The elemental "ought" in the "is" of the newborn. The concept of responsibility implies that of an ought—first of an ought-to-be of something, then of an ought-to-do of someone in response to the first. The intrinsic right of the object is prior to the duty of the subject. Only an immanent claim can objectively ground for someone else an obligation to transitive causality. The objectivity must really stem from the object. Thus all proofs of validity for moral prescriptions are ultimately reduced to obtaining evidence of an "ontological" ought. If the chances for this were not better than those of the famous "ontological proof" for the existence of God, the theory of ethics would be in a bad way, as indeed it is today. For the crux of present theory is just the alleged chasm between "is" and "ought." It denies that from any "is" as such, in either its given or possible being, something like an "ought" can issue. Premised here is the concept of a naked "is," present, past, or future. Needed, therefore, is an *ontic* paradigm in which the plain factual "is" evidently coincides with an "ought"—which does not, therefore, admit for itself the concept of a "mere is" at all. Is there such a paradigm? Yes, we answer: that which was the beginning of each of us, when we could not know it yet, but ever again offers itself to the eye when we can look and know. For when asked: show us a single instance (one is enough to break the ontological dogma) where that coincidence of "is" and "ought" occurs, we can point at the most familiar sight: the newborn, whose mere breathing uncontradictably addresses an ought to the world around, namely, to take care of him. Look and you know. I say: "uncontradictably," not "irresistibly": for of course the force of this, as of any, "ought" can be resisted, its call can meet with deafness or can be drowned by other calls and pressures, like sacrifice of the first-born, Spartan child-exposure, bare self-preservation—this fact takes nothing away from the claim being incontestable as such and immediately evident. Nor do I say "an entreaty" to the world ("please take care of me"), for the infant cannot entreat as yet; and anyway, an entreaty, be it ever so moving, does not oblige. Thus no mention also is made of sympathy, pity or whichever of the emotions may come into play on our part, and not even of love. I mean strictly just this: that here the plain being of a *de facto* existent immanently and evidently contains an ought for others, and would do so even if nature would not succor this ought with powerful instincts or assume its job alone.

"But why 'evident'?" the theoretical rigorist may ask: What is really and objectively "there" is a conglomeration of cells, which are conglomerations of molecules with their physico-chemical transactions, which as such *plus the conditions of their continuation* can be known; but that there *ought* to be such a continuation and, therefore, somebody ought to do something for it, that does not belong to the finding and can in no manner be seen in it. Indeed not. But is it the infant who is seen here? He does not enter at all into the mathematical physicist's view, which purposely confines itself to an exceedingly filtered residue of his otherwise screened-off reality. And naturally, even the brightest visibility still requires the use of the visual faculty for which it is meant. Look, and you will see.

2. What the evidence of the newborn teaches about the nature of responsibility. It only remains to explicate *what* is seen here: which traits, besides the unquestionable immediacy itself, distinguish this evidence from all other manifestations of an ought in reality and make it not only empirically the first and most intuitive, but also in content the most perfect paradigm, literally the prototype, of an object of responsibility. We shall find that its distinction lies in the unique relation between possession and non-possession of being displayed by beginning life, which demands from its cause to continue what it has begun.

The newborn unites in himself the self-accrediting force of being-already-there and the demanding impotence of being-not-yet; the unconditional end-in-itself of everything alive and the still-have-to-come of the faculties for securing this end. This need-to-become is an in-between, a suspension of helpless being over not-being, which must be bridged by another causality. The radical insufficiency of the begotten as such carries with it the mandate to the begetters to avert its sinking back into nothing and to tend its further becoming. The undertaking thereto was implicit in the generating. Its observance (even by others) becomes an ineluctable duty toward a being now existing in its authentic right and in the total dependence on such observance. The immanent ought-to-be of the suckling, which his every breath proclaims, turns thus into the transitive ought-to-do of others who alone can help the claim continually to its right and make possible the gradual coming true of the teleological promise which it carries in itself from the first. They must do this continually, so that the breathing continue and with it also the claim renew itself continually, until the fulfillment of the immanent-teleological promise of eventual self-sufficiency releases them from the duty. Their power over the object of responsibility is here not only that of commission but also that of omission, which alone would be lethal. They are thus responsible totally, and this is more than the common human obligation toward the plight of fellow humans, whose basis is something other than responsibility. In its most original and massive sense, responsibility follows from being the cause of existence; and all those share in it who endorse the fiat of procreation by not revoking it in their own case, viz., by permitting themselves to live—thus, the coexisting family of man.

With every newborn child humanity begins anew, and in that sense also the responsibility for the continuation of mankind is involved. But this is much too abstract for the prime phenomenon of utter concreteness we are considering here. Under that abstract responsibility there may have been, let us assume, the duty to produce "a child," but none possibly to produce *this* one, as the "this" was entirely beyond anticipation. But precisely *this* in its wholly contingent uniqueness is that to which responsibility is now committed—the only case where the "cause" one serves has nothing to do with appraisal of worthiness, nothing with comparison, and nothing with a contract. An element of impersonal guilt is inherent in the causing of existence (the most radical of all causalities of a subject) and permeates all personal responsibility toward the unconsulted object. The guilt is shared by all, because the act of the progenitors was generic and not thought up by them (perhaps not even known); and the later accusation by children and children's children for neglected responsibility, the most comprehensive and practically most futile of all accusations, can apply to everyone living today. So also the thanks.

Thus the "ought" manifest in the infant enjoys indubitable evidence, concreteness, and urgency. Utmost facticity of "this-ness," utmost right thereto, and utmost fragility of being meet here together. In him it is paradigmatically visible that the locus of responsibility is the being that is immersed in becoming, surrendered to mortality, threatened by corruptibility. Not *sub specie aeternitatis*, rather *sub specie temporis* must responsibility look at things; and it can lose its all in the flash of an instant. In the case of continually critical vulnerability of being, as given in our paradigm, responsibility becomes a continuum of such instants.

How this archetype of all responsibility sheds light on other, more public occasions for it, including the most pressing ones of the present state of things, and how its lessons on the essence of responsibility can benefit ethical theory, that is a subject for further arduous thought.

NOTES

1. For a most powerful critique, see Max Scheler, *Der Formalismus in der Ethik und die materiale Wertethik* (Halle, 1916).
2. Kant himself, of course, has rescued the mere formality of the categorical imperative by a "material" principle of conduct (ostensibly inferred from it, but, in fact, added to it): respect for the dignity of persons as "ends in themselves." To this, the charge of vacuity does not apply!
3. The same word for two so different meanings is no mere equivocation. Their logical connection is that the substantive meaning anticipates the full force of the formal meaning to fall on the agent in the future for what he did or failed to do under the substantive mandate.
4. Compare what I have said about the "ontological imperative" in "Responsibility Today: The Ethics of an Endangered Future," *Social Research* 43.1 (Spring 1976), p. 94.
5. Strictly speaking, of course, this holds for the education of children too, but there as we indicated—with the perennial "new beginning" afforded by the resources of personal spontaneity—antecedent deed has not the same finality of "results."
6. See "Responsibility Today . . .", p. 89-93, for a discussion of the discrepancy, in modern technology, between the tremendous time-reach of our actions and the much shorter reach of our foresight

concerning their outcome, and how to deal with it morally, i.e., responsibly. See also H. Jonas, *Philosophical Essays: From Ancient Creed to Technological Man* (Englewood Cliffs, N.J.: Prentice-Hall, 1974), p. 10, 18.

Commentary

Response to Hans Jonas

Daniel Callahan

A COMMON OBSERVATION about technological developments is that "what can be done will be done." But is that true? So far as we know, the Cobalt Bomb has not been developed, and no one has attempted to build a nuclear weapon which could destroy the world. Nor again, so far as we know, has anyone tried to develop a biological pathogen which could end all human life. Perhaps one might quibble about the technical feasibility of such possibilities—but they are at least conceivable, and there is no special reason to think they could not be developed. Yet they probably will not be. Apart from sheer insanity, such weapons would pose as great a threat to those who developed and used them as to those enemies they might be deployed against. This is not to deny that many things that can be developed will be developed; it is only to deny that a rigid law of technological inevitability can be postulated.

There is, however, an equally pervasive proposition about scientific and technological development which merits much closer attention than it has so far received. It can be put in the following way: if there is a conceivable, and potentially feasible, scientific or technological development that would significantly improve the human condition, then there is a *moral obligation* to pursue that development. Thus if it is possible to "conquer" cancer, a known source of misery and death, it is obligatory that work be carried on to realize that goal. Most recently, it has been contended by proponents of research on recombinant DNA that it would be *morally* remiss not to pursue a line of research which promises a great theoretical knowledge, as well as potentially enormous medical and agricultural benefits. To be sure, in the latter case there has been a major controversy about whether the potential benefits might be more than offset by the possible hazards of the research. Yet there seem few willing to deny the putative positive obligation to seek the fruits the research might realize if it can be done without harm.

Hans Jonas's essay on obligation provides a good occasion to consider whether, and under what circumstances, there is such a moral obligation to pursue scientific research. I pose this question in the context of Jonas's essay for three reasons. First, because it seems critical to determine what obligations those who wield scientific and technological power may now be said to have. Second, because I have some doubts about the extent to which the archetype of parental responsibility to a child can usefully be generalized to the problem of the responsible use of technological power. Third, because Jonas's reflections on that fundamental change in the perception of human goals and ends signalled by a denial of both reason and meaning in history raise afresh the question of the moral obligations of the scientific and technological community.

Let me first take up the third point. Assume that Jonas is correct in asserting that now "Only for the changeable and perishable can one be responsible, for what is threatened by corruption, for the mortal in its mortality." (p. 192) Assume also that Jonas is correct in his contention that the first moral commandment is to preserve "the *existence* of mankind." (p. 182) Yet if both those positions are accepted, we seem to be left in a curious situation. We must, on the one hand, work to keep alive "the possibility of there being responsibility in the world" (p. 182), while, on the other, living with the realization that history is going nowhere, that our ontology is "not that of eternity, but of time" (p. 192). Why, then, one might ask, is the whole venture worth it? If it is possible that the continued existence of mankind will realize some valuable essence or meaning, a *telos* to be achieved, then we are in the familiar arena of working to achieve valuable goals. But if we are told that we have a fundamental obligation to keep things going while simultaneously being told that they are not going anywhere, that surely, as Jonas holds, creates a wholly novel setting for the theory and exercise of responsibility.

What in particular does that imply about the obligation to pursue scientific and technological research which might improve the human condition? On the face of it, it would seem to imply such an obligation, at least for certain forms of research. There would surely be an obligation to pursue that technological research whose purpose it is to undo or ameliorate the survival-threatening results of earlier research and application. There would also appear to be an obligation to pursue that research attempting to forestall future dangers to survival—research on alternative sources of energy, social and scientific research designed to control population growth, and research on ways of increasing food supplies.

But would there be an obligation to pursue research the purpose of which is improve the quality of human life, individually and collectively—that is, to make life better, over and above mere survival? That would not seem to follow. If transcendence is no longer to be sought or hoped for, and history has no direction, then it is not clear why, with an endlessly unfolding horizontal temporality, *improvement* in the lives of individuals or the species is to be sought either. At least it does not seem an entailment that improvement *ought* to be sought—and it is hard to determine from Jonas's essay whether it would even be desirable to seek improvement. What, in the kind of cosmos and under the ontology he sketches, would count as "improvement"? It is hard to know what the idea of improvement could even mean in such a context. Apart from keeping the human venture going, there appear to be no goals toward which human life should strive. How would we go about choosing which possibilities to realize? It may be, then, that it is the mere process and fact of survival which is itself the purpose of human action, and the object of its obligation. Alternatively, it could be that any purposes are permissible as long as they do not threaten the possibility of survival. Jonas provides us with no clues on those points.

These omissions become all the more tantalizing when one

attempts to determine what the responsibility of those with scientific and technological power might be in the world Jonas delineates. Though this is not a problem Jonas directly addresses in his essay, it strikes me as a very obvious question to ask. For it is Jonas's initial assertion that it is precisely the* wielding of "contemporary (and foreseeably still rising) technological *power*" (p. 169) that has changed "the nature and scope of human action." (Ibid.) But who is it who actually wields this power, and what are their special responsibilities? That is not an easy question to answer, for a variety of reasons. In the first place, most technological power is now under state or governmental control. The power of technology is, on the whole, wielded by the political apparatus, which makes use of the power for its political, social, and cultural purposes. In the second place, however, the origin of the power resides within the scientific and technological communities. It is those communities which create the power in the first place, but the use of which can be and usually is *soon* removed from their direct control. In asking about the responsibility of those with technological power, one must really ask about the responsible uses of that power both by the larger political community and by the smaller community of science and technology.

I want to suggest that, while the archetype of obligation presented by the parent-child relationship cannot itself be directly employed to deal with the responsible uses of technological power, the archetype in conjunction with Jonas's model of the politician may be a promising combination. While Jonas concludes his essay with a hint that it may be possible to make use of this archetype more broadly, he even more clearly points to its possible limitation: its singularity. Only if one could show that the scientist stands in relationship to the world in a way analogous to the way in which the parent stands in relationship to the child would one be in a position to make use of the archetype.

If one accepts some of the stronger claims of science, this might not be as difficult an analogy to establish as might first appear to be the case. The strongest of all claims is that the future of mankind utterly depends upon unceasing scientific and technological development. This claim can be put in two ways. One is that, given human aspirations for a better life combined with growing scarcities of natural resources, we will be increasingly dependent upon ever more ingenious and sophisticated technology to avert disaster. The other is that, even if we learn how to scale down aspirations for more technology, we will still be dependent upon technology to insure a minimal standard of living; and even that modest goal will require a constant technological improvisation. Even if, for example, a great moral conversion should sweep the human race, such that it abjured further consumption of nonrenewable resources, the cost of that conversion would be the necessity to develop far more elaborate recycling technologies than we presently possess.

Under either version of the strongest scientific claim, the outcome is the same: the contemporary and foreseeable world is marked by a "radical insufficiency" (to use Jonas's characterization of the newborn infant), and scientific knowledge and technological application provide the only known means to meet that insufficiency. We can carry the analogy a step further. If our primary commitment ought to be to the survival of humankind, as Jonas contends, then that humankind ought also to invoke in those who have technological power an "ineluctable duty" (again, Jonas's term for parental responsibility) to work for its survival.

Perhaps I am moving too rapidly here. Let me, then, formulate a question. Can it be said that those who have technological power stand in the same relationship to mankind that the parent stands in relationship to the child? If we assume a "radical insufficiency" on the part of humankind in terms of its ability to survive without unceasing technological development, then the analogy would seem to hold. However, there are some difficulties in making it a strict analogy. The child is brought into the world by the procreative action of its parents; and it then exists before them in all of its needy immediacy. But the present scientific community did not bring our present world into existence, and that same world is even less the result of any individual scientist. Yet even if the *present* scientific community cannot be held responsible for the *present* world, might it not be argued that it is the historical scientific community which, more than any other, has made our world what it is? We would not, for instance, have a world population problem (with its attendant requirement for increased food supplies) had not science learned how to reduce death rates.

But there is still something lacking in plausibility in that argument. It was not the scientific community alone which created the world in which we live, but the use by political and cultural forces of scientific power which made the full difference. It is impossible to separate the responsibility of science for the contemporary world from the responsibility of those who made use of and deployed the fruits produced by that community. Someone or other is responsible for the "radical insufficiency" of the present and foreseeable world, but it turns out to be exceedingly difficult to trace that responsibility to any single source.

Another move may, however, be possible. In the parent-child relationship, the parents are responsible for the coming-into-being of the child, and that is one source of their obligation to the child. But Jonas does not rest his case on that point. The more important consideration, I gather, is that "the plain being of a *de facto* existent immanently and evidently contains an ought for others, and would do so even if nature would not succor this ought with powerful instincts or assume its job alone." (p. 195) In short, it is not why the infant is here, but *that* it is here which is decisive. We may, then, return to the scientific analogy. Whether and in what respect science is responsible for our world coming-to-be in its present form is less important than that the world now exists in a condition of "radical insufficiency," an insufficiency which can only be managed by more science and technology.

At this point the analogy of the political leader becomes potentially important. I will use Jonas's language. "First comes the 'ought-to-be' of the object, second the ought-to-do of the subject who, in virtue of his power, is called to its care." (p. 176) In the case of the statesman, he "will see his fame (which he may have quite at heart) precisely in that it can be said of him that he has acted for the good of those over whom he had power: i.e., *for* whom he had it. This, that 'over' become 'for,' sums up the essence of responsibility." (p. 179) In many respects, the scientist is like the statesman. There is no obligation that any given individual become a scientist. The language Jonas uses to describe that act of the statesman in voluntarily taking on power would just as aptly describe the scientist. It is "a unique privilege of human spontaneity. Unasked, needlessly, without a prior mandate or agreement (which may later add their legitimation) does the aspirant vie for power so as to burden himself with responsibility." (p. 179)

I am, of course, making some assumptions in drawing this analogy, but I think all can be defended. First, the scientist must and does vie for power these days—he must do well in school, prove himself to his mentors and to the peer community which he enters, find funds in a competitive grant system to carry on his work and do well enough in that work to advance his career. If there is any doubt that mastering the scientific world requires a vying for power, a rereading of James D. Watson's *The Double Helix* should dispel that notion (as will any conversation with any scientist seeking a grant). It is not necessary to see anything suspicious or despicable in that vying for power, it is necessary for my purposes here only to note it as a fact. Second, the scientist is also now widely held to be responsible for the uses of the power which he takes into his hands. I say "widely held" for it is certainly the case that there are still some scientists, particularly in basic research, who disclaim moral responsibility for either the results of that basic research or the technological applications to which they may be put. But that is an increasingly uncommon view, and one no longer tenable. Thus it seems valid to say, as much of the scientist as of the statesman, that "Having appropriated the ownerless responsibility, its holder is henceforth owned by it and no longer by himself. The highest and most presumptuous freedom of the self leads into the most imperious and unrelenting bondage." (p. 180)

There may be one significant flaw in this line of thought. The statesman wields considerable personal power as an individual, and has as a consequence considerable personal responsibility. This is rarely true of the contemporary scientist, who normally works as part of a team and in the context of a general community of scientists upon whom he can and must draw for that auxiliary knowledge needed to carry out his own work. Moreover, frequently enough, the scientist cannot exactly know (and often not even vaguely know) just what the consequences of his research will be. The statesman, by contrast, normally acts with a specific consequence in mind—he chooses this or that specific course of action because of the political and social effects he desires to achieve. The applied scientist may be in a comparable situation on occasion, e.g., in working to develop a pesticide designed to deal with a specific insect in a specific way. But many scientists are not in that position.

Let me return to my starting point. Jonas does not provide one with any indication about whether he thinks scientists have an obligation to make the world better. Indeed, if we are caught in a horizontal world which has no *telos*, no meaning in and of itself, then there would seem to be no obligation whatever on anyone's part to make life better. This is not to say that a choice to make things better would not be a valid choice; it is only to say that it is hard to see how it could be an obligatory choice. At most, then, the scientist is only obliged to do what he can to insure the survival of humankind. But that in itself is a large obligation, especially if it is true (as many scientists and others contend) that only more and better technology can insure that survival.

We are still left with a major difficulty, however. If the "radical insufficiency" of the world requires science and technology to insure the survival of humankind, in that sense, then, humanity itself can be likened to the child. At the same time, though, the scientist and the scientific community as a whole cannot quite be likened to the parent. There is no obligation for any given individual to become a scientist; he is more like the statesman who can choose to take on power but is not required to do so. And unlike the powerful statesman, the individual scientist is in a much weaker position in knowing what the consequences of his thinking and action will be. That is exactly why the subject of the responsibility of the scientist is a vexing and difficult one. In general, it is possible now to say that scientists and the scientific community have serious moral obligations. It is the detailing of those obligations which poses the hard questions, simply because the power is so diffused within the scientific community and diffused still further by the relationship between science and the political society in which it exists. That is a problem we have only barely begun to come to grips with.

Toward an Evolutionary Ethic

Bernard Towers

SINCE THIS PAPER is written from a Teilhardian standpoint, and since Teilhard de Chardin has often, mistakenly in my opinion, been judged to be in the tradition of eighteenth- and nineteenth-century philosophers of Progress,[1] it is important that I state at the outset my view that, with Teilhard properly understood, the doctrine of "progress" in its traditional sense has received a revolutionary twist that puts us into a totally new milieu from which to understand not only the nature of the evolutionary process itself but also the possibility of deriving from it a viable ethic of behavior. In a recent paper, currently in press, I wrote as follows:

> Where does this place us now, with regard to mankind's current explosive phase of technological evolution, and the ethical dilemmas to which that technology gives rise? All that I can hope to do, in the limited time at my disposal, is to alert you to the nature of the problem as I see it from the standpoint of what used to be called "natural philosophy." There is a vast amount remaining to be discovered and analysed about the process of evolution, that process concerning which "a whole host of our contemporaries is not yet modern" (to use one of Teilhard's phrases). Where are we to place mankind (especially in his recent expansionist phase) in the cosmic process? Must trends that we discern during the scientific era prolong themselves in an exponential way, or is it possi-

ble that the Law of Increasing Complexity-Consciousness, operating as it must through the fourth dimension of *time*, operates through cycles of *contracting and expanding time* (seen as a measure of change)? This would seem to be the way of it when we study the record of remote events ("remote," I mean, in geological not in historical time). Phases of explosive evolution, with wide divergence of often bizarre and always rapidly-progressing forms, crop up from time to time. And then there is a retrenchment, with a slowing of the rate of change and a gradual selection of those groups that prove themselves better "fitted" to survive, prove it by actually surviving. It is characteristic of the evolutionary process that with the achievement of each layer of increasing complexity in organization, the speed of change has itself increased. This is said to be one of the causes of our current distress: mankind has not yet had time to adjust to the vast technological changes that have come about in recent centuries. But we should recognize, in my view, that expansionist phases of the past have always been self-limiting, and that there is no reason to think that the present phase of evolution, now in the full swing of "noogenesis" (i.e. development of what Teilhard termed the noosphere) will not shortly enter a natural phase of retrenchment. Indeed it seems to me to be already doing so. The Industrial Revolution has done its job, and shown us how to harness power and improve the material standard of living of increasing millions of people. There is no reason to think that, given goodwill (a big given!), honest politicians (even bigger!) and skilled diplomats, the present, American standard of living (standard, at least, for all but the very poor) should not become the norm on a world-wide scale. As to what would happen then, with increasing comfort and leisure for untold numbers, various scenarios have been postulated. The one that seems to me to be the most probable is that sketched out by Gunther Stent in his book *The Coming of the Golden Age: A View of the End of Progress* (1969, American Museum of Natural History; Natural Press, New York). Arguing from detailed analyses of the recent history of the biological sciences—and especially from his intimate knowledge of Monod's field of molecular biology—and from the history of art and music with their ever more frenetic exploitation of "novelty", he concludes that we are approaching (and in many instances have already reached) the limits of exploitation permitted during the expansionist phase of post-Renaissance civilization. With the end of the customary notion of "progress" (seen as fundamentally expansionist) we shall enter a phase of inward-turning self-assessment, contemplation, and sheer enjoyment such as we see in some popular movements today. That will be, for Stent, the coming of "The Golden Age." In Teihard's evolutionary scheme it will represent a visible manifestation of that process of *enroulement* ("infolding") which he always saw as more fundamental to the evolutionary process than the traditional *déroulement* ("unfolding") of nineteenth-century thinkers. Both phases are necessary, but unfolding is of itself meaningless unless it leads to an infolding where the more "conscious" component of complexity-consciousness can manifest itself.[2]

This interpretation of Teilhard will seem strange to those commentators who diminish (in my view) his vision of the future as the parochial attempt of a French aristocrat to find the future in further growth and exploitation of Western science and Western Catholic Christianity. Teilhard did, it is true, represent as the second coming of Christ that "omega-point" towards which he postulated that mankind, and the cosmos within which he evolved, would ultimately converge. His insights into the ways in which that process might occur went much deeper, and incorporated a much more open, tolerant, and pluralistic ethic, than his own Catholic church could possibly admit. That is why he was plagued all his life with problems with church authorities; and why his posthumously published writings still attract so much official skepticism. He did not see himself as leading a new philosophical or religious movement. Rather he thought himself just one of the stones in the foundations of a new ethic, an ethic of *process* rather than "progress," which all parts of mankind must help construct for themselves.

This present essay represents an attempt to add a little more bulk to the foundations. A new arena of ethical philosophy must be constructed if we are ever to cope with the increasing complexity and sophistication of medical technology. We are already deep into a crisis situation as technology impinges more and more on the conduct of our individual lives and on that of society. My above-quoted interpretation of Teilhard is more truly teilhardian than one that would merely place him as an apostle of nineteenth-century progress strangely bound to traditional Catholic Christianity.

In view of much recent publicity about both evolution and ethics, I feel constrained at this point to state that I have no intention of entering the current debate on socio-biology, at least not in its present form.[3] The angry exchanges between the *environmentalist determinists* and the *genetic determinists* seem to me to be singularly unrewarding. Interplay between the forces of "nature and nurture" is a constant theme in studies of the morphogenesis of both soma and psyche seen in terms of both ontogeny and phylogeny. It seems to me that Wilson takes account of each of these four variables, and that, despite his leanings towards strict determinism, he has raised the level of inquiry to new heights with his recent book. That the debate should have been reduced to the level it has by a group determined to polarize it for political ends is lamentable. Although it may finally result in an increase in awareness (or, to use Teilhardian terms, in complexity-consciousness), it seems to me that there are better ways of achieving that primary "goal" of evolution.

One of the effects of acrimonious debate of this kind is that it emphasizes mechanisms rather than history. It diverts attention from the fact, repeatedly emphasized by Teilhard de Chardin, that the process of evolution (operating under the constraints of both genetic and environmental determinants) has, in fact, led to the development of those increasingly complex nervous systems without which conscious awareness and ultimately ethical decision-making would not have been possible. The science of paleoneurology has progressed rapidly in the period since Teilhard's death. His observations and predictions about the unidirectional trend, in evolution, towards increase in relative size and complexity of the central nervous system have been validated in all groups studied to date.[4] The argument in my paper for this conference is that if philosophers and scientists are ever to engage in fruitful discussion about basic ethical concepts, then they must first agree about the evolution of that human brain which alone makes such discussion possible. The difficulty with this suggestion is that it is not at all clear that most or even many modern philosophers and theologians are prepared, in fact, to take the theory of biological evolution really seriously. In the paper already referred to, I made two quotations from *The Phenomenon of Man* central to the argument. They were as follows:

1) What makes and classifies a "modern" man (and a whole host of our contemporaries is not yet "modern" in this sense) is having become capable of seeing in terms not of space and time alone but also of duration, or—and it comes to the same thing—of biological space-time; and above all having become incapable of seeing anything otherwise—anything—*not even himself*.[5] 2) One might well become impatient or lose heart at the sight of so many minds (and not mediocre ones either) remaining today still closed to the idea of evolution, if the whole of history were not there to pledge to us that a truth once seen, even by a single mind, always ends up by imposing itself on the totality of human consciousness.[6]

The principal thrust of that paper was that philosophers, more than most, appear today to have minds "still closed to the idea of evolution"; closed at least in the sense that many apparently give only what I called "notional assent" to the idea of evolution rather than give real assent to it. The difference implied by these terms is that while it is true that virtually all modern philosophers are prepared to acknowledge intellectually that the theory of biological evolution, first enunciated with clarity and strength by Charles Darwin only a little over a century ago, is valid, yet there are relatively few who appear to have felt or experienced its reality to the extent that would make them "modern" according to Teilhard's definition of the word, as given in the passage quoted above.

That my assessment of the current climate of philosophical thinking is not unjust is borne out, in fact, by the very title of this present meeting: "Foundations of Ethics and Its Relationship to Science: Values and the Biomedical Sciences." This wording appears to suggest that the appropriate mode is first to establish the metaphysical bases of ethical theory, and then to see how that theory, or those theories, should be applied to the theory and practice of science and medicine. I shall argue that this is to put the cart before the horse. Just as Aristotle's physics necessarily antedated and was logically prior to his metaphysics, so must modern science (and in particular the science of biological evolution) lay the groundwork for, and establish the mode of, modern ethics. The bioethicist must first discover and learn and inwardly digest, what it is that the biological scientist and the medical practitioner have to tell him about the way things move in nature, rather than attempt to instruct him, on the basis of some ethical theory or other (whether normative, utilitarian, formalist, situationist, or whatever), about how things are or how they ought to be.

Why should it be that few of us would be prepared to accept the logic of this more proper order of things? Well, for a start, "the art is long, and life is short," as the Hippocratic practitioners of medicine maintained. Is it not better (or at any rate much easier), if we are to philosophize at all, that we take, as our basis of experience of the world, those sights and sounds, those "observations" that happen to have come our way in life, rather than try to tackle observable reality as known through the bewildering complexities of modern science? Old philosophical and cultural traditions show remarkable resilience. It has not been easy to persuade philosophers that they really should take notice of such an upstart as modern science.[7] Scientific inquiry is indeed a newcomer in the world of scholarship, and its very successes have made the endeavor the object of suspicion to many. Daniel J. Boorstin pointed out, in the first of his 1975 Reith lectures, just how recently, in the history of man, came the switch from *discovery* to *exploration* as a valid and even necessary activity, for "the cautious quest for what they knew (or thought they knew) was out there into an enthusiastic reaching for the unknown."[8] There are more scientists alive today than have ever existed in the past three centuries; nevertheless, relatively few members of the human race have, to date, shown themselves to be *explorers* in the modern sense. The risks are great when one casts off from the safe world of *being* onto the ocean of uncertainty represented by *becoming*. Teilhard de Chardin, the palaeontologist, is said to have described himself as "a pilgrim of the future on the way back from a journey made entirely in the past."[9] That is the statement of a modern explorer *par excellence*, a "modern man" who did learn to see in terms of "duration" or of "biological space-time," and to see everything so, *including himself*.

Boorstin observed, in his second lecture, that:

The great awakening of modern man was his finding out that life was not really as repetitious as it had always seemed. This proved to be one of the most difficult steps in human development. It was not easy to grasp the fact that experience was not merely a series of similar events, but an unfolding scene of exploration. In the world of biology, it was not until the late 19th century that learned men of Western Europe began to believe that novelty was really possible. . . .Until then, biology had described a world of re-birth. . . . But the idea of evolution changed biology into a world of revolutions.

Biology has indeed changed, from a *stasis* to a *dynamis*. But what of history? of philosophy? Is it absurd to suggest that since these latter are the creatures of man, and if man is himself a part of the evolutionary process, it is time for us to recognize that, in so far as the practice of philosophy is relevant or even possible, it must be done in terms of *process*? We ourselves are the product of process, a process of which we are privileged to form not only *a* part but the keenest, most advanced part, with the greatest power yet achieved, in the history of that process, to direct its future course. Not everyone, of course, feels, or is even prepared to say he *knows*, the truth of that statement. Especially is this so in *academia*: university colleagues seem trapped more than others in the logical ordered world of "again and again" as Boorstin calls it. That was the pre-evolutionary world of thought within which classical philosophies of all varieties were con-ceived. But increasingly today, and especially amongst the young, with their concern for ecology and for possible reciprocal meanings of and for the environment and ourselves, one detects a sensitivity for the process of evolution such as has never before been experienced *en masse*. It was towards an understanding of that process that Teilhard directed his life's energies. His explora-tions[11] carried him into new and uncharted seas, to describe which caused him to engage in those endless neologisms and poetic expressions which have made him the bane of many in both science and philosophy. As I have expressed it in the past, he is essentially a "pioneer" rather than a "master."[12]

Pioneers always receive more criticism than they subsequently appear (if they turn out to have been right even part of the time) to deserve. This is true, whether we are dealing with pioneers in the arts or in the sciences. It is rarely acknowledged that the vast majority of scientists cannot at all be classed as "pioneers" or "explorers." They are "discoverers," busy discovering what is already predictable within the confines of the particular scientific paradigm within which they feel comfortable. Science then becomes, as Peter Medawar called it in his 1967 book of that title, "the art of the soluble" (London: Methuen). If it was wrong in the past to think of scientists, as a class, as "cave-dwellers" who were not "refined, like classical men" (see note 7), it is equally wrong to think of them as being essentially "progressive" or "liberal" in their approach to their work or in their approach to life. Within their ranks are to be found all kinds, from dullest to brightest, and from the fastest bound reactionary to the most daring kind of free "explorer."[13] Teilhard was very bright, and was imbued with the spirit of exploration.[14] This was how he viewed the evolutionary process itself, as a voyage into uncertainty, where there would be many failures, to be compensated for by an occasional (but inevitable, on the basis of his "law of complexity-consciousness") success. He called the process one of "groping," and in that word conveyed a great deal. The struggle within the evolutionary process at the biological level is always one of "groping." At close range it appears random. Groping movements are often—usually, in fact—fruitless. But when a "solution" or set of solutions is arrived at, it or they are immediately grasped, provided only that the biological group concerned is "aware" enough to recognize it then, and not yet hidebound enough to fail so to do. The universe itself seems to evolve by increase in complexity and increase in consciousness, as if by instinct. At least it does so in that part of it of which we are most aware, namely, our own planet and its immediate surrounds, and at any rate since that "period of singular time," as the astronomers call it, some ten thousand million years ago, when the present expansionist phase (which is all we know, all we probably ever shall know, and maybe all there is to know) began. In the nineteenth century, and in much of the twentieth, evolution was viewed as essentially random, with individual groups "borrowing" energy for a time to increase their own complexity, only to lose it later and thereby add to the general increase in entropy, or randomness, to the general state of "mixed-up-ness." Bertrand Russell stated it thus in 1935:

> The same laws which produce growth also produce decay. Some day, the sun will grow cold, and life on the earth will cease. The whole epoch of animals and plants is only an interlude between ages that were too hot and ages that will be too cold. There is no law of cosmic progress, but only an oscillation upward and downward, with a slow trend downward on balance owing to the diffusion of energy. This at least is what science at present regards as most probable, and in our disillusioned generation it is easy to believe. From evolution, so far as our present knowledge shows, no ultimately optimistic philosophy can be validly inferred.[15]

That such a view, wherein biology is made subservient to a restricted nineteenth-century understanding of the laws of thermodynamics (especially the second law), is false, even within the prebiological era, was clear to Teilhard. It has recently been argued by Layzer that matter in itself, when seen in "duration," inevitably tends to arrange itself into groupings and hierarchies of increasing order, of increasing complexity, of increasing information. Layzer expresses views nearly consonant with those of Teilhard. Thus he says, in concluding his article on "The Arrow of Time": "The present moment always contains an element of genuine novelty and the future is never wholly predictable. Because biological processes also generate information and because consciousness enables us to experience those processes directly, the intuitive perception of the world as unfolding in time captures one of the most deep-seated properties of the universe."[16]

This as I said, comes near to a Teilhardian view of the universe seen in duration. One of the phrases used ("consciousness") seems unduly restricted according not only to Teilhardian use but to biological use generally; a second ("unfolding in time") is characteristic of some earlier evolutionary theories, but misses an essential Teilhardian insight which is nevertheless implicit in Layzer's argument. Let us look at these both singly and together since they are indeed interrelated. Ordinary men, and philosophers amongst them, tend naturally and rightly to think of themselves as "conscious beings." The phenomenon of consciousness or conscious awareness seems, during much of history, to have been imputed only to human beings, and indeed to be a distinguishing character òf such a being. Thus, in the seventeenth and eighteenth centuries, under the influence of Cartesian dualistic thought, animal experimentation was conducted without any regard to the manifestations of pain displayed by the subjects (or rather objects) of the experimental procedures. It was argued that since animals were not possessed of a "soul," the seat of emotion, intellect, and free-will, their cries and writhings indicated no more than that the experiments were interfering with the internal organization of the "machine." By contrast, a human subject would respond with genuine consciousness because there was a "soul in the machine." Relicts of this relatively modern philosophy are everywhere to be seen still today. But to a modern biologist, whether neurophysiologist, ethologist, experimental psychologist, or (subsuming all of these) evolutionary scientist, nothing is more obvious than that other animal forms are "conscious" or aware. It is also clear that there are levels of conscious-awareness which in general proceed from higher to lower mammals, from mammals to birds and reptiles, and from land-forms to water-dwelling vertebrates. Analysis of the degree of "psychism" of animal forms, and comparison between the freer type of awareness of vertebrates with the more restricted and stereotyped awareness of the the majority of invertebrate species, was of fundamental importance to Teilhard. Moreover, the anatomical correlate of increasing complexity of organization of the nervous system, with increasing levels of conscious-awareness, was clear to him; it formed a major plank in the platform from which he viewed the world-in-process.[17] It was, of course, within the biosphere that man evolved. He inherited many of the "advanced" features of his nearest mammalian relatives, and through them, and the progenitors common to them both, the degrees of complexity-in-organization appropriate to prior forms. But with man there emerged a reflective consciousness, or "consciousness raised to the power of two," which gave to him the power of thought. It is this *reflection* which becomes, for Teilhard, the basis of his theory that, while evolution may represent, for long periods and in general, an "unfolding" of the kind implied by Layzer in the passage quoted above, a meaning perhaps inherent in the word "evolution" itself, nevertheless, in its ultimate significance evolution always involves an "infolding" rather than an "unfolding," an "involution" rather than an "evolution." Here is how Teilhard refers to the period, in the evolutionary history of the *Hominides* of the "threshold of reflection": "From our experiential point of view, reflection is, as the word indicates, the power acquired by a consciousness to turn in upon itself, to take possession of itself *as of an object* endowed with its own particular consistence and value: no longer merely to know, but to know that one knows."[18] But this cannot happen to the brain considered as an isolated organ. The development of such a power as reflection requires the collaboration of many other parts or systems of the whole organism. This is why, incidentally, we say it is the person who is conscious, not his brain, and this is why our current and arbitrary tying of consciousness or personhood to the brain, or any one part of it, will probably seem, to future generations, as absurd as was the linking of the pineal gland with the soul by the Cartesians. It is man who has evolved and is evolving, not simply his brain. Thus Teilhard says,

> It is true that in the end, from the organic point of view, the whole metamorphosis leading to man depends on the question of a better brain. But how was this cerebral perfectioning carried out—how could it have worked—if there had not been a whole series of other conditions brought together at just the same time? If the creature from which man issued had not been a biped, his hands would not have been free in time to release the jaws from their prehensile function, and the thick band of maxillary muscles which had imprisoned the cranium could not have been relaxed. It is thanks to two-footedness freeing the hands that the brain was able to grow; and thanks to this, too, that the eyes, brought closer together on the diminished face, were able to converge and fix on what the hands held and brought before them—the very gesture which formed the external counterpart of reflection. In itself this marvelous conjunction should not surprise us.[19]

It is through considerations such as these, where prehuman conscious-awareness is seen as a necessary precursor to human self-consciousness, that Teilhard is led to extend his idea of consciousness not only to all living things (where most biologists might follow him, since "reactivity-to" or "awareness of" the environment is regarded as an intrinsic property of living matter) but indeed to all matter, at least to the extent that particles might be in a state of "co-inherence" with other particles. His theory is that if there were not built into matter (even in its simplest form) the possibility of combination and co-inherence with other matter; and further, that if there were not built into Matter-in-Time an inherent tendency to form, by such advancing integration, increasingly complex systems, then self-reflective consciousness as we know it in man would never have been possible. Indeed, none of the higher primates would have been possible, nor any of the thousands of millions of other forms of highly complex arrangements of matter—because everything is the product of a process-in-time which the record shows tends always to generate information, improbabilities, "negentropy," wherein higher and higher levels of awareness can become actualized. At the human level, we find not only the power but the responsibility to continue the trend towards increased complexity-consciousness. The *power* is clearly there in nature, as it has always been. The *responsibility* comes because, for all that *we* are utterly dependent on *nature* for survival, yet, nevertheless, because of the power over nature that we have already achieved, many parts of *nature* are utterly dependent upon *us*, upon our conscious reflection, upon that "love" which Teilhard saw as the ultimate manifestation of the force that draws things together. That was the force he called "radial" energy, which operates to create the "within" of things. Thermodynamic energy he called "tangential," because it tends towards dispersion. Both forms of energy are intimately interwoven throughout the "duration" of the universe. Teilhard says it, as usual, in dramatic form:

> To think, we must eat. That blunt statement expresses a whole economy, and reveals, according to the way we look at it, either the tyranny of matter or its spiritual power. . . Once again: 'To think, we must eat'. But what a variety of thoughts we get out of one slice of bread! Like the letters of the alphabet which can equally well be assembled into nonsense as into the most beautiful

poem, the same calories seem as indifferent as they are necessary to the spiritual values they nourish.[20]

And so to the question posed by the title of this conference: "Foundations of Ethics and Its Relationship to Science." Must we in science wait upon the ethicists of today, in the hope that they might settle their arguments about the metaphysical bases of ethics (arguments that have continued unabated since at least the time of Plato), so as to tell us how we should conduct our affairs? Or will ethicists be prepared to give ear to the science of biological evolution as developed by one who was also something of a philosopher and who was versed, at least, in theology?[21]

Maurice B. Visscher has recently argued, in a paper on "Science and Value," as follows: "As a physiologist, I see the really unique evolutionary advance in *Homo sapiens* over higher mammals to be in his superiority in abstract projective rationality. I speak of his capacity, not necessarily his performance. A fuller use of reason would of necessity involve the use of science in arriving at decisions as to ethical desiderata and as to how to educate children so that socially desirable forms of individual and group conduct would become attractive norms."[22] Visscher wants to encourage the teaching of the science of human and animal behavior, as a basis for elucidating ethical desiderata. Teilhard would agree, but would go much further, since he would incorporate an ethical stance that emanates from the phenomena themselves. In his 1948 essay entitled "The Human Rebound of Evolution" he says,

It is enough for me to cite the twofold respect for things and for personality in the individual. Clearly whatever we may seek to build will crumble and turn to dust if the workmen are without conscience and professional integrity.[23] And it is even more abundantly clear that the greater our power of manipulating inert and living matter, the greater proportionately must be our anxiety not to falsify or outrage any part of the reflective conscience that surrounds us. Within a short space of time, owing to the acceleration of social and scientific developments, this twofold necessity has become so clearly urgent that to refer to it is to utter a commonplace. In recent years voices of alarm have been raised in many quarters pointing to the fast-growing gulf between technical and moral progress in the world today. The perils of the situation are plain to everyone. But do we yet fully recognize its deep significance?

Many people, I am convinced, still regard the higher morality which they look for and advocate as no more than a sort of compensation or external counter-balance, to be adroitly applied to the human machine from outside in order to off-set the overflow of Matter within it. But to me the phenomenon seems to go far deeper and to have far wider implications. The ethical principles which hitherto we have regarded as an appendage, superimposed more or less by our own free will upon the laws of biology, are now showing themselves—not metaphorically but literally—to be a condition of survival for the human race. In other words Evolution, in rebounding reflectively upon itself, acquires morality for the purpose of its further advance.[24]

The process of evolution, as understood in the Teilhardian scheme, not only acquires a morality, it demands it of those who will survive as a species. In a later (1950) essay Teilhard wrote:

When responsibility is restored to the setting of a world that is recognised and accepted once and for all as being by nature convergent, then it is automatically and immediately *universalized* and *intensified*, to the very dimensions of cosmic evolution and in exact step with it. And I need hardly point out that by that very fact it becomes *organic*.

So long as we thought that all we were confronted with was a set of rules (to be respected or disregarded), more or less arbitrarily decreed by man for the use of other men, we could believe that some escape from them or some violation of them was still possible. As soon, however, as we realise with excitement that socialization[25] is gradually enclosing us in a network not of conventions but of organic bonds, we begin mentally to appreciate the true greatness and gravity of man's condition.

One can always, you see, reach a compromise with the juridical and so rub along together; but thwart the organic, and there can be no pardon.[26]

Where then do we find our ethical guidelines? In the evolutionary process itself, seen as a process of both divergence and convergence, but with convergence assuming greater and greater significance as the "arrow of time" (see Layzer, note 16) continues on its irreversible trajectory. We must be open, pluralistic, and opportunistic in our decision-making in all areas of medical ethics. But we must always be motivated by the force of radial energy, by love for man and for the world. And the prime rule for the physician must be, as always, *primum non nocere* (first, do no harm). Perhaps it comes, in the end, to Augustine's *ama, et fac quod vis* (love and do what you will). We need such an ethic, today more than ever in history.

We may need it, but how might we ever see it happen? Perhaps the very pressures of crowded urban living will force us to love if we would survive. At the 1976 *Habitat: the United Nations Conference on Human Settlements*, held in Vancouver, B.C., the Prime Minister of Canada concluded his opening address, after specific reference to "this extraordinary scholar" (Teilhard), as follows:

> It is clear that in order to survive, we will be forced to socialize ourselves more and more. What is actually meant by 'socializing'? From a human viewpoint, it means loving one another. We will have not only to tolerate one another, but also love one another in a way which will require of us an unprecedented desire to change ourselves. Such a change will be more drastic than a major mutation of our species.
>
> The only type of love which would be effective in the tightly packed world we already live in would be a passionate love. The fact that such a statement sounds slightly absurd is a measure of the extent of the change we must make if we are to save ourselves.
>
> "Love one another, or you will perish," writes Teilhard in 'L'Energie Humaine,' adding that we have reached a critical point in human evolution in which the only path open to us is to move toward a common passion, a 'conspiracy' of love.
>
> The conspiracy of men with men and the conspiracy of the universe with an ever more just humanity: In this lies the salvation of human settlements.[27]

NOTES

1. See P.B. Medawar's Herbert Spencer Lecture for 1963, "Onwards from Spencer: Evolution and Evolutionism," *Encounter* 120 (Sept. 1963): 35-43. Reprinted as "Herbert Spencer and the Law of Gen-

eral Evolution," P. B. Medawar, *The Art of the Soluble* (London: Methuen, 1967).

2. Bernard Towers, "Ethics and Evolution," in *Proceedings of the Third Trans-disciplinary Symposium on Philosophy and Medicine*, ed. H. Tristram Engelhardt, Jr., and Stuart Spicker (Holland: Reidel, 1977), pp. 164-5.

3. E. O. Wilson, *Sociobiology: The New Synthesis* (Cambridge: Harvard University Press, 1975). For the most recent round to date in the controversy, see L. Allen et al., "Sociobiology—Another Biological Determinism (Sociobiology Study Group of Science for the People)," and E. O. Wilson, "Academic Vigilantism and the Political Significance of Sociobiology," *Bioscience*, 26 (March 1976): 182-90. References to earlier rounds are given in these two articles.

4. H. J. Jerison, "Paleoneurology and the Evolution of Mind," *Scientific American*, 234, no. 1 (Jan. 1976): 90-101, and H. J. Jerison, *Evolution of the Brain and Intelligence* (New York: Academic Press, 1973).

5. Pierre Teilhard de Chardin, *The Phenomenon of Man* (London: Collins, 1959), p. 219.

6. Ibid., p. 218.

7. See F. M. Cornford, *Microcosmographia Academica: Being a Guide for the Young Academic Politician*, 5th ed. (Cambridge: Bowes and Bowes, 1953), p. 5, for a brilliant account of how natural science was viewed in the University of Cambridge as recently as one life span ago.

8. Daniel J. Boorstin, *The Exploring Spirit: America and the World Then and Now* (New York: Random House, 1976), p. 3.

9. Neville Braybrooke, ed., *Teilhard de Chardin: Pilgrim of the Future* (New York: Seabury Press, 1964).

10. Daniel J. Boorstin, *The Exploring Spirit*, pp. 19-20.

11. "Explorations" is used in the sense employed by Boorstin (see note 8 *supra*) to distinguish this activity from that of *discovery*. As Boorstin says (p. 6), "The etymology of the word 'discover' is obvious. Its primary meaning is to uncover, or to disclose to view. The discoverer, then, is a *finder*. He shows us what he already knew was there. . . .The word 'explore' has quite different connotations. Appropriately, too, it has a disputed etymology. Some say it comes from *ex* (out) and *plorare* (to cry out), on the analogy of 'deplore.' The better view appears to be that it comes from *ex* (out) and *plorare* (from *pluere*, to flow). Either etymology reminds us that the explorer is one who surprises (and so makes people cry out), or one who makes knowledge flow out."

12. Bernard Towers, "Scientific Master versus Pioneer: Medawar and Teilhard," *The Listener*, 73 (1965): 557-63. Reprinted in Bernard Towers, *Concerning Teilhard, and Other Writings on Science and Religion* (London: Collins, 1969).

13. This is not to suggest that any one type is "better" or more desirable than any other. Inhomogeneity of the genetic pool is essential to future development, if inherent potential is ever to be even partially actualized.

14. For a complete listing of books and articles, in all languages, dealing with Teilhard, see the semi-annual *Archivum historicum Societatis Jesu*. For a useful bibliography of sources both primary and secondary, see Alice V. Knight, *The Meaning of Teilhard de Chardin: A Primer* (Old Greenwich, Conn.: Devin-Adair Co., 1974), pp. 149-65.

15. Bertrand Russell, *Religion and Science* (London: Thornton Butterworth, 1935), p. 81. For a critique of these views see Bernard Towers, "Evolutionary Trends and Human Potential," in *New Values: New Man. Proceedings of the 1970 International Future Research Conference* (Kodansha, Japan, 1971).

16. David Layzer, "The Arrow of Time," *Scientific American*, 233, no. 6 (Dec. 1975): 56-69.

17. See also recent developments in the science of paleoneurology (note 4 *supra*).

18. Pierre Teilhard de Chardin, *The Phenomenon of Man* (London: Collins, 1959), p. 165.

19. Ibid., p. 170.

20. Ibid., pp. 63-64.

21. Donald P. Gray, "The Phenomenon of Teilhard," *Theological Studies*, 36 (1975): 19-51. In this review article Gray gives a fair indication of the extent to which Teilhard's insights have begun to affect theologians and some philosophers, but he is rather silent on the extent to which teilhardian thinking increasingly affects the scientific world. He concludes with a section on Teilhard as a "terrestrial man," and as a bridge-builder between disciplines. He says, "He remains one of the significant voices pointing the way to a human future capable of providing necessary meaning for present commitment. Today we tend to see him as one of a larger chorus, not so much any more as one standing alone. For many, however, he has made it possible to see that there were others and to hear and understand what they were saying."

22. Maurice B. Visscher, "Science and Value," *Persp. Biol. Med.*, 18 (1975): 299-305.

23. In this connection it is interesting to note the extent to which the lie (a relatively minor evil in more restricted groups) is fast becoming an inhibiting major vice in large social organisms, so that one might say that (like hatred—and the *taedium vitae*) it tends to constitute a major obstacle to the formation of a Noosphere. (Footnote by Tielhard de Chardin in original.)

24. Pierre Teilhard de Chardin, "The Human Rebound of Evolution," *Rev. Quest. Scientifiques* (1948). Reprinted in *The Future of Man* (London: Collins, 1964). pp. 204-205.

25. This is not, of course, meant in the narrow political sense, but as a manifestation of that "hominization" which is central to Teilhard's thinking.

26. Pierre Teilhard de Chardin, "The Evolution of Responsibility," *Psyche* (1950). Reprinted in *Activation of Energy* (London: Collins, 1970), pp. 213-14.

27. Pierre Elliott Trudeau, "Man's Salvation: A Conspiracy of Love," *Los Angeles Times*, June 7, 1976.

5

The Poverty of Scientism and the Promise of Structuralist Ethics

Gunther S. Stent

THE IDEOLOGY OF SCIENTISM, the belief that the methods and insights of science are applicable to the entire sphere of human activity, aims to validate moral acts on scientific grounds. Indeed, this perspective sees scientific knowledge as the only kind of authentic knowledge. From this viewpoint, the only rational alternative would be an ethical nihilism under which everything is permitted, since the traditional theological grounding of ethics is seen as a morass of irrational superstitions belonging to a prescientific age.[1] This perception is widespread, and underlies the broad popular appeal of scientism, despite its more or less general rejection by contemporary philosophers and the often-repeated exposure of its potentially dangerous political consequences as a rational basis for the totalitarian state.[2] Thus acceptance of scientistic beliefs is usually the unstated but implicit ethical premise held by the opposing sides in current debates—"establishment" versus "science-for-the-people," "progress" versus "ecology" and "zero-population-growth."

In considering the scientistic approach to ethics it is useful to distinguish two different types of scientism—hard-core and soft-core. Believers in hard-core scientism take the view that moral norms and values can, or even must, be justified on scientific grounds. Believers in soft-core scientism may acknowledge that valid moral values can be justified on nonscientific grounds, but they still insist on the primacy of science as a guide to moral action.

Hard-core Scientism

Biology is the branch of science which obviously seems most relevant for hard-core scientism. For example, lessons gained from the study of evolution, such as the idea that survival of the species is an authentic value, are thought to have ethical relevance; hence "fitness" in the Darwinian sense is an objectively "good" quality. Herbert Spencer was one of the main nineteenth-century apostles of this particular version of hard-core scientism, which still has many adherents today. Thus, Spencer thought that the "good" can be identified with the concept of "more highly evolved," or simply with progress *tout court*.[3]

Another biological discipline often cited as a source of authentic moral values is ethology which concerns animal behavior. Here, moral goodness is assigned to those righteous features of human behavior, such as altruism, mother-love, or male supremacy, for which parallels, or sometimes merely similarities, can be found in the animal world, and for whose functional adaptiveness in nature credible explanations can be offered. Moreover, moral badness is assigned to features of human behavior, such as cannibalism or killing fellow members of one's species, which animals are alleged to avoid in the wild and exhibit only under the sociopathological conditions of captivity.[4] Although the ethological approach to ethics is most often used for trivial, a posteriori rationalizations of values generally held anyway and traditionally justified on other, nonscientistic grounds,[5] a not quite so trivial reversal of that procedure has surfaced recently. Here the ethological sanction of conventional morals is stood on its head; and traditionally negatively valued aspects of human behavior, such as aggression[6] or homosexuality,[7] are declared to be either morally neutral, or even to have positive value, on the grounds that animals also exhibit them in nature for apparently adaptive reasons.

On first sight, the diverse versions of hard-core scientism all appear to represent a logical short-circuit. For the authority of science and the claim for the authenticity of its knowledge depends critically on the very belief that scientific statements, being based on impersonal observations and measurements, are objective and value-free. But it is obviously logically invalid to derive conclusions that predicate values from value-free premises. Thus, in the case of the evolutionistic moral codes based on species survival or higher complexity, no moral value judgment can logically follow from the objective observations that live specimens of *Homo sapiens* exist or that *Homo* is more complex than the frog *Rana*. Moral values can be derived from these observations only if they are combined with nonobjective, nonscientific, value-laden premises, such as "human survival is good" or "biological complexity is good." It seems likely that the logical error of the evolutionistic moral code has its roots in the semantically troublesome "fitness" concept of Darwinian natural selection theory. Whereas in ordinary English discourse "fitness" connotes value, in the context of evolutionary theory, particularly under the mathematical formalisms of neo-Darwinian population genetics, "fitness" is supposed to be a value-free algebraic parameter that refers to the contribution made by a particular hereditary trait to the differential reproduction rate of the organism which manifests it. But even within the purely descriptive scientific domain, the "fitness" concept is troublesome, as evidenced by the current dispute among students of molecular evolution concerning the role that natural selection, as opposed to random genetic drift, is likely to have played in organic evolution.[8] Moreover, the attempt to derive value from ethological insights appears as merely a bizarre extension to the lower orders of Rousseau's romantic notion of the noble savage, or a scientistic yearning for the Good Old, pre-Fall Days in Eden.

On second sight, however, the derivation of value from scientific statements may not be logically invalid after all, but for reasons that can give little comfort to the adherents of hard-core scientism. For it is held by some contemporary philosophers[9] that the kind of impersonal and objective science on behalf of which authority is claimed is only an ideal and does not, in fact, exist. Since scientists are human beings rather than Martians, since they and the phenomena they observe necessarily interact, and since they use language to communicate their results, it follows that scientific statements, particularly in biology,[10] are rarely free of terms which imply functions, roles, and values. For instance, it is entirely possible that, protestations of neo-Darwinian population geneticists notwithstanding, the concept of "fitness" cannot be purged of all value content without losing its explanatory power for evolutionary processes. In other words, many scientific statements may be what Patrick Heelan has called "manifest images."[11] Although in this case hard-core scientism would not fail on logical grounds, the idol of the uniquely authentic scientific knowledge that inspires scientism in the first place would turn out to stand on feet of clay.

Soft-core Scientism

Since adherents of soft-core scientism do not claim to justify moral norms or values on scientific grounds, they escape the logical dilemma of the hard-core. But the more restricted claim of soft-core scientism for the primacy of science as a guide to moral action also fails, if not on logical, then on empirical or practical grounds. First, quite apart from the fact that this milder version of scientism usually neglects the subjective realm of the affects, it turns out that its adherents seem to have trouble bearing constantly in mind the admittedly nonscientific basis of the moral code.

I offer here one concrete example of this difficulty, based on a recent personal experience at a conference on "Biology and the Future of Man," held at the Sorbonne.[12] I was one of several biologists who took part in a panel discussion ostensibly devoted to defining the stage in embryonal development at which human life can be said to begin. Although this topic seemed to concern a purely technical question, it turned out to be supercharged with moral content, for the French parliament was then considering a bill to legalize abortion; in view of the extensive coverage given to the conference by the news media, it was obvious that our discussion was meant to influence the outcome of the debate in the *Assemblée Nationale*.

One of my fellow panelists was the cytogeneticist, Jerome Lejeune, a leader of the French "right-to-life" movement opposing the abortion bill. Lejeune maintained that human life begins at the moment of fertilization of the ovum by the sperm, since it is at that moment that the future person acquires a genetic individuality. Hence, abortion at any time is murder and must not be sanctioned by law in a civilized state. Most of the other panelists took the view that human life really begins only at some later developmental stage, prior to which there cannot exist any moral obstacles to artificial termination of pregnancy. Some thought life begins at the stage at which the heart muscles begin to beat rhythmically; others favored the stage at which electrical signals can first be detected in the brain; and still others thought life really begins only with parturition.

Although from the political point of view the debate was evidently effective, in that the abortion bill was eventually passed, from a philosophical point of view the discussion was quite futile. Neither Lejeune's genetic nor his opponents' physiological arguments addressed the underlying moral issue, namely, the generally accepted proscription of the taking of human life. Both Lejeune and his adversaries based their arguments on biological knowledge gained from the study of animal development, without considering that there are no moral restrictions against killing the nonhuman subjects of such studies. That is, the panelists did not seem to recognize that whereas it may be possible to have a strictly value-free scientific discussion on the subject of the most meaningful or heuristically useful definition of the beginning of the profane life of a vertebrate, mammalian, or even primate embryo, it is quite another matter to define the beginning of the sacred life of a human embryo. Any such discussion must begin with a consideration of why human life is morally protected in the first place and must confront the deep problem of the special status we confer on fellow humans, as compared to other denizens of the living world. This lack of recognition of the true nature of the problem under discussion was particularly vexing because the panel was seated in the Great Amphitheater of the Sorbonne, facing a statue of René Descartes. After all, three centuries earlier, Descartes had not only laid the philosophical foundations for physiology by advancing the fruitful notion that the human body is a machine, but he had also taken pains to point out that since moral principles do not apply to machines, man, to whom moral principles do apply, must be more than an automaton in human shape. And what makes man more than a machine is that he has a soul. Hence, when asking within a moral context when human life begins, the panelists—Cartesians one and all—should have been trying to focus on that moment when the embryo acquires a soul, or, in modern parlance, becomes a person. And that problem cannot be settled on genetic or physiological grounds.

A second, more serious deficiency of soft-core scientism is that it embraces the dubious empirical proposition that the realization of moral aims is necessarily impeded by acts that are motivated by objectively false beliefs. Indeed, a more extreme version of this proposition makes the demonstrably false claim that to escape doom a society must not base its organization on scientific falsehoods. This claim is itself false because one can point to many societies of the past which operated in a reasonably successful and stable manner while making value judgements based on witchcraft, astrology, prophecy, and other practices that we now know to be scientifically unsound. The reason why objectively false beliefs can promote the realization of moral aims is that social relations are complex, multi-causal, and highly non-linear phenomena and that any aim must be seen as an optimization rather than maximization of value parameters. This fact is generally recognized by cultural anthropologists since Bronislaw Malinowski[13] pointed out that the function of myths and rites is to strengthen the traditions that help to maintain a social way of life. Thus, although the false belief of the Hopi Indians that they can bring about rain by dancing may have been harmful for their agriculture, the rain dance itself provided for a communal cohesion whose benefits may have outweighed the potential gains in crop yield which abandonment of that false belief might have produced.

These considerations are relevant for the current hubbub in the United States and Britain about research on the hereditary basis of intelligence, whose totalitarian miasma can be traced to this feature of soft-core scientism. The opposing sides in this dispute both appear to accept the validity of the proposition that if there *were* a significant variation in the genetic contribution to intelligence between individuals, or between racial groups, then this factor ought to be taken into account in the organization of society. Since to the opponents of such research the mere consideration of the notion of hereditary determinants of intelligence, let alone taking it into account in social action, is an ethically inadmissible underpinning of racist ideology, they seem to feel morally obliged to deny outright the possibility of any connection between heredity and intelligence. Just like Christian Morgenstern's Palmström, they reason "pointedly, that which must not, cannot be."[14]

The proponents of research in hereditary determinants of intelligence, on the other hand, appear to be convinced that the failure to give due recognition to the existence of hereditary differences has pernicious social consequences and that, therefore, every effort must be made to identify the genetic basis of intelligence in a scientifically valid manner. This conclusion is not, however, rationally self-evident. For instance, let us consider Society A, which falsely believes that there is no hereditary contribution to intelligence (if that belief were really false, that is) and utilizes its educational resources less efficiently than Society B, which "tracks" its pupils according to a scientifically validated familial or ethnic prognosis (if such a prognosis were possible, that is). Cultural anthropologists might easily conclude under these circumstances that the losses sustained by Society A due to its falsely based educational system are more than outweighed vis-à-vis Society B by a greater communal cohesion, fostered by the (false) belief in innate human equality.

The most serious deficiency of soft-core scientism, however, derives from its overestimation of the power of science to provide an authentic understanding of just those phenonema which are most relevant for the ethical domain. That is, the physical sciences whose propositions are the most solidly validated have the least bearing on the realization of moral aims, whereas the propositions of the human sciences, which have the most bearing on the realization of moral aims, are conspicuously devoid of objective validation. Biology occupies an intermediate position between these two extremes, with respect both to the validity and the moral relevance of its propositions. Although this difference between the laws of, say, physics and sociology is, of course, generally recognized, the deeper epistemological reasons why the "hard" sciences are more authentic than the "soft" sciences are less widely appreciated.[15]

Pareto Distributions

In doing his work the scientist has to recognize some common denominator, or structure, in an ensemble of events; this structure is the phenomenon which is to be explained in terms of a scientific law. An event that is unique, or at least that aspect of an event which makes it unique, cannot, therefore, be the subject of scientific investigation: an ensemble of unique events has no common denominator, is not a phenomenon, and there is nothing in it to explain. Such events are random, and the observer perceives them as noise. Since every real event incorporates some element of uniqueness, every ensemble of real events contains some noise. The basic problem of scientific observation, therefore, is to recognize a significant structure of an ensemble of events above its inevitable background noise. Most of the phenomena for which successful scientific theories had been worked out prior to about one hundred years ago are relatively noise-free. Such phenomena were explained in terms of deterministic laws, which assert that a given set of initial conditions (antecedent situation) can lead to one and only one final stage (consequent). Toward the end of the nineteenth century the methods of mathematical statistics came to be trained on previously inscrutable phenomena involving an appreciable element of noise. This development gave rise to the appearance of indeterministic laws of physics, such as the kinetic theory of gases and quantum mechanics. These indeterministic laws envisage that a given set of initial conditions can lead to several alternative final states. An indeterministic law is not devoid of predictive value, however, because to each of the several alternative final states there is assigned a probability of its realization. Indeed, a deterministic law can be regarded as a limiting case of a more general indeterministic law in which the chance of the occurrence of one of the alternative final states approaches certainty. The conventional touchstone of the validity of both deterministic and indeterministic laws is the realization of their predictions in future observations. If the predictions are realized, then the structure which the observer believes to have perceived in the original phenomenon can be considered to have been real.

But, as was pointed out by Benoit Mandelbrot,[16] many of those noisy phenomena which continue to elude successful theoretical understanding are not only inaccessible to analysis by deterministic theories, but have also proven refractory to explanation in terms of indeterministic theories. According to Mandelbrot, it is the statistical character of the noise presented by these phenomena, or their spontaneous activity, which renders them scientifically opaque. In almost all systems for which it has so far been possible to make successful indeterministic scientific theories, the spontaneous activity displays a statistical distribution such that the mean value of a series of observations converges rapidly toward a limit. That limit can be subjected to analysis of the classical deterministic type. For instance, in the successful kinetic theory of gases, the spontaneous activity of a gas satisfies this condition. Here the energy of individual molecules is subject to a very wide variation (thermal unrest), but the mean energy per molecule converges to a limit and is, therefore, for all practical purposes determined. But many of the phenomena for which it has not been possible to make successful scientific theories so far turn out to possess a spontaneous activity which displays quite a different kind of distribution, which is called "Pareto" distribution after the turn-of-the-century Italian economist who first observed it for the spread in incomes. For such phenomena the mean value of a series of observations converges only very slowly, or not at all, toward a limit. And here, it is very much more difficult to ascertain whether any structure the observer believes to have perceived is real, or whether the phenomenon is merely a figment of his imagination.

As Mandelbrot has pointed out, the "softness" of the human sciences arises from the predominance of Pareto distributions in the basic phenomena to which they must address their analysis. In economics, for instance, firm sizes and income and price fluctuations follow Pareto's law. In sociology, the sizes of "human agglomerations" have a similar distribution, which demonstrates that such common-sense terms as "cities," "towns," and "villages" are ambiguous, impressionistic structures. That our vocabulary contains these terms, nevertheless, is a reflection of our habit of providing a specific description of a world whose events are intuited in terms of converging mean-value statistics.

Hence, it is because of the intrinsically refractory statistical character of the phenomena in want of explanation that it is possible only in exceptional cases to ascertain whether the propositions of the human sciences represent reality or figments of the imagination. It is for just that reason that the human sciences are "soft," and their laws generally beyond the reach of validation. This is not to suggest by any means that the human sciences are worthless enterprises and that no attention need be paid to the insights they provide. On the contrary, we cannot do without them; just as we cannot do without morality. But these considerations do show that the scientistic claims on behalf of an authoritative role of science guiding moral action can themselves be doubted on scientific grounds.

Structuralism

That the human sciences are, in fact, unlikely to provide the authentic guide to the realization of moral aims envisaged by soft-core scientism has come to light with the emergence of the "structuralist" approach to the human mind and the decay of positivism as the philosophical infrastructure of modern science.[17] Structuralism transcends the limitation on the methodology, indeed on the agenda of permissible inquiry, of the human sciences imposed by positivism. Structuralism admits, as positivism does not, the possibility of innate knowledge not derived from direct experience. It represents, therefore, a return to Cartesian rationalist philosophy. Or, more exactly, structuralism embraces this feature of rationalism as it was later reworked by Kant for his philosophy of critical idealism. Kant held that the mind constructs reality from experience by use of innate categories, and thus, to understand man, it is indispensable to try to fathom the nature of his deep and universal cognitive endowment. Accordingly, structuralism not only permits propositions about behavior that are not directly inducible from observed data, but it even maintains that the relations between such data, or surface structures, are not by themselves explainable. According to this view the causal connections that determine behavior do not relate to surface structures at all. Instead, the overt behavorial phenomena are generated by covert deep structures, inaccessible to direct observation. Hence, any theoretical framework for understanding man must be based on the deep structures, whose discovery ought to be the real goal of the human sciences.

Universal Grammar

Linguistics is one of the human sciences in which the structuralist approach is currently very prominent. The older, positivist approach to linguistics addressed itself to the discovery of structural relations among the elements of spoken language. That is, it was concerned with the surface structures of linguistic performance, the patterns which can be observed as being in use by speakers of various languages. Since the patterns which such classificatory analysis reveals differ widely, it seemed reasonable to conclude that these patterns are arbitrary, or purely conventional, one linguistic group having chosen to adopt one, and another group having chosen to adopt another convention. There would be nothing that linguistics could be called on to explain, except for the taxonomic principles that account for the degree of historical relatedness of different peoples. By contrast, the structuralist approach to linguistics, according to its main modern proponent, Noam Chomsky, starts from the premise that linguistic patterns are not arbitrary.[18] Instead, all men are believed to possess an innate, a priori knowledge of a universal grammar, and that despite their superficial differences, all natural languages are based on that same grammar. According to that view, the overt surface structure of speech, or the organization of sentences, is generated by the speaker from a covert deep structure. In his speech act, the speaker is thought to formulate first his proposition as an abstract deep structure that he transforms only secondarily according to a set of rules into the concrete surface structure of his utterance. The listener in turn fathoms the meaning of the speech act by just the inverse transformation of surface to deep structure. Chomsky holds that the grammar of a language is a system of transformational rules that determines a certain pairing of sound and meaning. It consists of a syntactic component, a semantic component, and a phonological component. The surface structure contains the information relevant to the phonological component, whereas the deep structure contains the information relevant to the semantic component, and the syntactic component pairs surface and deep structures.

So far, it does not seem to have been possible to identify clearly those aspects of the grammar of any one natural language which are universal, and hence shared with all other natural languages, in contrast to those aspects which are particular, and hence responsible for differentiating that language from other languages. Some success has been achieved at the sound level, where a limited number of universal "distinctive features" has been identified. Each feature takes on one of a very few discrete values (such as "present" or "absent") in a given sound element of speech. In other words, every symbol of a phonetic alphabet can be regarded as a set of these features, each with a specified value. Thus it should be possible to construct a universal phonetic script which would allow, in principle at least, a speaker of any natural language to pronounce correctly a written text in any other natural language.

Much less success has been achieved so far at the philosophically more interesting meaning level. Here the concept of a universal grammar would suggest the existence of an ensemble of universal semantic "distinctive features" and laws regarding their interrelations and permitted variety. That is, every meaningful concept would be fathomable as a set of semantic features, each with a specified value. From this point of view, it should be possible to construct a universal "semantic script," texts of which all speakers of natural languages would understand. Unfortunately, it has proven difficult to put forward any specific proposals for or examples of the putative "semantic features," except to conclude that they must be of a highly abstract nature. In any case, if both the surface level of sound and the deep level of meaning are universal aspects on which all natural languages are based, then it must be the transformational components of grammar that have become greatly differentiated during the course of human history, since the building of the Tower of Babel. But the presumed constancy through time of the universal aspects cannot be attributable to any cause other than an innate, hereditary aspect of the mind. Hence, the general aim of structuralist linguistics is to discover those universal aspects.

The great strength of the structuralist human sciences is that they do offer a theoretical approach to understanding human behavior. Their great weakness, however, is that it is not possible to validate the propositions which they offer regarding the mental deep structures. The reason for this is not only the refractory statistical character of the surface structures, or phenomena to be observed, which is no less troublesome for the positivist than for the structuralist approach, but also the transformational relation between surface and deep structures, with which the positivist approach need not contend. Propositions about the deep structures are nearly impossible to falsify by empirical study of the surface structures, since it is almost always feasible to reconcile any apparent contradiction between theoretical prediction and observed fact by an appropriate adjustment of the transformational rules. Thus, the structuralist schools active in the human sciences do try to explain human behavior within a general theoretical framework, in contrast to their positivist counterparts who cannot, or rather refuse to try to do so. But there is no way of validating the structuralist theories in the manner in which the theories of physics can be validated through critical experiments or observations.

Biology and the Kantian a priori

As it turns out, however, the structuralist approach to the mind can draw support from the insights of modern biology. To secure this support, it is not necessary to embrace the position of extreme materialism which envisages that all conscious thought is "reducible" to neurophysiology. Instead, it suffices to hold the minimal position compatible with any scientific approach to the mind-body problem, namely, that there exists some isomorphism between cerebral and mental events. One example of a provision of support by biological insights for a structuralist tenet has been the resolution of an old dilemma posed by Kant's epistemology. As Kant set forth, sensations become experience, that is, gain meaning only after they are interpreted in terms of a priori concepts, such as time and space. Other a priori concepts, such as induction (or causality), allow the mind to construct reality from that experience. But if, as Kant alleges, we bring such concepts as time and space to sensation and causality to experience a priori, how is it that these transcendental concepts happen to fit our world so well? Considering all the ill-conceived notions we might have had about the world prior to experience, it seems nothing short of miraculous that our innate concepts just happen to be appropriate. Here the positivist view that all knowledge is derived from experience a posteriori would seem much more reasonable. It turns out, however, that the way to resolve this dilemma posed by the Kantian a priori has been open since Darwin put forward the theory of natural selection in the mid-nineteenth century. As Konrad Lorenz[19] has pointed out, the positivist argument that knowledge about the world can enter our mind only through experience is valid if we consider only the ontogenetic development of man from fertilized egg to adult. But once we take into account also the phylogenetic development of the human brain through evolutionary history, it becomes clear that individuals can also know something of the world innately, prior to and independent of their own experiences. After all, there is no biological reason why such knowledge cannot be passed on from generation to generation through the ensemble of genes that determines the structure and function of our nervous system. For that genetic ensemble came into being through the process of natural selection operating on our remote ancestors. According to Lorenz, "Experience has as little to do with the matching of a priori ideas with reality as does the matching of the fin structure of a fish with the properties of water." In other words, the Kantian notion of a priori knowledge is not implausible at all, but fully consonant with present mainstream evolutionary thought. The a priori concepts of time, space, and causality happen to suit the world because our brain—and hence, in view of its isomorphism with the brain, our mind—was selected for evolutionary fitness, just as were innate behavioral acts.

In addition to being fully consonant with modern evolutionary thought, the notion of Kantian a priori, and its latter-day, neo-Kantian structuralist elaboration, finds support from recent neurological findings which indicate that, in accord with those tenets, information about the world reaches the brain, not as raw data but as highly processed structures that are generated by a set of stepwise, preconscious informational transformations of the sensory input.[20] These neurological transformations proceed according to a program that preexists in the brain, and, in their initial stages, at least, consist of abstracting the vast amount of experiential data continuously fathered by the senses. In order to abstract, the brain destroys selectively portions of the input data and thus transforms these data into manageable categories, or structures that are meaningful.

One set of such neurological findings concerns the manner in which the nervous system of higher vertebrates, including man, transforms the light rays entering the eyes into a visual percept. This transformation begins in the retina at the back of the eye. There, a two-dimensional array of about a hundred million primary light receptor cells—the rods and the cones—converts the radiant energy of the image projected via the lens on the retina into a pattern of electrical signals, much as a television camera does. Since the electrical response of each light receptor cell depends on the intensity of light that happens to fall on it, the overall activity pattern of the light receptor cell array represents the light intensity existing at a hundred million different points in the visual space. The retina not only contains the input part of the visual sense, however, but also performs the first stage of the abstraction process. This first stage is carried out by another two-dimensional array of nerve cells, namely, the million or so ganglion cells. The ganglion cells receive the electrical signals generated by the hundred million light receptor cells and subject them to information processing. The result of this processing is that the activity pattern of the ganglion cells constitutes a more abstract representation of the visual space than the activity pattern of the light receptor cells. Instead of reporting the light intensity existing at a single point in the visual space, each ganglion cell signals the light-dark contrast which exists between the center and the edge of a circular receptive field in the visual space, with each receptive field consisting of about a hundred contiguous points monitored by individual light receptor cells. In this way, the point-by-point fine-grained light intensity information is boiled down to a somewhat coarser field-by-field light contrast representation. As can be readily appreciated, such light contrast information is essential for the recognition of shapes and forms in space, or visual perception.

For the next stage of processing the visual information leaves the retina via the nerve fibers of the ganglion cells. These fibers connect the eye with the brain, and after passing a way station in the forebrain the output signals of the ganglion cells reach the cerebral cortex at the lower back of the head. Here the signals converge on a set of cortical nerve cells. Study of the cortical nerve cells receiving the partially abstracted visual input has shown that each of them responds only to light rays reaching the eye from a limited set of contiguous points in the visual space. But the structure of the receptive fields of these cortical nerve cells is more complicated, and their size is larger than that of the receptive fields of the retinal ganglion cells. Instead of representing the light-dark contrast existing between the center and the edge of circular receptive fields, the cortical nerve cells signal the contrast which exists along straight line edges whose length amounts to many diameters of the circular ganglion cell receptive fields. A given cortical cell becomes active if a straight line edge of a particular orientation—horizontal, vertical, or oblique—formed by the border of contiguous areas of high and low light intensity is present in its receptive field. For instance, a vertical bar of light on a dark background in some part of the visual field may produce a vigorous response in a particular cortical nerve cell, and that response will cease if the bar is tilted away from the vertical or moved outside the receptive field. Thus the process of abstraction of the visual input begun in the retina is carried to higher levels in the cerebral cortex. At the first abstraction stage the data supplied by the retinal ganglion cells concerning the light-dark contrast within small circular receptive fields are transformed into the more abstract data structure of contrast present along sets of circular fields arranged in straight lines.

Toward a Structuralist Ethics

These findings thus support the structuralist dogma that explanations of behavior must be formulated in terms of deep structures and transformational processes. This biologically grounded reemergence of the Kantian concept of a priori knowledge in the guise of structuralist epistemology provides encouragement for developing also a neo-Kantian structuralist ethics. The purpose of such a project is not the scientistic objective to extend the authority of science to the ethical domain, but merely to illuminate the metaethical question of how morals are possible at all. Although science cannot justify moral values and is only of limited use for their realization, it may, all the same, be able to give an account of their biological basis. This account would not, of course, consist of functionalist explanations of the social role that morals play in human intercourse or the nature of the evolutionary "fitness" which morality may have conferred on *Homo sapiens*. There has been no shortage of such explanations since the rise of Darwinism a century ago, which, as I have said, have provided a cornerstone for the foundations of hard-core scientism.[21] Rather, instead of Darwin's recognition of the role of natural selection in evolution, the point of departure of this project would be Kant's recognition that the peculiar obligatoriness of moral principles can be explained only by their unrestricted universality, that is, by their independence of any existential facts. Thus, contrary to the tenets of utilitarianism, it is not to promote happiness, or to serve progress, but to accede to the demand of human reason that action be in accord with universal law that we feel obligated to obey moral principles. It is man's innate knowledge of this law, whose origin—it goes without saying—can readily be consigned to the evolutionary history of *Homo sapiens,* which gave rise to the possibility of a social existence in the first place. Moreover, the nature of that universal law determined the kind of social structures which eventually arose.

Some idea of what structuralist ethics would be like can be gained by extending Chomsky's approach to the nature of language to the ethical domain. Just as one of Chomsky's empirical starting points for the development of the transformational grammar concept was the creative aspect of human language, which provides a speaker with the capacity to produce a limitless number of meaningful statements, so any account of the nature of morality must begin with the empirical fact that there seems to be no limit to the number of significantly different social situations for which individuals can produce value judgments that appear reasonable to other men. So the empirical premise of structuralist ethics would be that moral judgments arise by a generative process involving transformational operations on a subconscious mental deep structure. This approach, therefore, acknowledges the subjective and intuitive nature of moral judgments. But despite their subjectivity, moral judgments would not be viewed as arbitrary or completely idiosyncratic, not for the trivial or functionalist reason that they must not be dysfunctional or give rise to unviable forms of social organization, but because they reflect an innate, a priori, universal ethical deep structure which all humans share. These universal deep structures would be more or less equivalent to Kant's concept of the categorical imperative, which he took to govern human action independently of any desired ends, including happiness. However, the neo-Kantian feature of the structuralist approach to morality is that it would posit a more complicated, or transformational, relation between the universal categorical imperative and particular moral judgments than the direct connection evidently envisaged by Kant.

From that neo-Kantian point of view, the overt ethical surface structures would consist of the concrete moral code of which a person is consciously aware and to which he can give verbal expression. This surface structure is reflected in the moral judgments made by that person, and hence is accessible to direct observation through his acts and statements. One obvious empirical fact, relevant to these surface structures, is that they can differ significantly between diverse social groups and among members of the same social group. The reason for these differences is that the particular moral code held by any individual is the product of a twofold historical process, namely, of the ethnic history of his social group and of his personal, ontogenetic history. The covert ethical deep structure, on the other hand, would consist of an abstract moral code, of which the person is not consciously aware and to which he cannot in general give verbal expression. This ethical deep structure is innate and common to all men, as members of the species *Homo sapiens*. The abstract ethical deep structure gives rise to the concrete moral code of the surface structure through a transformational process. According to this view, the empirically observable differences in extant moral codes would be attributable to differences in the rules by which particular individuals carry out the deep-to-surface transformational processes. In line with model psychological concepts, the primary course of the personal set of transformational rules would be the assimilation of parental moral authority by the child, just as in the acquisition of speech, the child assimilates the syntactical and phonological components of the grammar of its native language from the examples provided by parental speech. The child is able to assimilate these moral transformational rules only because, thanks to an innate possession of the universal, abstract, ethical deep structure, he already knows the abstract essence of human morality of which his own ethical system will be a particular concrete realization. In particular, it is thanks to the deep structure that the child has an a priori, intuitive understanding of the meaning of the unanalyzable, undefinable concepts of moral values, such as "good."

Thus, according to this structuralist concept, the extant moral systems all share certain fundamental features, of which the very notion of moral value is one of the most basic, because they are all rooted in the same universal ethical deep structure. Hence, the discovery and elucidation of the ethical deep structure ought to be the central goal of what J. M. Gustafson defined as "ethics," namely, "a human intellectual discipline which develops the principles which account for morality and moral action and the normative principles and values that are to guide human action."[22]

But just as the structuralist linguists have been more successful in demonstrating the plausibility of the existence of a universal grammar than in spelling out just what abstract linguistic principles it contains, so it is easier to adduce arguments in favor of the existence of a universal, deep ethical structure than to describe its abstract moral content. Kant thought, of course, that he had managed to identify that content, by proposing that there is one fundamental categorical imperative from which all specific moral duties can be derived, namely: "Act only according to that maxim which you can will to be universal law." It seems highly plausible that some such criterion of universalizability of the moral code is indeed contained in the deep ethical structures, in view of the empirical fact that the "golden rule," which is manifestly an expression of that principle, forms part of almost all the great religions. But it seems equally plausible that despite the fact that the criterion of universalizability may well be, as Kant claimed, a logical necessity for requiring universal obedience to a rule of action, this criterion cannot be contained in the deep structures in the strong form enunciated by him. For any such all-inclusive generalization would place too severe a limitation on the creative aspect of morality and limit the variety of social situations under which rational value judgments can be produced. Thus, it is clear that there are few if any moral rules that we would want to be followed without exception, for whose justifiable contravention we cannot imagine scenarios.

Here we reach what would appear to be the most significant aspect of the ethical deep structure, namely that its open-ended creative possibilities appear to be achieved at the expense of logical consistency. Whatever may be the abstract moral content of the deep structure, its nature is such that the transformations to which it is subject give rise to a set of judgments that are not necessarily logically compatible and hence are not necessarily reconcilable rationally. Indeed, the irreconcilable yet unavoidable coexistence of an authoritative science and an autonomous morality is most plausibly attributable to that feature of our a priori knowledge. Thus, from the structuralist viewpoint, the moral dilemmas and paradoxes with which we are wrestling today are not simply the result of unenlightened or irrational human attitudes but are, instead, reflections of the fundamental inconsistency of the ethical deep structure which underlies our morality in the first place. Thus the resolution of these dilemmas, if possible at all, is not likely to be achieved by merely calling attention to their existence or by any simple remedy short of changing human nature. But whether such a change is possible, or even desirable, as has long been maintained by Buddhism and some other Eastern philosophies, or whether we can only continue to muddle along as best we can with our paradoxical endowment is, in my opinion, the central ethical question of the future.

NOTES

I thank Georges Kowalski and Gonzalo Manévar for helpful suggestions and discussions during the writing of this essay.

1. Jacques Monod, *Chance and Necessity* (New York: Alfred A. Knopf, 1971).
2. Helmut Schoeck and James W. Wiggins, eds., *Scientism and Values* (Princeton, N.J.: Van Nostrand Co., 1960).
3. Herbert Spencer, *Principles of Ethics*, 2 vols. (London: Williams and Norgate, 1892-3). C. H. Waddington, in his *The Ethical Animal* (London: Allen and Unwin, 1960), finds that Spencer's ethical "theories have been so completely discredited that at this time little further needs to be said about them" (p. 23). But Waddington then produces a casuistic variant of Spencer's hard-core evolutionist ethics, namely, one that holds that although the notion of "good" cannot be simply identified with progress, a particular set of moral values can be judged to be good if it promotes "anagenesis," or evolutionary improvement (p. 202).
4. Konrad Lorenz, *On Aggression* (New York: Harcourt, Brace & World, 1966).
5. A (undoubtedly unintended) caricature of this approach can be found in Wolfgang Wickler, *Die Biologie der Zehn Gebote* (München: Piper Verlag, 1971).
6. Desmond Morris, *The Naked Ape* (New York: McGraw Hill Book Co., 1967).
7. Richard P. Michael, "Bisexuality and Ethics," in *Biology and Ethics*, F. J. Ebling, ed. (London: Academic Press, 1969), pp. 67-72.
8. James F. Crow, "The Dilemma of Nearly Neutral Mutations: How Important Are They For Evolution and Human Welfare?" *Journal of Heredity*, 63 (1972) 306-16.
9. T. S. Kuhn, *The Structure of Scientific Revolutions* (Chicago: University of Chicago Press, 1964).
10. Ernst Mayr, "Teleological and Teleonomic, a New Analysis," *Boston Studies in the Philosophy of Science* 14 (1974), 91-117.
11. Patrick Heelan, "Medical Praxis and Manifest Images of Man," in *Science, Ethics and Medicine*, H. T. Engelhardt, Jr. and Daniel Callahan, eds. (Hastings-on-Hudson: Institute of Society, Ethics and Life Sciences, 1976), pp. 218-24.
12. C. Galpérine, ed., *Biology and the Future of Man* (Paris: The Universities of Paris, 1976), pp. 377-415.

13. Bronislaw Malinowski, "Anthropology," in *Encyclopedia Britannica,* 13th ed. (New York: Encyclopedia Britannica Inc., 1926), Vol. 29, pp. 131-40.
14. Christian Morgenstern, "The Impossible Fact," in *Gallows Songs and Other Poems,* trans. Max Knight (München: Piper Verlag, 1972), p. 25.
15. Gunther S. Stent, *The Coming of the Golden Age. A View of the End of Progress* (Garden City, N.Y.: The Natural History Press, 1969), pp. 115-21.
16. Benoit Mandelbrot, *Les objets fractals* (Paris: Flammarion, 1975).
17. Gunther S. Stent, "Limits to the Scientific Understanding of Man," *Science* 187 (1975), 1052-57.
18. Noam Chomsky, "The Formal Nature of Language," in E. H. Lenneberg, *Biological Foundations of Language* (New York: John Wiley, 1967), pp. 397-442. *Language and Mind* (New York: Harcourt, Brace and World, 1968).
19. Konrad Lorenz, "Kant's Doctrine of the *a priori* in the light of contemporary biology," in *General Systems,* L. Bertalanffy and A. Rappaport, eds. (Ann Arbor: Soc. Gen. Systems Research, 1962).
20. Gunther S. Stent, "Cellular Communication," *Scientific American* 227 (September 1972), 42-51.
21. A collection of recent examples of this genre can be found in *Biology and Ethics,* F. J. Ebling, ed. (London: Academic Press, 1969).
22. J. M. Gustafson, unpublished draft manuscript prepared for discussion at the Hastings Center.

Commentary

Deep Structures and an
Evolutionary Ethic

Patrick Heelan

BERNARD TOWERS, with Pierre Teilhard de Chardin, believes that
the "phenomena" delineated by evolutionary biological science
justify the claim that organic complexity is accompanied by a
psychic "inside." This "Law of Increasing Complexity-Consciousness," as Teilhard called it, results in a conscious thrust toward
"convergence" or the unification of matter, that becomes reflexively conscious in the higher primates, especially in man. It
moves men towards the overarching good of consciously establishing a unity of matter over the globe; this goal is a social goal
and will be achieved only when a single world-wide tech-
nologically based society exists where all share in peace and
stability, the personal and social goods that all desire. Teilhard,
Julian Huxley, and Towers agree on this thesis as a *scientific* (or
"phenomenological") thesis rooted in the evolutionary biological
fact, with an *obverse* in the realm of biophysical complexity and
a *reverse* in the realm of conscious, goal-oriented phenomena. It
is then argued that an open, pluralistic ethic flexibly adapted to
diverse and changing circumstances is needed to guarantee the
achievement by man of full development, that is, of the emergence of the eschatalogical global society.

"Where do we find our ethical guidelines?" asks Towers. "In
the evolutionary process itself, seen as a process of divergence
and convergence."

Such an argument Gunther Stent would have found vitiated by the naturalistic fallacy of "hard-core scientism." The naturalistic fallacy is the fallacy of concluding that what is, must be or ought to be so, where what is, is taken to be what science describes it to be in scientific terms. Such a conclusion is illegitimate because the explanatory categories of science are related to impersonal processes of measurement or analogies of such processes, in which moral or goal-intended criteria do not occur as descriptive. Descriptive categories of (what I have called elsewhere)[1] "scientific images" are not goal-oriented or person-oriented, consequently, what is, in a scientific way, is so not because it is related to a goal. An electron possesses a single negative charge; but does not possess it within a structure of obligation or moral satisfaction. If we do say at times, using a peculiar form of words, that an electron "*must* have a single negative charge," what we mean is that a person must not or ought not to call X an electron, if X has not a single negative charge, for the "must" and "ought" falls on a person—not on a thing like an electron. "Must" and "ought" have a place, however, as descriptive categories in (what I have called elsewhere)[2] "manifest images," where it is proper to describe things in terms of their intended functions or moral roles. If, then, the distinction between "scientific" and "manifest images" as two well-differentiated taxonomic classes holds firm, the naturalistic fallacy would indeed preclude the validity of an ethical conclusion from premises formulated exclusively within a scientific image though not within premises that involve manifest images. Since the theory of evolution is the basis for a scientific, not a manifest image, Stent's implied criticism of Towers would seem to be correct.

However, it is not clear to me that the premises used by Towers do in fact belong exclusively to a scientific image, despite the fact that physical complexity and at least the behavorial consequences of social consciousness are both subject to scientific analysis. For the law of complexity-consciousness requires that the *obverse* include not merely physical complexity, but also behavorial complexity—or whatever in short can be described and explained in scientific and non-personal terms. The *reverse* is consciousness considered as a structure of reflexively motivated, goal-intended, or at least goal-directed, actions. Consciousness in this sense belongs to manifest images. What the law of complexity-consciousness says then is that scientific images have a mutuality—a pairing—with goal-oriented manifest images and that the realization of the latter depends on the realization of the former as on a set of necessary, perhaps even sufficient, conditions. The establishment of this thesis is assumed by Towers.

The thesis of *complexity-consciousness* is at first sight analogous to the structuralist thesis as expressed by Gunther Stent, which affirms a certain "isomorphism of cerebral and mental events," with the physical providing the *deep structure* that controls the variety of *surface mental or conscious structures*. For Towers, however, the physical basis of complex organization doesn't stop at the neurological, but embraces the technology of industry, transport, and communications. For him, the present locus of evolutionary pressures are in this wider physical domain; selective pressures are exerted through this larger base that acts as the deep structure controlling the cognitive and moral skills that are made possible by this physical base. Since the physical complexity of the deep structure changes with historical changes in cultural life, Towers's structuralist thesis is one of varying deep structure. Between Gunther Stent and Towers there is a *community* of structuralist thinking. But since Towers affirms a flexible and varying deep structure his position is less easy to articulate through philosophical or scientific analysis.

For Towers, as for Teilhard, the central problem is to make plausible the thesis that there is a psychic "convergence" of mankind over the global surface. Fifty years ago, it seemed to people like Teilhard that Western scientific industrial society with its historical roots in Christendom would conquer the world and spread its technology and institutions (and, some hoped, Christian values and beliefs) over all mankind. But despite the fact that its historical roots are in Western Christendom, scientific-technological cultures can be appropriated as well by nonWestern nonChristian societies as by those that share the basic values and religious orientation of the West. Sociological studies of contemporary Japan and what we know about present-day China demonstrate clearly that Westernization and a fortiori Christianization can be effectively uncoupled from the activity of appropriating scientific and technological achievements. Is then, we may ask, the psychic thrust for "convergence" a phenomenon characteristic of what is Western and perhaps residual of a Judaic-Christian orientation in society, or is the claim that it stems from the ferment produced by scientific-technological culture as an evolutionary force in whatever society it finds itself? Towers would answer affirmatively to the latter alternative.

But for Teilhard, a secular vision of the future of man in one global society which is the product solely of human ingenuity and evolutionary forces would have lacked plausibility. The history of the past few decades has considerably weakened the case for an optimistic future for man based only on secular or scientific evidence; the fragility of the social fabric is dangerously manifest and there seems to be no sure indication that mankind is moving towards the establishment of a common, stable, civilizational complex. Teilhard in his time appreciated the fragility of that fabric, and he argued that a common stable civilizational complex would emerge only on one condition: that men responded to a common felt need for unity with a person, that is, for a common love of a personal love-center of the world. He furthermore postulated the fulfillment of this need, in (what he called) Omega; personal like a man, but greater than any man. Omega, he identified with Jesus Christ on the basis of an interpretation of the New Testament. Jesus Christ as Omega was, he claimed, the cause and condition of man's psychic structure of convergence. Thus, Teilhard found in the religious traditions of Christianity a divine confirmation of the scientific thesis of the "convergence" of matter.

It is my belief that the future of man is, as Teilhard saw it to be, a question with an essentially religious context: whether our personal stories or the stories of peoples or civilizations are worth pursuing into the future—by which I mean whether the future holds any guarantee of happy endings—is a question not exclusively for science, history, or even philosophy, but one that must involve a new framework that synthesizes science, history, and philosophy with religious inquiry. At the present time, possible answers to the question of necessary conditions for human fulfillment tend to divide men into two classes—the religious and the non-religious: the former affirming a personal love-center (in something like Teilhard's sense) to the world, and the latter denying such. Looking back it is understandable that Teilhard's religious faith was mixed inextricably with a certain chauvinism about Western values and institutions which he tied too closely to the Christian traditions of the Western church. He addressed, nevertheless, as I believe, the basic religious question which like a universal deep structure calls forth a personal response from men and sets the stage for a variety of religious faiths and religious institutions. Nevertheless, although needful of modification because of the broader horizons that have appeared in the past forty years, Teilhard's religious approach still offers a plausible solution which Towers's Teilhardianism without the religious dimension does not. I do not then believe one can be a Towers without being a Teilhardian all the way.

Turning now to Gunther Stent's paper, the structuralist thesis he affirms is that men have what he calls "innate knowledge," genetic in its physical basis and refined as all genetic materials are by evolutionary processes; this "innate knowledge" or "deep structure of knowledge" is not directly accessible but manifests itself in and through the variety of surface structures of knowledge into which it is transformed (or mapped); these surface structures of knowledge are publicly accessible systems of knowledge, pluralistic in character, and depend on the variety of cultures and environments to which people are exposed. To clarify his thesis, Stent uses as his models the neurophysiological basis of vision, the transformational grammar of Chomsky's linguistics, and the fluid hydrodynamics of the unconscious in Freud. The claim for innate knowledge in the sense used above is that certain skills are learned *easily*: for instance, natural languages, the recognition of lines, edges, object on ground, etc. Stent posits in his paper analogous deep structures of ethical conduct.

All such cases of innate knowledge account for, or claim to account only for, the easily learned skills. Besides easily learned skills, we are also in possession of many difficult skills which are often no less effective in doing what is desired than the former but which differ from the former in having a certain degree of artificiality, of remoteness, of human invention that the former do not have. It may be innate, for instance, that English comes easily to children born in our culture; Fortran is learned, however, with difficulty by natives of all cultures, yet Fortran can be used as well as English to state truths and goes a certain way beyond the capacities of all natural languages to express mathematical truths. It may be innate to recognize easily an object on a ground, but magnetic fields and mitochondria are not objects on grounds and to observe them one has to use artificial devices, like staining or recording instruments. An interesting aspect of these more difficult skills is that they always use the innate skills as media that carry messages about objects not easily observed. For instance, by staining and magnifying, mitochondria are made to appear as objects on grounds. By measuring with an appropriate instrument, a magnetic field is made to modulate a medium of needles, light gradients, or objects on grounds. Fortran is an artificial language, but it needs the resources of a natural language to interpret its formulas. (It is possible that some forms of mathematics are also innate in this sense—easily learned—and that other branches of mathematics are not innate but depend on the innate forms as necessary conditions for their emergence.)

What is specifically human is *not* that we possess deep structures—in neurophysiology, in visual pathways in the cortex, in language, in mathematics, perhaps—but that we can transcend the simple, easily learned activities to construct more difficult skills based on these and with a horizon that is simply not accessible through innate skills. As lines and edges are to plastic, three-dimensional objects outlined by these, so are plastic objects, e.g., dials, counters, photographs, to the entities of atomic physics and biochemistry.

To know *innately*, then, is not to know *objects* of a certain kind, but only to be predisposed to be aware of objects that manifest themselves through the media of lines, edges, light gradiants, textures, etc. Innate structures do not specify what is known but only that whatever is known is known through certain media signs. They say nothing about the content of our ontology, although they may explain what makes a primitive ontology *primitive* or a pathological ontology *pathological*. They speak only of certain kinds of necessary conditions—conditions in the medium of communication—without which we human beings cannot have an ontology.

Pursuing the structuralist analogy and its critique into ethics, one would be led to conclude that deep structures would influence the form of ethical conduct but not its content. Such forms, for example, have been studied by Piaget, Kohlberg, Bettelheim, and others, who have noted a certain sequence of surface ethical structures that characterize the moral development of a child. These may well be generated by a transformation law from a unique deep structure. But neither the existence of the sequence, nor its relation to an ethical deep structure, does anything to validate the content of the structures in sequence. Is altruism better than egoism? Is an altruism that embraces strangers better than one that embraces merely friends and relatives? The deep structure may well give certain necessary conditions of the possibility of one ethic or another, but it would be incapable of giving warrant or superior warrant to any one of them. The structuralist thesis, then, I believe to be curious and interesting, relative to necessary conditions of a certain kind for any ethic, but not relevant to the establishment of any ethical principle or system. This brings me to a question: can the structuralist principle rationalize the plurality of ethical principles we find in societies? I believe that the structuralist thesis is not an answer to this question. On merely formal matters, however, the structuralist thesis has many consequences to which Gunther Stent's paper has introduced us in a very articulate way.

NOTES

1. Patrick Heelan, "Medical Praxis and Manifest Images of Man," in *Science, Ethics and Medicine,* ed. H. Tristram Engelhardt, Jr., and Daniel Callahan (Hastings-on-Hudson: Institute of Society, Ethics and Life Sciences, 1976), pp. 218-24.
2. Ibid.

The Meaning of Professionalism: Doctors' Ethics and Biomedical Science

Stephen Toulmin

I.

What makes a profession a "profession?" What entitles us to describe an organization or institution as (say) a "professional society?" What is meant by calling an action or line of conduct "professional" or "unprofessional?" These questions are of some importance at the present time because, in many areas of life, the twentieth century has seen an expansion in the role of the professions so rapid that our ideas about the status, meaning, and implications of "professions" and "professionalism" have scarcely kept pace.

Rather than survey the whole subject, even in outline, the present paper will deal with certain selected topics only. The choice has been made with one specific goal: viz., to focus attention on a certain class of *conflicts of claim, duty and/or obligation* arising within the conduct of the professions. These conflicts affect all those contemporary professions that have a collectively sanctioned status, as providing services to individual persons. Hitherto, they have been defined and characterized most lucidly in relation to the law; but (as I shall argue) they arise as often, and as severely, in the practice of medicine also—especially since the alliance of clinical medicine with physiology, pharmacology, biochemistry, and the other so-called "biomedical sciences."

Indeed, one source of the recent growth in public distrust toward physicians can be understood better if we look and see how the success of that alliance has sharpened those particular conflicts. To put the central point bluntly: Some patients have come to doubt whether, in dealing with the conflicting claims on their consciences—of society, of the individual patient, and of "science"—present-day doctors still give "personal care" the same priority they did—or are perceived as having done—in the good old days of "general practice."

II.

We may begin by looking at the whole range of human activities—law, science, medicine, sport, or architecture, nursing, politics, plumbing, soldiering, or whatever—that can be said to have become "professionalized" during the last couple of centuries. Within this broad class, we are at once forced to draw some initial distinctions. There are, for instance, *quantitative degrees* of professionalization; so that biochemistry (say) is more fully professionalized than botany, and hospital nursing more professionalized than the care of the elderly, i.e., a greater proportion of biochemical research and hospital nursing is done by "professionals." But there are also *qualitative differences* in the respects in which professional activities of one kind or another are subject to formal regulation, organization, and public restriction or control, simply in virtue of being "professional"; so that law and medicine (say) are professionalized in a more thorough-going way than the natural sciences, i.e., they are subject to public restriction and control in many respects that science is not.

To mark these differences, let us take note of three respects in which an activity may or may not be "professionalized," and three corresponding conditions that such activities must satisfy, if they are to have a truly "professional" status. In order of stringency:

(1) Professionals engage in their chosen activities "for a living" rather than "for fun"—as amateurs or dilettantes;

(2) There is a recognized body of skills, constituting "the state of the art," with which professionals become familiar through training or apprenticeship, and a network of guild-type institutions, which act as custodians of those arts and supervise the accreditation procedures for entry into the profession;

(3) There are statutory bodies, established by legislation or official decree, which confer on professionals the privileges attaching to the exercise of the profession, in return for an acceptance by the professional "guild" of correlative responsibilities toward the public for maintaining the requisite standards of performance and conduct.

Sport is currently professionalized in respect (1), but not in (2) or (3). The professional football player (say) must acquire certain characteristic skills, but there are no formal accreditation procedures to be gone through when entering football as a profession. Much of science is currently professionalized in respects (1) and (2), but not in (3). Although most scientists are formally accredited through university or similar certification, there is currently no statutory system of public "licensure" to which anyone must submit before being legally permitted to "practice" as a scientist. (Notice that, in many jurisdictions, even beauticians are professionalized in this last respect, while scientists are not. Why is this? Until recently, it has been taken for granted that beauticians can do their individual clients more harm than scientists can, and are therefore in more need of public control. Who are a scientist's "clients," anyway?)

Consider the functions of professional organizations and associations within the operations of a profession, and we shall find a similar complexity. Corresponding to (1) above: such associations as the American Bar Association and the American Medical Association are legitimately concerned with the conditions of work in the professions, including its financial rewards. At the same time, (2): as trustees for the "guild," they also have the task of overseeing the quality of (say) legal or medical training. Though it is not their direct responsibility to operate the procedures of accreditation or licensure, they have an immediate interest in the character of those procedures, and thus in the quality of (e.g.) law schools and medical schools. Finally, (3): professional associations also have a part to play in negotiations with governmental authorities about matters of licensure and public regulation, and about the duties and privileges attaching to exercise of the profession. Any full-fledged profession, such as medicine, displays this multiplicity of functions. It reflects the two-sided bargain that physicians (say) have with the public authorities, through which certain rights and privileges are granted by statute in return for specific duties and responsibilities.

It is worth underlining the differences, in this last respect, between the respective positions of medicine and of science. Scientists are subject to no system of public licensure. The activity of "doing science" is exposed to no general statutory restraints, of the kind there are on practicing medicine. Anybody whose work and ideas begin to be discussed seriously by other current members of the scientific profession is thereby co-opted as a "scientist." In the strict legal sense of the term, the scientific profession is, as a result, an *irresponsible* profession. Its members are answerable for "quality control" over their collective activities only to one another: there is no statutory requirement, backed up by formal sanctions, for them to answer to the public. To some extent, the increasing financial dependence of scientific research on public funding since 1945 has, no doubt, created a situation in which informal controls operate. But one of the incidental by-products of the "peer review" system for federally-funded projects—if not its main charm to working scientists—is the way in which it *protects* the irresponsibility of the scientists concerned against any demand for direct public accountability. (Recall the indignant responses of the scientific community to some recent congressional questions about the federal support of scientific research.)

What is meant, accordingly, by describing an action, performance, or line of conduct, as "professional" or "unprofessional"? These terms have a number of familiar uses, some of them simply descriptive, others judgmental. To begin with non-judgmental uses: suppose we describe someone as doing a piece of glassblowing (say) in a highly "professional" manner. This will commonly be understood to mean that he is doing it with a skill and economy of effort normally found only in trained and experienced glassblowers. Conversely, if, as a mere amateur, I apologize for the "unprofessional" join that I have made between two glass tubes, I imply that, although the join may serve its purpose, it looks decidedly ham-fisted, at least by comparison with what we should get from a man who does glassblowing for a living.

Alternatively, the terms "professional" and "unprofessional" are used normatively or judgmentally, implying that the conduct in question is *worthy* or *unworthy* of a professional. The bases for such judgments are, once again, of three distinct kinds, reflecting the three kinds and degrees of "professionalization" noted earlier. At the strongest, (3): One can characterize conduct as fulfilling, or failing to fulfill, the responsibilities placed on members of the profession by their statutory "contract" with the rest of society. Thus, a defense attorney may be criticized for revealing confidential information about his client to the police, in breach of the ABA "code of professional responsibility," or a group of hospital physicians may be criticized similarly for having (say) organized a strike against their employing hospital without making provision for emergency medical care.

Less stringently, (2): these judgments may concern the skills and procedures inherent to the practice of the profession concerned (compare the glassblowing example) or alternatively— what is not always distinguished from those skills and procedures—the modes of life and conduct associated with the practice of that profession, as a matter of history and etiquette. So, a physician's colleagues may criticize his procedures as "unprofessional," either for being clumsy and risky, or because they perceive them as being "not respectable" in terms of the medical profession's current collective self-image. (Professions like medicine being by nature conservative, their professional associations tend to be *gerontocratic*, and this makes them particularly prone to confuse skill with respectability.)

Finally, and most loosely, (1): Normative judgments of "professional" or "unprofessional" conduct may concern the extent to which the conduct in question supports, or threatens to undercut, the special interests (especially the economic interests) of the profession itself. Thus, an A.M.A. negotiator (say) may be criticized by rank-and-file members as having acted "unprofessionally," for being—in their eyes—too much "in with" the

DHEW officials to whom he puts the Association's case on a supposedly adversarial basis.

III.

With these initial distinctions in mind, let us look at the various ways in which irresolubly conflicting claims may arise in the exercise of a profession. We may start by considering "ethical conflicts" as a general class. An individual agent is frequently subject to two or more duties, obligations, claims on his attention, or the like; and does the best he can to meet them, within the limits of his available time and energy. If he is uncommonly fortunate, or lives a particularly unadventurous life, he may succeed in meeting all these demands adequately, without running into actual, active conflicts. Still, given two or more claims, duties, or obligations, we can always conceive in theory of possible situations in which the resulting demands would conflict; and the passage of time alone will commonly bring such imagined situations to pass in practice, for some agent or other, so that, for him, the possible conflict becomes an actual, active one.

In many cases, this liability to ethical conflicts reflects the fact that an individual agent wears several different "hats," i.e., has several alternative, parallel statuses and/or roles, and stands in correspondingly different relationships to his fellow-humans. He may be, at one and the same time, a son, a personal friend, a judge, a Rotarian, a Harvard graduate (Class of '56), and a hockey-player; and the ethical claims to which he is accordingly subject—*qua* son, friend, judge, Rotarian, etc.—will occasionally point in different, even opposite, directions. So, it may be his painful duty, *qua* judge, to stand by without intervening while a Rotarian friend is sent to jail. (Conflicts of this "role-conflict" type are the stuff of which soap-operas are made.)

Are all real-life ethical conflicts of this kind? If all active conflicts of claim, duty, or obligation arose from role or status conflicts, so that all the ethical claims to which an agent was exposed on account of any *single* status, role, or relationship, were intrinsically harmonizable, that would perhaps take some of the sting out of them. Granted that anyone's obligations *qua* son are liable to conflict with his obligations *qua* judge (say), he would at any rate have the comfort of knowing that, taken separately, his duties or obligations *qua* son (or *qua* judge) were intrinsically consistent and free of internal conflict. The crucial ethical question for him would then be, quite simply, "Are my duties as a judge more important, in this situation, than my obligation as a son, or *vice versa?*"

A moment's thought is enough to destroy that hypothesis. We may perhaps be more liable, in practice, to encounter ethical conflicts in virtue of the different claims arising from multiple roles, than we are in virtue of the multiple claims arising from any single role; but that difference is only one of degree. The learned professions (for instance) organize their procedures and frame their codes of professional responsibility as best they can, so as to minimize the risk of recurrent conflicts of obligation. But an absolutely conflict-free code, capable of anticipating even the hardest of particular hard cases, is at best an ideal, and an unrealizable ideal at that. Even within the conduct of his profession (*qua* doctor, lawyer, teacher, or whatever) an agent is subject to a number of distinct standing claims; and, once again, only imagination and the passing of time are normally required before conflicts between these different claims become not merely potential but actual and active.

To sharpen up the point: these *intra-professional* conflicts may be of several different kinds. Consider the respective demands to be made of properly "professional" conduct on account of (1) group loyalty, (2) competence and/or respectability, and (3) basic, statutory responsibilities. These parallel claims will, in various conceivable situations, point in different, even opposite, directions. On one occasion, for instance, a lawyer's basic responsibility to his client (say, a citizens' interest group) may require him to argue in a sense contrary to the collective professional interests of lawyers—thus pitting type (3) against type (1); on another, to press his client's case by using tactics which, though skilled, are barely "respectable" by the current standards of the legal profession—type (3) against type (2). Both these kinds of conflicts pit claims of different types against one another, but ethical conflicts may equally well arise within any one type. Some familiar problems of medical technique, for instance, involve conflicts internal to type (2). In borderline cases, decisions about the properly "professional" treatment of a case, in the sense of the appropriately "skilled" treatment, are often ambiguous. From one point of view, a case may seem to call for chemotherapy, from another for surgery, and adopting either alternative may have the effect of ruling out the other. In such difficult cases, the physician exercises his judgment and gives his advice in full knowledge that, whichever course he advises, he may be open to retrospective criticism. (The different claims of professional loyalty and/or common interest—(type 1)—may be similarly ambiguous on occasion, so that the best way of promoting the status of the profession becomes a matter of judgment and opinion.)

The crucial issues for this present paper, however, have to do specifically with *conflicting claims within type (3)*. The question to be discussed is, "In what circumstances, if any, will the code of professional responsibilities operative in (say) medicine or law prove internally ambiguous, and so land practitioners in inherent ethical conflicts?" As to that, my conclusion will be, *firstly*, that there can be no "code of responsibilities" that will define the ethical claims resting on any member of a profession clearly, unambiguously, and without conflict in all cases; and, *secondly*, that an indispensable ingredient in the application of any such code is a set of common understandings about the relative significance and priorities of the various kinds of claims involved.

At this point (I shall argue) we face today some unanswered questions about the relative significance and priorities of the physician's duties, obligations, and other claims toward his patient, toward society, and toward "biomedical science."

In earlier days, there was little doubt that the present patient's immediate welfare was the paramount consideration. Once society imposed further duties on the physician, e.g., to report certain communicable diseases, a first source of possible ethical conflicts was created, to the extent that such reports might involve breaches of the patient's confidence. But more serious problems have been created as a byproduct of the modern alliance between medical practice and science, an alliance which has put the profession's priorities in question, and introduced ambiguities into the public's perception of medicine and the physician. For how do doctors who are also involved in—or with—the activity of scientific research determine the relative urgency of the professional claims facing them, on the one hand as physicians, on the other hand as scientists?

Before confronting these problems directly, we may glance briefly at one last introductory topic. Historically speaking, the natural sciences have differed from most other professional activities in one further important respect: viz., that science has been a more nearly "single-valued" and "single-minded" enterprise than (say) nursing, medicine, or legal practice. True, the seventeenth-century founders of modern science acknowledged two basic values, not just one. Francis Bacon preached the need to pursue both "light" and "fruit"—both intellectual discovery and practical utility—and it was widely assumed that the resulting claims, though theoretically distinct, would never conflict in practice. From around the year 1700, however, it became apparent that the Newtonian way of doing science—giving paramount importance to "light," and deferring the claims of "fruit"—could yield results that far outweighed those likely to flow from Bacon's mixed procedures. Over the next two hundred or two hundred and fifty years, accordingly, the tasks of natural science were defined in progressively more singled-valued terms, while the life of science came to be lived in a correspondingly single-minded way.

In recent years, notably since Hiroshima, both scientists and laymen have had some second thoughts about the Newtonian priorities; yet most scientists—not least, biomedical scientists—still take for granted the general validity of the Newtonian procedures. It was, for instance, a fundamental criticism of President Nixon's "Conquest of Cancer Campaign" that effective cancer therapy must rely on improving our understanding of the fundamental processes of cell biology; so that any pursuit of new therapeutic methods, in advance of better theoretical grasp, would inevitably be an ineffective, Canute-like attempt to control something that we do not yet properly understand.

The life of science likewise retains to this day much of the "monastic" character so felicitously described by John Ziman some years ago. The apprentice scientist sees his primary, if not exclusive, commitment as being toward his discipline, i.e., toward the development of progressively more powerful methods of theory and experiment; all other—especially all more worldly—values are secondary to this task. (Just as a novice in a medieval monastery would prefer to become a saint, rather than a cardinal, so too today's scientific apprentice would prefer to win a Nobel Prize, rather than become something irrelevant to his discipline, like science advisor to the President of the United States.) It can even be argued—as Gerald Holton did in a recent Hastings publication—that this "single-valuedness" is one of the significant attractions of natural science, and determines in many cases which talented high school graduates will select themselves out at college as future "scientists." For, in devoting himself high-mindedly and single-mindedly to the pursuit of better scien- tific understanding, the young scientist can opt out of such "inex- act" and inherently ambiguous discussions as are inescapable in (say) ethics, politics, and technology; and this can be a genuine motive, for those who are psychically vulnerable and highly intelligent, for embracing a scientific career.

On the face of it, other professional activities lack this feature of natural science. The everyday tasks of nurses, lawyers, and physicians, are essentially multi-valued, and confront them ines- capably with moral quandaries and ethical ambiguities of kinds that do not—or did not, until very recently—confront workers in the natural sciences. Yet, in some other ways, the urge to legis- late such ethical conflicts out of existence is not confined to science. Other professions, equally, find it hard to accept the fact that the very fabric of their enterprises embodies the permanent possibility of ethical conflict. To see how these conflicts arise and must be dealt with in practice, we may usefully look first at law, then at medicine.

IV.

We may take as our model a recent book by Professor Monroe Freedman of Hofstra University, called *Lawyers' Ethics in an Adversary System*. Freedman sets out to demonstrate the un- avoidable ethical conflicts that are inherent to the American Bar Association's Code of Professional Responsibility, when it is applied in the context of the actual practice of law. His discus- sion, notably the chapter entitled "Perjury: the Criminal Defense Lawyer's Trilemma," has two special merits for our argument here. Firstly, he shows in an elegant yet forceful manner that the sources of conflict are not the inadvertent result of bad drafting, but inescapable features of the lawyer's practical situation, while, at the same time, he indicates his own priorities by coming down firmly in favor of the conclusion that the lawyer's duty to his individual client is paramount. Secondly, he has aroused a heated controversy merely by drawing attention to the possibility of inherent conflicts, and pursuing its implications to unavoidable but unwelcome conclusions—for which he has been attacked as bringing the law itself into discredit. In both respects (I believe) Freedman's approach to the problems of legal ethics has something to teach us about the problems of professional ethics—including medical ethics—more generally.

One can summarize briefly a whole series of points that Freedman makes, and illustrates, carefully and at considerable length. The practicing attorney is subject to obligations, duties, or other ethical claims, towards three different parties, viz., his immediate client, the court before which he is pleading, and society at large. (1) Working as advocate for his client within an adversary system of justice, he is required to present the client's case before the court in the best available light. (2) Acting as "an officer of the court" who "participates in a search for truth," he is required to present himself to the court in a way "characterized by candor." (3) In his capacity as a citizen, he should use any knowledge he acquires in the course of his profession to the best interest of the public and his fellow citizens.

Even when we leave aside the claims of society, the lawyer is subject to three distinct claims in his relations to the client and the court; and these claims may easily conflict.[2]

> As soon as one begins to think about these responsibilities, it becomes apparent that the conscientious attorney is faced with what we may call a trilemma—that is, the lawyer is required to know everything [relevant to his client's case], to keep it in confidence, and to reveal it to the court . . .

Hence, Freedman argues, there arise situations in which—against all that we might prefer to believe—it is a criminal lawyer's bounden duty to act in ways that violate our intuitive sense of what is right and proper: e.g., to present testimony which he has good reason to suppose is perjured, or to conceal from the police and other interested parties information concerning other crimes, when it is obtained from the client in confidence. (His chosen illustration is a notorious murder case at Lake Pleasant, New York.)

While all these conclusions are controversial, he finds good judicial authority to support them:[3]

> Justice White has observed that although law enforcement officials must be dedicated to using only truthful evidence, "defense counsel has no comparable obligation to ascertain or present the truth. Our system assigns to him a different mission . . . [we] insist that he defend his client whether he is innocent or guilty."

> Such conduct by defense counsel does not constitute obstruction of justice. On the contrary, it is "part of the duty imposed on the most honorable defense counsel," from whom "we countenance or require conduct which in many instances has little, if any, relation to the search for truth." . . . Chief Justice Warren, too, has recognized that when the criminal defense attorney successfully obstructs efforts by the government to elicit truthful evidence in ways that violate constitutional rights, the attorney is "merely exercising . . . good professional judgment," and "carrying out what he is sworn to do under his oath—to protect to the extent of his ability the rights of his client." Chief Justice Warren concluded: "In fulfilling this responsibility the attorney plays a vital role in the administration of criminal justice under our Constitution."

In these troublesome cases, accordingly, the defense lawyer may be obliged (e.g.) to conceal material facts, to destroy the credibility of a witness whom he personally believes to be truthful, to countenance perjured testimony, or to present his client's line of defense with more zeal than proportion. Any or all of these lines of conduct may be forced on him by his essential duties as an advocate: particularly, as a consequence of the confidential relationship between lawyer and client.

Why does Freedman give such priority to the claims of confidentiality, with all that they imply in difficult cases? His discussion of the adversary system, and the underlying values that determine its priorities, is worth reading in full on account of its wider relevance. To give a single excerpt:[4]

In a society that honors the dignity of the individual, the high value that we assign to [judicial] truth-seeking is not an absolute, but may on occasion be subordinated to even higher values.

The concept of a right to counsel is one of the most significant manifestations of our regard for the dignity of the individual. No person is required to stand alone against the awesome power of the People of New York or the Government of the United States of America. Rather, every criminal defendant is guaranteed an advocate—a "champion" against a "hostile world," the "single voice on which he must rely with confidence that his interests will be protected to the fullest extent consistent with the rules of procedure and the standards of professional conduct."

By setting out his painful conclusions, and defending them so clearly and with such copious authority, Monroe Freedman stirred up a hornet's nest. He first presented them publicly in 1966, in a lecture on legal ethics for the Criminal Trial Institute in Washington, D.C., of which he was then Co-Director:[5]

I discussed what my colleagues and I had found to be the three hardest questions faced by the criminal defense lawyer. Those questions were: (1) Should you put a witness on the stand when you know the witness is going to commit perjury? (2) Should you cross-examine a prosecution witness whom you know to be accurate and truthful, in order to make the witness appear to be mistaken or lying? (3) Should you give your client advice about the law when you know the advice may induce the client to commit perjury? I concluded, with admitted uncertainty, that the adversary system . . . often requires an affirmative answer to these questions.

A brief report of my lecture . . . in the *Washington Post* . . . [produced] two different but oddly similar reactions. First, a very liberal federal judge wrote to me, saying that I had done a disservice to the profession and to the rights of criminal defendants by publicly airing such issues. Second, several very conservative federal judges, led by Chief Justice Warren Burger . . . unsuccessfully attempted to have me disbarred and dismissed from my position as a Professor of Law at George Washington University. In fact, only one day after the *Washington Post* story appeared, I received a registered letter from the United States District Court Committee on Admissions and Grievances, informing me that disciplinary proceedings had been begun against me, on the complaint of several federal judges that I had "expressed opinions" in apparent disagreement with the Canons of Professional Ethics.

We may ignore the grotesque aspects of this episode—the fact that disciplinary proceedings were initiated on the basis of a brief newspaper report alone, etc.—and focus on the central point. Whatever Freedman's conclusions may have been, they were evidently not *in disagreement with* the Canons of Professional Ethics. On the contrary, his lecture took for granted the *general acceptability* of those canons, and set out to explore, rather, their *specific implications* in hard cases: in particular, the ethical conflicts unavoidably built in to the practical application of the lawyers' professional code. Most strikingly, this episode shows[6]

the resistance within the profession to candid analysis of serious questions of legal ethics . . . [and] the extraordinary difficulty, if not impossibility, of resolving the dilemmas presented by conflicting ethical values.

("Prior to that episode," he adds, "I had not intended to write about professional ethics. Indeed, my first article on the subject was induced in part by the extraordinary effort to use disciplinary proceedings to prevent discussion of the issues. I was therefore tempted for a time to dedicate this book 'To the Chief Justice of the United States, but for whose efforts this book would never have been written.' ")

To sum up: What is indispensable in the practical employment of a professional code of conduct, or Canons of Professional Responsibility, is a body of shared understanding about the *values underlying* the code, and the *consequent priorities* to be placed on different considerations when the canons conflict. As to these priorities, Freedman makes his own position crystal-clear: the defense lawyer's paramount obligation is to his immediate client. Granted, he also has specific duties toward the court, as well as more general obligations to society at large; but those other claims cannot override his duty to the client, except in extreme situations. Only where, for instance, the client demands that the attorney become an actual party to his own perjury will he be placing the attorney in an ethically impossible position; but, even in that event, the correct course will normally be for the attorney to withdraw from the case as tactfully as he can, without betraying the confidentiality of the client's communications.

V.

The sub-title of this paper, "Doctors' Ethics and Biomedical Science," was chosen in order to underline the analogies between medicine and law, and thus put us in a position to reapply Monroe Freedman's analysis for our own broader purposes. So let us now consider the physician's standing professional duties, obligations, and other ethical claims, and ask how, in what respects, and in what kinds of case, conflicts may arise between them. This question would bear a detailed examination, along the lines of Professor Freedman's analysis of the A.B.A. Canons of Professional Responsibility, taking the American Medical Association's various pronouncements on medical ethics and professional responsibility and showing how, in particular hard cases, the accepted canons of medical practice *inescapably* give rise to ethical conflicts. Here, I shall explore just a few of the resulting issues, notably those that spring from the new alliance between medicine and science. (For fuller discussion of, e.g., the ethics of "randomized clinical trials," see Charles Fried's recent book, *Medical Experimentation: Personal Integrity and Social Policy*.[7])

The physician is subject to standing claims not just toward one, but toward several parties. Evidently enough, his primary obligations are toward the individual patient with whose medical condition he is immediately concerned. But he has formal duties also, toward the public health authorities or, where relevant, toward the institution within which he practices—clinic, hospital, university, or group practice—and even, in the case of an industrial, prison, or other institutional clinic, toward the organization within which it is located. (There are, indeed, recurrent role conflicts to be faced in all institutional settings, to the extent that the physician is also recognized, or recognizes himself, as a member of the custodial or administrative staff.) In addition, the physician has less formal obligations to the entire medical profession; and, more widely, to the biomedical scientists whose research interests are nowadays perceived—either by the physician himself or by others—as being in harmonious alliance with his therapeutic goals.

Toward the immediate patient, again, the doctor has not one but several parallel obligations. To begin with, he is in a position of privileged communication with the patient. This imposes on him a strict duty of confidentiality, which may even come into conflict with what is ostensibly his overriding duty, viz., to give his patient the best examination, advice, and treatment currently available within the accepted armamentarium of medicine. For instance, a patient's clearly diagnosed condition may be treatable only if the physician reports to some third party embarrassing facts that the patient has revealed to him within their confidential relationship. And what if, after the doctor has given his advice, the patient values his privacy so highly that he decides to forego the treatment? Clearly, the doctor should use his best efforts to persuade the patient to reconsider this decision; but, if his efforts fail, the duty of confidentiality may seemingly prevent him from giving the patient the treatment he needs. To paraphrase this point in Monroe Freedman's deliberately paradoxical style:

> It may be the physician's bounden duty to *refrain from treating* a patient's clearly diagnosed pathological condition.

(It is a measure of the difficulty that this conflict presents to the medical profession that the A.M.A. and the B.M.A. are inclined to resolve it in opposite ways. The American Medical Association is prepared to tolerate breaches of confidentiality, in cases where the physican conscientiously believes them to be necessary "in the patient's best interests": the British Medical Association insists on the patient's autonomy, and so regards confidentiality as paramount.)

Toward the public health authorities, the physician has—to recall—statutory obligations which require him to act in breach of the patient's confidence in certain carefully specified cases: e.g., the obligation to report certain communicable diseases. The traditional priorities of medicine being what they are, however, these compulsory disclosures should be kept to the absolute minimum. Though the attending physician is legally required to reveal these facts to the public health authorities, and also may feel morally bound to disclose them in confidence to members of the patient's immediate household—if only, so that they may protect themselves from infection—that in no way lifts the duty to limit further communication.

So, even within his traditional role of "general practitioner," the physician is confronted by ethical conflicts which may, in extreme situations, face him with agonizing decisions. *How is he to resolve these difficulties?* If that question is taken to mean, "How can he escape from the conflict?" the answer is, "He cannot!" If it is taken to mean, "How can he decide which of the conflicting claims is paramount?" the answer is, "Only by being clear about the values and priorities involved." In this respect, Freedman's argument about priorities in legal ethics has a clear parallel in medicine. To modify and reapply a passage quoted above:

> In a society that honors the dignity of the individual, the high value that we assign to [medical] truth-seeking is not an absolute, but may on occasion be subordinated to even higher values.

A physician can give his patient the personal service to which he is entitled—and so act in an effective manner as the patient's "champion" against the "dread power" of death, disease, and disablement—only if he acknowledges the patient's autonomy, and seeks to retain his trust, by respecting not only the confidentiality of any information the patient reveals to him, but equally the patient's right to decline or ignore his advice. (In this respect, the doctor plays the same part on his client's behalf vis-à-vis the mortal threats of disease that the lawyer plays vis-à-vis the awesome power of the state.) True, unless the patient is in the legal position of a "ward," e.g., an infant or a committed lunatic, any physician who gives him treatment to which he has not consented opens himself up to the charge of *battery*. (Shrewd attorneys for disgruntled patients have, in fact, been discovering that it may well be easier to sustain a charge of battery than one of malpractice.) But, even aside from questions of tort malfeasance, the same order of priorities could be defended on ethical grounds. To modify and reapply another of Freedman's conclusions:

> A physician shall not knowingly reveal a confidence or secret of the patient, or use a confidence or secret to the disadvantage of

the patient, or to the advantage of a third person, without the patient's consent.

Notice that this injunction holds good equally, regardless of the possibility that the "third person" in question is a professional colleague—whether fellow physician or biomedical scientist—in whom the doctor himself has implicit trust.

At this stage, we can locate the point at which the "biomedical alliance" between practicing physicians and scientific researchers—and, still more, the widespread tendency to equate physicians with biomedical scientists—creates occasions for public disquiet. The higher priority a physician allows his "obligations to science," either in the persons of his scientific colleagues or in his own ulterior motives, the more doubts his patients are liable to have about the singlemindedness of the care they are receiving; and the greater sense they are liable to have, conversely, that in the physician's eyes they are "interesting cases of disease X," rather than individual human beings with all their human needs and dignity. Correspondingly: to the extent that a physician is in continuing interaction or involvement with biomedical research, as well as medical practice, the more liable he will be—even inadvertently—to "use the patient's confidence or secret . . . to the advantage of a third person": *sc.*, either a scientist colleague, or else himself in his scientific role.

Why should the patient mind? That is not the point. The point is that the patient is entitled to mind. In Kantian language, he is entitled to "moral autonomy"—to be treated "as an end in himself, not as a means only." This implies that "his" doctor, quite as much as "his" attorney, must fully respect his decisions about the use to be made of any information he gives in the privacy of his office or consulting room.

Surely the accepted requirement, of the patient's consent to any wider disclosure, is sufficient safeguard? Would that it were! Even apart from more basic ethical conflicts, the present state of health-care delivery in the United States can make it hard for some people to obtain adequate medical services, except within the context of a research program. For instance, one powerful reason why prisoners volunteer to participate in pharmaceutical research—such as that conducted within Southern Michigan State

Prison at Jackson by Parke Davis and Upjohn—is their knowledge that this is the only way they can get a physical examination in which they feel any trust. (Similarly, at the recent National Minorities Conference on Human Experimentation, many speakers argued that the poor are in much the same position as prisoners, and spoke, rhetorically but in all seriousness, about the problem of shielding their people from "the onslaughts of researchers." We may, no doubt, suspect some spirit of exaggeration in the use of such language; but it is a morally relevant fact that these particular patients should perceive their involvement in biomedical research as to that extent coerced.)

Are these not special—and admittedly scandalous—cases, from which we ought not generalize? That response should not pass without careful scrutiny and reflection. Even if prisoners and the poor did have access to the same medical care as the free and well-to-do, the more basic ethical conflicts still remain to be dealt with. As to these, we may well question whether the distinction between "free and informed" and "coerced" consent is powerful enough to resolve these fundamental issues. It has frequently been argued, for instance, that any prison is an "inherently coercive environment," so that consent by prisoners to participate in human experimentation is always of questionable force. Taken on its own terms, this is an impressive argument; but, in return, we might ask whether *sickness itself* is not also "inherently coercive"; and whether, in virtue of the natural authority a physician exercises toward anyone in that condition, the patient will not inevitably feel constrained to participate as a research subject for any scientific project in which he perceives "his" doctor as having an interest. That argument provides *both* sufficient grounds for public anxiety over the current close alliance between medical practice and biomedical research, *and also* reasons to re-examine with care the institutional relations between—particularly, the traditional buffers between—the work of the physician and that of the scientist.

Are not these fears and doubts exaggerated? The present paper will be criticized for making heavy weather of ethical issues that all competent physicians understand and cope with perfectly well in their day-to-day practice. On a certain pragmatic level, this response may have some merit. A great deal of good old-style medical practice is no doubt still going on around the country; and the doctors involved would no doubt think not twice, but a dozen times, before proposing that *their* patients become research subjects. But it is the principle of the thing that I am concerned with here; and I do not believe that it is generally recognized just how radical this issue is, nor what the full price would be for letting the barriers between general practice and biomedical research be lowered still further.

Several times recently, for instance, the Deputy Director for Science at the National Institute of Health, Dr. DeWitt Stetten, has spoken out against what he sees as unreasonable public prejudices toward biomedical research; and in doing so he has predicted that, in another fifty or a hundred years, public feelings about human experimentation will change, and all sick people will automatically—and happily—be research subjects. In that future stage of mankind, it will be unnecessary to seek "informed consent," because by that time we shall be proud to lend our diseased bodies to science.[8] Yet one of the chief things that arouses the "unreasonable prejudices" that Dr. Stetten wishes to allay is just this kind of patronizing attitude on the part of biomedical scientists; and it is a proper insistence on being treated with human dignity, as individuals or ends-in-themselves, rather than as "research fodder," that prompts prisoner advocates, minority spokesmen, and others, to perceive medical researchers (so to say) as "predators." (Notice that Dr. Stetten's argument is based on a highly subjective view of ethics, viz., on the premise that "ethical objections" are concerned merely to present the current state of "public feelings," which he sees as highly labile; rather than as drawing attention to objective risks and basic human rights, which will remain relevant to the problems of medicine and law for the foreseeable future.)

The need to keep the radical nature of these ethical conflicts clearly in view is also the reason why this present argument is framed in very general terms, instead of dealing with the much more specific methodological and ethical quandaries arising in the actual course of clinical research. (In any event, Professor Fried discusses several of these quandaries in an interesting and powerful way in his book; and argues—like a good lawyer—against current claims that the concept of *personal care* is itself in course of becoming incoherent and superannuated.[9]) The heart of the present paper thus comprises, not any criticism of the detailed procedures of biomedical research, nor even any demand for a detailed scrutiny of the organization and operations of contemporary hospitals, but an attempt to focus in on the *constellations of professional attitudes* that physicians bring to their work; and it suggests the desirability of re-affirming the traditional responsibilities that the physician has brought to his individual clients, regarded as human agents and patients. Indeed, what may be most needed today is a spokesman who is prepared, even at the risk of paradox, to assert the paramount ethical claims of personal care in medicine in the same absolute terms that Monroe Freedman employs in the sphere of legal ethics.

Recall our earlier analogy between the awesome power of the state and the dread power of death and disease. Faced by the dark and threatening mysteries of sickness and possible death, the individual patient needs from his physician the same protection that an advocate gives to the individual faced by a criminal charge—viz., the "single voice on which he must rely with confidence that," whatever else may be the case, "his interests will be protected to the fullest extent." (This was the traditional role of the general practitioner, with his single-minded commitment to the welfare of his immediate client.) The extent to which the professional, whether attorney or physician, gives priority to the client's needs and justifies his confidence, shows how far he still fully respects "the dignity of the individual," which Freedman sees as the paramount value of our society; and it is that dignity which is threatened by any tendency for biomedically-minded physicians to view their patients, not as individuals, but as "cases."

Even so, is this not a short-term, temporary problem, without deeper implications for the ethics of medicine? One might be tempted to suppose that the issues raised in this paper were merely transition problems, arising for us in our generation only as a result of the new intersection between medical practice and biological theory. And it is true that the argument presented here is framed in terms that encourage that supposition. Yet it is worth remarking in addition that (as Eric Cassell emphasized in discussing an earlier version of the paper) the problems raised here have had formal counterparts at every stage in the development of the physician's art. Ever since the time of Hippocrates, in fact, the physician has had not one set of ethical claims to consider—viz., those to his patient—but two sets—viz., those to his patient and those to "the art." Now, it is a matter for debate to say exactly what was meant, in earlier epochs, by references to the physician's duties to his art, or to characterize the types of situation in which there might arise, even for the true Hippocratean physician, conflicts between the two parallel sets of ethical claims upon his consideration. Still, even from the beginning, one can see well enough in general terms that the art of medicine was the possession of a "collective," to be transmitted from generation to generation by the process of apprenticeship, and so on; and that this very fact necessarily created, for all those involved, relations of mutual dependence and consequent ethical obligations, which might have to be weighed in some kind of scale against the claims of an individual patient.

Seen in this broader historical perspective, our topic here ceases to be merely a local mid-twentieth-century affair, and can be understood as an inescapable and persisting problem. The emergence of biomedical science into its contemporary prominence has, no doubt, brought this problem into fresh prominence, and has aggravated public anxiety about it. But the form that it takes for us today—as a seeming conflict between the particular demands of therapy and the general demands of science—is only one, contemporary specification of a more general type of problem, which must arise in other specific forms for medical professionals in any generation. Just *how* it will arise for physicians working in this or that particular culture and epoch is a question to be looked at in detail by historians and sociologists of medicine: the answer will depend on a great many other facts about the economic and social development of the society in question, about the political expectations of people-at-large within that society, about the state of the medical art at that time and place, and so on. Only by taking all these things into account, can we hope to reconstruct an adequate picture of the "collective professional self-perception" of medical practitioners within the milieu concerned, of which their attitudes toward possible conflicts between the claims, duties and obligations of their individual members are one expression.

There is, in fact, a significant new kind of history of medicine to be written, which would throw helpful light on the issues discussed here. Such a history would comprise, precisely, an analysis of the changes that have taken place in the collective self-perception of the medical profession over the centuries. (The same kind of history could also be written, with advantage, about the development of natural science, law, and other more or less "professionalized" enterprises.) Where exactly in the scheme of things have doctors (or lawyers, or scientists) seen their enterprise as "fitting in" to different milieus? To what basic goals has it been perceived as directed? Whose good were these goals viewed as promoting? (And so on, and so on.) If we understood better where these collective "self-perceptions" come from, how they are shaped, and what can modify them, all the questions that arise about the internal ethical dilemmas of the professions would be that much the easier to state, and to resolve.

VI.

A final point is worth adding, since it indicates one additional reason why any blurring of the distinction between medical practice and biomedical science is corrosive of the public trust. Early in this paper, two different kinds of "professions" were distinguished: those such as law and medicine, which have a statutory basis and are subject to public regulation, and those in which the practitioners are not answerable to any public body, only to one another. By these standards, the natural sciences are *irresponsible*; scientists, unlike physicians, are answerable for the quality of each other's work only to one another.

Is the general public sensitized to such fine distinctions? There is no reason to be too skeptical about their perceptions: on the contrary, we need not be particularly "street-wise" to detect a widespread awareness of just that difference. Even apart from all archaic myths about "the mad scientist," people-at-large certainly recognize that they have even less power to monitor what scientific researchers do to them than they have to check up on the ways in which their doctors treat them—which is little enough in any event! What provokes anxiety about the "biomedical alliance," accordingly, is not just the existence of *inherent ethical conflicts*, between the doctor's duties to his patient, to society, and to "science." In addition, it is the recognition that any subordination of medical standards to the requirements of scientific research will tend to subordinate a *legally responsible* enterprise to a *legally irresponsible* one.

To say this is not a call for any general change in the legal status of natural science, so as to make it statutorily "responsible" in the way that medicine is. In an ethically complex and difficult situation, I would myself argue—as a completely general matter—that the reasons for maintaining the present status of science outweigh those for bringing it under such public control. But the issues involved are too large to embark on here, and they resist easy generalization. The ethics of field botany is one thing, the ethics of high-energy physics another, the ethics of human pathology something different again. So, even if a case could be made out for the "licensing" of biomedical research workers who do not hold an M.D. degree, this would still not oblige us to extend that requirement to *all* scientific research—both that which does, and that which does not, involve human experimentation, and so puts human research subjects at risk.

There are, in fact, reasons for regarding biomedical science, especially, but not solely, those parts of biomedical science that involve human experimentation, as a special case. We do not need to settle the ethics of the scientific enterprise in general, in order to be clear that the ethics of biomedical science forms a legitimate area for social concern and public involvement; and to satisfy ourselves that political and social issues about (e.g.) the representation of the lay community on institutional review boards, and the like, are urgent and proper topics for public debate.

NOTES

1. Monroe H. Freedman, *Lawyers' Ethics in an Adversary System* (Indianapolis and New York: Bobbs-Merrill, 1975).
2. Ibid., p. 28.

3. Ibid., pp. 3-4.
4. Ibid.
5. Ibid., pp. viii-ix.
6. Ibid.
7. Charles Fried, *Medical Experimentation: Personal Integrity and Social Policy* (Amsterdam: North-Holland and New York: American Elsevier, 1974), esp. ch. 6, pp. 141 ff.
8. See, e.g., his contribution to the public discussion organized by the National Academy of Sciences in Washington, D.C., early in 1975, as printed in *Experiments and Research with Humans: Values in Conflict* (Washington, D.C.: National Academy of Sciences, 1975). The specific reference here is to the public presentation by Dr. Stetten at a meeting on science and ethics organized at the University of Chicago on the occasion of the dedication of the papers of the late Professor James Franck to the Regenstein Library.
9. Fried, *Medical Experimentation*, ch. 4, pp. 79 ff.

Commentary

The Fragmentation of Value

Thomas Nagel

THE CONFLICTS BETWEEN DISPARATE VALUES, claims, and interests described in Stephen Toulmin's paper are not limited to the
professions. They belong to a broader category of practical and
moral problems that merits attention: the problems created by a
disparity between the fragmentation of value and the singleness
of decision.

Members of the professions serve the interests of their clients
in ways that cannot be immediately and directly evaluated by the
clients, because they involve special knowledge and uncertainty
and delay in the achievement of results. Therefore clients cannot
regulate professional activity in detail. Professional codes are
designed for the conspicuous self-regulation of such activities and
services, so that the public can submit to professional ministra-
tions with reasonable confidence. If the justification for that
confidence is sometimes doubted in the case of medicine, it is
because the public recognizes the variety of claims on a physician, from within and without, and sees that the patient's interests
have a great deal to compete with. A realistic professional code
will reflect these conflicts. It may turn out, however, that they
are not most fairly dealt with by a system of professional self-
regulation. Leaving aside the economic interests of physicians,
the main competitors of the individual patient's interests are
medical research and medical education, both of which serve the

interests of future patients but may involve risk and sacrifice of comfort to the one who is serving as a subject. Some such distribution of burdens is necessary, but its shape is too often determined by factors like poverty and ignorance. Some people have no choice about the terms under which they will undergo medical treatment. There is a case for external regulation both of how patients may be used for research and training, and of which patients are thus used.

But I am going to discuss the problem of practical conflict more generally, with only occasional reference to the biomedical professions. By a practical conflict I do not mean merely a difficult decision. Decisions may be difficult for a number of reasons: because the considerations on different sides are very evenly balanced; because the facts are uncertain; because the probability of different outcomes of the possible courses of action is unknown. A difficult choice between chemotherapy and surgery, when it is uncertain which will be more effective, is not an example of what I mean by practical conflict, because it does not involve conflict between values which are incomparable for reasons apart from uncertainty about the facts. There can be cases where, even if one is fairly sure about the outcomes of alternative courses of action, or about their probability distributions, and even though one knows how to distinguish the pros and cons, one is nevertheless unable to bring them together in a single evaluative judgment, even to the extent of finding them evenly balanced. An even balance requires comparable quantities.

The strongest cases of conflict are genuine dilemmas, where there is decisive support for two or more incompatible courses of action or inaction. In that case a decision will still be necessary, but it will seem necessarily arbitrary. When two choices are very evenly balanced, it doesn't matter which choice one makes, and arbitrariness is no problem. But when each seems right for reasons that appear decisive and sufficient, arbitrariness means the lack of reasons where reasons are needed, since either choice will mean acting against some reasons without being able to claim that they are *outweighed*.

Whether the conflict is a true dilemma or just a decision involving disparate values, it seems reasonable to propose, as Toulmin does, that to deal with it one must establish priorities among the conflicting claims. However, it is not clear how this can be done, or even what form the priorities would take. (It is unlikely, for example, that an absolute ranking of values into an order of precedence could be correct: even if X usually takes priority over Y, some large weight of Y will outweigh some small weight of X.) And the problem cannot even be addressed until we know more about the claims or values that give rise to the conflicts we are trying to resolve. My own view is that a general system of priorities, whether or not it involves the reduction of apparently disparate values to a common denominator, is not the appropriate method for dealing with these problems. But I shall argue for the point only after saying something about the sources of practical conflict, and how they can be classified.

There are five fundamental types of value that give rise to basic conflict. Conflicts can arise within as well as between them, but the latter are especially difficult. (I have not included self-interest in the group; it can conflict with any of the others.)

First, there are specific obligations to other people or institutions: obligations to patients, to one's family, to the hospital or university at which one works, to one's community or one's country. Such obligations have to be incurred, either by a deliberate undertaking or by some special relation to the person or institution in question. Their existence depends in either case on the subject's relation to others, although the relation does not have to be voluntary. (Even though young children are not at liberty to choose their parents or guardians, parental care creates some obligation of reciprocal future concern.)

The next category is that of constraints on action deriving from general rights that everyone has, either to do certain things or not to be treated in certain ways. Rights to liberty of certain kinds, or to freedom from assault or coercion, do not depend on specific obligations that others have incurred not to interfere, assault, or coerce. Rather, they are completely general, and restrict what others may do to their possessor, whoever those others may be. Thus a doctor has both specific obligations to his patients and general duties to treat anyone in certain ways.

The third category is that which is technically called utility. This is the consideration that takes into account the effects of what one does on everyone's welfare—whether or not the components of that welfare are connected to special obligations or general rights. Utility includes all aspects of benefit and harm to all people (or all sentient beings), not just those to whom the agent has a special relation, or has undertaken a special commitment. The general benefits of medical research and education obviously come under this heading.

The fourth category is that of perfectionist ends or values. By this I mean the intrinsic value of certain achievements or creations, apart from their value *to* individuals who experience or use them. Examples are provided by the intrinsic value of scientific discovery, of artistic creation, of space exploration, perhaps. These pursuits do of course serve the interests of the individuals directly involved in them, and of certain spectators. But typically the pursuit of such ends is not justified solely in terms of those interests. They are thought to have an intrinsic value, so that it is important to achieve fundamental advances, for example, in mathematics or astronomy even if very few people come to understand them and they have no practical effects. The mere existence of such understanding, somewhere in the species, is regarded by many as worth substantial sacrifices. Naturally opinions differ as to what has this kind of worth. Not everyone will agree that reaching the moon or Mars has the intrinsic value necessary to justify its current cost, or that the performance of obscure or difficult orchestral works has any value apart from its worth to individuals who enjoy them. But many things people do cannot be justified or understood without taking into account such perfectionist values.

The final category is that of commitment to one's own projects or undertakings, which is a value in addition to whatever reasons may have led to them in the first place. If you have set out to climb Everest, or translate Aristotle's *Metaphysics*, or master the *Well-Tempered Clavier*, or synthesize an amino acid, then the further pursuit of that project, once begun, acquires remarkable importance.[1] It is partly a matter of justifying earlier investment of time and energy, and not allowing it to have been in vain. It is partly a desire to be the sort of erson who finishes what he begins. But whatever the reason, our projects make autonomous claims on us, once undertaken, which they need not have made in advance. Someone who has determined to master the *Well-*

Tempered Clavier may say "I can't go to the movies, I have to practice"; but it would be strange for him to say that he had to master the *Well-Tempered Clavier*.

These commitments should not be confused with self-interest, for self-interest aims at the integrated fulfillment over time of *all* one's interests and desires (or at least those desires one does not wish to eliminate). Special commitments may, in their pursuit, be inimical to self-interest thus defined. They need not have been undertaken for self-interested reasons, and their pursuit certainly need not be controlled by self-interest.

Obligations, rights, utility, perfectionist ends, and private commitments—these values enter into our decisions constantly, and conflicts among them, and within them, arise in medical research, in politics, in personal life, or wherever the grounds of action are not artificially restricted. What would it mean to give a system of priorities among them? A simpler moral conception might permit a solution in terms of a short list of clear prohibitions and injunctions, with the balance of decision left to personal preference or discretion, but that will not work with so mixed a collection. One might try to order them. For example: never infringe general rights, and undertake only those special obligations that cannot lead to the infringement of anyone's rights; maximize utility within the range of action left free by the constraints of rights and obligations; where utility would be equally served by various policies, determine the choice by reference to perfectionist ends; and finally, where this leaves anything unsettled, decide on grounds of personal commitment or even simple preference. Such a method of decision is absurd, not because of the particular order chosen but because of its absoluteness. The ordering I have given is not arbitrary, for it reflects a degree of relative stringency in these types of values. But it is absurd to hold that obligations can never outweigh rights, or that utility, however large, can never outweigh obligation.

However, if we take the idea of outweighing seriously, and try to think of an alternative to ordering as a method of rationalizing decision in conditions of conflict, the thing to look for seems to be a single scale on which all these apparently disparate considerations can be measured, added, and balanced. Utilitarianism is the best example of such a theory, and interesting attempts have been made to explain the apparent priority of rights and obligations over utility in utilitarian terms. The same might be tried for perfectionist goals and personal commitments. My reason for thinking that such explanations are unsuccessful, or at best partially successful, is not just that they imply specific moral conclusions that I find intuitively unacceptable (for it is always conceivable that a new refinement of the theory may iron out many of those wrinkles). Rather, my reason for doubt is theoretical: I do not believe that the source of value is unitary—displaying apparent multiplicity only in its application to the world. I believe that value has fundamentally different kinds of sources, and that they are reflected in the classification of values into types. Not all values represent the pursuit of some single good in a variety of settings.

Think for example of the contrast between perfectionist and utilitarian values. They are *formally* different, for the latter takes into account the number of people whose interests are affected, and the former does not. Perfectionist values have to do with the mere level of achievement and not with the spread either of achievement or of gratification. There is also a formal contrast between rights or obligations and any ends, whether utilitarian or perfectionist, that are defined in terms of the outcome of actions—in terms of how things are as a result. The claims represented by individual obligations begin with relations between individuals, and although the maintenance of those relations in a satisfactory form must be part of any utilitarian conception of a good state of affairs, that is not the basic motive behind claims of obligation. It may be a good thing that people keep their promises or look after their children, but the reason a person has to keep his own promises is very different from the reason he has to want other people unconnected with him to keep their promises— just because it would be a good thing, impersonally considered. A person does not feel bound to keep his promises or look after his children because it would be a good thing, impersonally considered. There certainly are things we do for such reasons, but in the motive behind obligations a more personal outlook is essential. It is your *own* relation to the other person or the institution or community that moves you, not a detached concern for what would be best overall.

Reasons of this kind may be described as agent-centered or subjective (though the term "subjective" here should not be misunderstood—it does not mean that the general principles of obligation are matters of subjective preference which may vary from person to person). The reasons in each case apply primarily to the individual involved, as reasons for *him* to want to fulfill his obligations—even though it is also a good thing, impersonally considered, for him to do so.

General rights are less personal in their claims, since a right to be free from interference or assault, for example, does not derive from the possessor's relation to anyone in particular: everyone is obliged to respect it. Nevertheless, they are agent-centered in the sense that the reasons for action they provide apply primarily to individuals whose actions are in danger of infringing such rights. Rights mainly provide people with reasons not to do certain things to other people—not to treat them or interfere with them in certain ways. Again, it is objectively a good thing that people's rights not be violated, and this provides disinterested parties with some reason for seeing that X's rights are not violated by Y. But this is a secondary motive, not so powerful as the reason one has not to violate anyone's rights directly. (That is why it is reasonable for defenders of civil liberties to object to police and judicial practices that violate the rights of criminal suspects, even when the aim of those policies is to prevent greater violations by criminals of the rights of their victims.) In that sense the claims deriving from general rights are agent-centered: less so than those deriving from special obligations, but still definitely agent-centered in a sense in which the claims of utility or perfectionist ends are not. Those latter claims are impersonal or outcome-centered; they have to do with what happens, not, in the first instance, with what one does. It is the contribution of what one does to what happens or what is achieved that matters.

This great division between personal and impersonal, or between agent-centered and outcome-centered, or subjective and objective reasons, is so basic that it renders implausible any reductive unification of ethics—let alone of practical reasoning in general. The formal differences among these types of reasons correspond to deep differences in their sources. We appreciate the force of impersonal reasons when we detach from our personal situation and our special relations to others. Utilitarian considerations arise in this way when our detachment takes the form of adopting a general point of view that comprehends everyone's view of the world within it. Naturally the results will not always be clear. But such an outlook is obviously very different from that which appears in a person's concern for his special obligations to his family, friends, or colleagues. There he is thinking very much of his particular situation in the world. The two motives come from two different points of view, both important, but fundamentally irreducible to a common basis.

I have said nothing about the still more agent-centered motive of commitment to one's own projects, but since that involves one's own life and not necessarily any relations with others, the same points obviously apply. It is a source of reasons that cannot be assimilated either to utility, or perfectionism, or rights, or obligations (except that they might be described as obligations to oneself).

My general point is that the formal differences among types of reason reflect differences of a fundamental nature in their sources, and that this rules out a certain kind of solution to conflicts among these types. Human beings are subject to moral and other motivational claims of very different kinds. This is because they are complex creatures who can view the world from many perspectives—individual, relational, impersonal, ideal, etc.—and each perspective presents a different set of claims. Conflict can exist within one of these sets, and it may be hard to resolve. But when conflict occurs between them, the problem is still more difficult. In the professions, conflicts between personal and impersonal claims are ubiquitous. They cannot, in my view, be resolved by subsuming either of the points of view under the other, or both under a third. Nor can we simply abandon any of them. There is no reason why we should. The capacity to view the world simultaneously from the point of view of one's relations to others, from the point of view of one's life extended through time, from the point of view of everyone at once, and finally from the detached viewpoint often described as the view *sub specie aeternitatis* is one of the marks of humanity. This complex capacity is an obstacle to simplification.

Does this mean, then, that basic practical conflicts have no solution? The unavailability of a single, reductive method or a clear set of priorities for settling them does not remove the necessity for making decisions in such cases. When faced with conflicting and incommensurable claims we still have to do something—even if it is only to do nothing. And the fact that action must be unitary seems to imply that unless justification is also unitary, nothing can be either right or wrong and all decisions under conflict are arbitrary.

I believe this is wrong, but the alternative is hard to explain. Briefly, I contend that there can be good judgment without total justification, either explicit or implicit. The fact that one cannot say why a certain decision is the correct one, given a particular balance of conflicting reasons, does not mean that the claim to correctness is meaningless. Provided one has taken the process of practical justification as far as it will go in the course of arriving at the conflict, one may be able to proceed without further justification, but without irrationality either. What makes this possible is *judgment*—essentially the faculty Aristotle described as practical wisdom, which reveals itself over time in individual decisions rather than in the enunciation of general principles. It will not always yield a solution: there are true practical dilemmas that have no solution, and there are also conflicts so complex that judgment cannot operate confidently. But in many cases it can be relied on to take up the slack that remains beyond the limits of explicit rational argument.

This view has sometimes been regarded as defeatist and empty since it was expressed by Aristotle. In reply, let me say two things. First, the position does not imply that we should abandon the search for more and better reasons and more critical insight in the domain of practical decision. It is just that our capacity to resolve conflicts in particular cases may extend beyond our capacity to enunciate general principles that explain those resolutions. Perhaps we are working with general principles unconsciously, and can discover them by codifying our decisions and particular intuitions. But this is not necessary either for the operation or for the development of judgment. Secondly, the search for general principles in ethics, or other aspects of practical reasoning, is more likely to be successful if systematic theories restrict themselves to one aspect of the subject—one component of rational motivation—than if they try to be comprehensive.

To look for a single general theory of how to decide the right thing to do is like looking for a single theory of how to decide what to believe. Such progress as we have made in the systematic justification and criticism of beliefs has not come mostly from general principles of reasoning but from the understanding of particular areas, marked out by the different sciences, by history, by mathematics. These vary in exactness, and large areas of belief are left out of the scope of any theory. These must be governed by common sense and ordinary, prescientific reasoning. Such reasoning must also be used where the results of various more systematic methods bear on the matter at hand, but no one of them determines a conclusion. In civil engineering problems, for example, the solution depends both on physical factors capable of precise calculation and behavioral or psychological factors that are not. Obviously one should use exact principles and methods to deal with those aspects of a problem for which they are available, but sometimes there are other aspects as well, and one must resist the temptation to either ignore them or treat them by exact methods to which they are not susceptible.

We are familiar with this fragmentation of understanding and method when it comes to belief, but we tend to resist it in the case of decision. Yet it is as irrational to despair of systematic ethics because one cannot find a completely general account of what should be done as it would be to give up scientific research because there is no general method of arriving at true beliefs. I am not saying that ethics is a science, only that the relation between ethical theory and practical decisions is analogous to the relation between scientific theory and beliefs about particular things or events in the world.

In both areas, some problems are much purer than others, that is, their solutions are more completely determined by factors that admit of precise understanding. Sometimes the only significant factor in a practical decision is personal obligation, or general utility, and then one's reasoning can be confined to that (however precisely it may be understood). Sometimes a process of decision is artificially insulated against the influence of more than one type of factor. This is not always a good thing, but sometimes it is.

The example I have in mind is the judicial process, which carefully excludes, or tries to exclude, considerations of utility and personal commitment, and limits itself to claims of right. Since the systematic recognition of such claims is very important (and also tends over the long run not to conflict unacceptably with other values), it is worth isolating these factors for special treatment. As a result, legal argument has been one of the areas of real progress in the understanding of a special aspect of practical reason. Systematic theory and the search for general principles and methods may succeed elsewhere if we accept a fragmentary approach. Utilitarian theory, for example, has a great deal to contribute if it is not required to account for everything. Utility is an extremely important factor in decisions, particularly in public policy, and philosophical work on its definition, the coordination problems arising in the design of institutions to promote utility, its connections with preference, with equality, and with efficiency, can have an impact on such decisions.

This and other areas can be the scene of progress even if none of them aspires to the status of a general and complete theory of right and wrong. There will never be such a theory, in my view, since the role of judgment in resolving conflicts and applying disparate claims and considerations to real life is indispensable. Two dangers can be avoided if this idea of noncomprehensive systematization is kept in mind. One is the danger of romantic defeatism, which abandons rational theory because it inevitably leaves many problems unsolved. The other is the danger of exclusionary overrationalization, which bars as irrelevant or empty all considerations that cannot be brought within the scope of a general system admitting explicitly defensible conclusions. This yields skewed results by counting only measurable or otherwise precisely describable factors, even when others are in fact relevant. The alternative is to recognize that the legitimate grounds of decision are extremely various and understood to different degrees. This has both theoretical and practical implications.

On the theoretical side, I have said that progress in particular areas of ethics and value theory need not wait for the discovery of a general foundation (even if there is such a thing). This is recognized by many philosophers and has recently been urged by

John Rawls, who claims not only that the pursuit of substantive moral theory, for example the theory of justice, can proceed independently of views about the foundation of ethics, but that until substantive theory is further developed, the search for foundations may be premature.[2]

This seems too strong, but it is certainly true of any field that one need not make progress at the most fundamental level to make progress at all. Chemistry went through great developments during the century before its basis in atomic physics came to be understood. Mendelian genetics was developed long before any understanding of the molecular basis of heredity. At present, progress in psychology must be pursued to a great extent independently of any idea about its basis in the operation of the brain. It may be that all psychological phenomena are ultimately explainable in terms of a theory of the central nervous system, but our present understanding of that system is too meager to permit us even to look for a way to close the gap.

The corresponding theoretical division in ethics need not be so extreme. We can continue to work on the foundations while exploring the superstructure, and the two pursuits should reinforce each other. I myself do not believe that all value rests on a single foundation or can be combined into a unified system, because different types of values represent the development and articulation of different points of view, all of which combine to produce decisions. Ethics is unlike physics, which represents one point of view, that which apprehends the spatio-temporal properties of the universe described in mathematical terms. Even in this case, where it is reasonable to seek a unified theory of all physical phenomena, it is also possible to understand a great deal about more particular aspects of the physical universe—gravitation, mechanics, electromagnetic fields, radiation, nuclear forces—without having such a theory.

But ethics is more like understanding or knowledge in general than it is like physics. Just as our understanding of the world involves various points of view—among which the austere viewpoint of physics is the most powerfully developed and one of the most important—so values come from a number of viewpoints, some more personal than others, which cannot be reduced to a common denominator any more than history, psychology, philology, and economics can be reduced to physics. Just as the types of understanding available to us are distinct, even though they must all coexist and cooperate in our minds, so the types of value that move us are disparate, even though they must cooperate as well as they can in determining what we do.

With regard to practical implications, it seems to me that the fragmentation of effort and of results that is theoretically to be expected in the domain of value has implications for the strategy to be used in applying these results to practical decisions, especially questions of public policy. The lack of a general theory of value should not be an obstacle to the employment of those areas of understanding that do exist; and we know more than is generally appreciated. The lack of a general theory leads too easily to a false dichotomy: either fall back entirely on the unsystematic intuitive judgment of whoever has to make a decision, or else cook up a unified but artificial system like cost-benefit analysis,[3] which will grind out decisions on any problem presented to it. (Such systems may be useful if their claims and scope of operation are less ambitious.) What is needed instead is a mixed strategy, combining systematic results where these are applicable with less systematic judgment to fill in the gaps.

However, this requires the development of an approach to decisions that will use available ethical understanding where it is relevant. Such an approach is now being sought by different groups working in applied ethics, with what success we shall not know for some time. I want to suggest that the fragmentation of value provides a rationale for a particular way of looking at the task, and an indication of what needs to be done.

What we need most is a method of breaking up or analyzing practical problems to say what evaluative principles apply, and how. This is not a method of decision. Perhaps in special cases it would yield a decision, but more usually it would simply indicate the points at which different kinds of ethical considerations needed to be introduced to supply the basis for a responsible and intelligent decision. This component approach to problems is familiar enough in connection with other disciplines. It is expected that important policy decisions may depend on economic factors, political factors, ecological factors, medical safety, scientific progress, technological advantages, military security, and other concerns. Advice on all these matters can be obtained by responsible officials if there is anyone available whose job it is to think about them. In some cases well-established disciplines are involved. Their practitioners may vary widely in understanding of the subject, and on many issues they will disagree with one another. But even to be exposed to these controversies (about inflation or nuclear power safety or recombinant DNA risk) is better than hearing nothing at all. Moreover it is important that within most serious disciplines there is agreement about what is controversial and what is not. Anyone with an important decision to make, whether he is a legislator or a cabinet officer or a department official, can get advice on different aspects of the problem from people who have thought much more than he has about each of those aspects, and know what others have said about it. The division of disciplines and a consensus about what dimensions of a problem have to be considered are very useful in bringing together the problems and such expertise as there is.

We need a comparable consensus about what important ethical and evaluative questions have to be considered if a policy decision is to be made responsibly. This is not the same thing as a consensus in ethics. It means only that there are certain aspects of any problem that most people who work in ethics and value theory would agree should be considered, and can be professionally considered in such a way that whoever is going to make the decision will be exposed to the relevant ideas currently available. Sometimes the best ideas will not be very good, or they will include diametrically opposed views; but this is true everywhere, not just in ethics.

It might be suggested that the best approach would be to emulate the legal system by setting up an advocacy procedure before a kind of court whose job would be to render decisions on ethically loaded policy questions. (The recent proposal of a science court shows the attractions of the legal model: its non-democratic character has great intellectual appeal.) But I think the actual situation is too fluid for anything like that. Values are relevant to policy in too many ways, and in combination with too many other kinds of knowledge and opinion, to be treatable in this manner. Although some legal decisions are very difficult, courts are designed to decide clear, narrowly defined questions to which a relatively limited set of arguments and reasons is relevant. (Think of the function of a judge in striking material from the record or refusing to admit certain data or testimony in evidence: such restrictions do not in general apply to legislative or administrative deliberations.) Most practical issues are much messier than this, and their ethical dimensions are much more complex. One needs a method of insuring that where relevant understanding exists, it is made available, and where there is an aspect of the problem that no one understands very well, this is understood too.

I have not devised such a method, but clearly it would have to provide that factors considered should include, among others, the following: economic, political, and personal liberty, equality, equity, privacy, procedural fairness, intellectual and aesthetic development, community, general utility, desert, avoidance of arbitrariness, acceptance of risk, the interests of future generations, the weight to be given to interests of other states or countries. There is much to be said about each of these. The method would have to be more organized to be useful, but a general position on the ways in which ethics is relevant to policy could probably be agreed on by a wide range of ethical theorists, from relativists to utilitarians to Kantians. Radical disagreement about the basis of ethics is compatible with substantial agreement about what the important factors are in real life. If this consensus, which I believe already exists among ethical theorists, were to gain wider acceptance among the public and those who make policy, then the extensive but fragmented understanding that we possess in this area could be put to better use than it is now. It would then be more difficult simply to ignore certain questions, and even if the ethical considerations, once offered, were disregarded or rejected, the reasons or absence of reasons for such rejection would become part of the basis for any decision made. There is a modicum of power even in being able to state a prima facie case.

This conception of the role of moral theory also implies an answer to the question of its relation to politics, and other methods of decision. Ethics is not being recommended as a decision procedure, but as an essential resource for making decisions, just as physics, economics, and demography are. In fundamental constitutional decisions of the Supreme Court, one branch of ethics plays a central role in a process that takes precedence over the usual methods of political and administrative decision. But for most of the questions that need deciding, ethical considerations are multiple, complex, often cloudy, and mixed up with many others. They need to be considered in a systematic way, but in most cases a reasonable decision can be reached only by sound judgment, informed as well as possible by the best arguments that any relevant disciplines have to offer.

NOTES

1. See Gilbert Harman, "Practical Reasoning," *Review of Metaphysics*, XXIX (1976): 432-63.
2. John Rawls, *A Theory of Justice* (Cambridge: Harvard University Press, 1971), pp. 51-60. See also "The Independence of Moral Theory," *Proceedings and Addresses of the American Philosophical Association* (1974-75): 5-22.
3. See Lawrence Tribe, "Policy Science: Analysis or Ideology?" *Philosophy and Public Affairs*, 2 (1972): 66-110.

7

Error in Medicine

Eric J. Cassell

A NINETY-YEAR-OLD MAN who had been healthy and active was awakened in the middle of the night by the urge to urinate. When he did so, he was frightened to discover the toilet bowl turn red with blood and clots. He telephoned his doctor and was admitted to the urology service of a modern medical center. The initial tests and X-rays revealed an unusual form of cancer of the bladder.

In the morning, the man's physician helped him choose a specialist. Because the case was unusual and interesting, he suggested that the attending surgeon be a man much favored by the residents of the service, for then the case would provide maximum teaching benefits and the patient receive good care.

Pre-operative evaluation revealed the man to be in relatively good health except for mild hypertension and varicose veins. It was suggested that he receive small doses of heparin during and after surgery to prevent pulmonary emboli, a complication common in post-operative bedridden patients of his age. Such therapy was new at the time and viewed by the surgeons who had had no experience with it as exposing the patient to a risk of bleeding, despite the published evidence to the contrary.

The operation (partial removal of the bladder) went extremely well and offered promise that cancer would not soon recur or be the cause of death.

The first post-operative day was uneventful except that the

295

patient had considerable pain. On the second day, morphine was given because of the severe pain, and that evening the patient was found by the internist to be stuporous and breathing poorly. He wrote a note on the chart suggesting that morphine be discontinued because of its depressant effect and told the nurse not to give the next dose until the resident had seen the note and stopped the morphine. On the next day, still receiving morphine, the patient was neither alert nor breathing well. The internist discontinued the morphine, and the discussion with the surgical resident that followed was sharp and angry on both sides. The following day was Sunday and the internist did not see the patient. That night he was notified that the patient had been transferred to the intensive care unit.

A review of the chart revealed that the morphine had been restarted in a smaller dose and that the patient had gone into respiratory arrest and shock. The resident (the same one who restarted the morphine) had worked long and vigorously to reestablish effective respiration and blood pressure and correct the associated metabolic abnormalities. Blood chemistries revealed that the patient's kidneys were not functioning well, but the report of similar tests done when he was first admitted could not be found for comparison.

The attending surgeon could not be reached (and had not responded to earlier calls). His attraction for the house staff, it turned out, was not only his competence but also the fact that he often turned his cases over to them and then stayed out of the way.

In the intensive care unit, the patient was appropriately monitored and his respiratory problem effectively managed. The physician in charge of the unit decided to start peritoneal dialysis to take over the function of the patient's kidneys, despite the fact that the degree of kidney failure was not severe nor endangering him.

Although the patient was able to leave the intensive care unit, his renal function worsened and did not return. Numerous consultants saw the patient and the case was discussed frankly with the family, and, to the degree possible, with the patient. Repeated peritoneal dialyses were required which, although ultimately seen as pointless, were also seen as difficult to discontinue. He developed massive swelling of the lower extremities, interpreted as thrombosis of the inferior vena cava. Ultimately the peritoneum became infected and he finally died of pulmonary emboli and pneumonia. Autopsy confirmed the thrombosis of the inferior vena cava, peritonitis, pneumonia, and pulmonary emboli.

The case is illustrative of the many facets of medical error. It was marked by mistakes throughout, except for late in the illness. It is an example of what may be a medical maxim. In a difficult case, when errors start, each will give rise to more. Were a malpractice suit to be brought (that did not happen because the family was grateful for the attentive care), the jury would undoubtedly have found for the plaintiff. The suit could have been based on more than one technical error, easily proven, and virtually impossible to defend.

The small dose heparin regimen should have been employed to prevent thrombosis. Since that opinion had been entered on the chart by the medical consultant, when the surgeons decided against the heparin, their opinion and the reasons for it should have been entered on the chart. The morphine should have been discontinued and certainly should not have been restarted. The events leading to the respiratory arrest should have been documented in the doctor's notes. The absence of initial laboratory results entered on the chart would have attested to inadequate pre-operative evaluation of the function of the remaining kidney. There were undoubtedly other errors which I have forgotten. As many technical errors as there were, there were also errors of judgment. They ranged from the initial choice of operation, to the decision to start peritoneal dialysis. In those instances, perhaps no technical mistakes were committed, but clearly a reasoned analysis of the case and the arguments for or against alternative actions were lacking at each step.

Although fortunately the example does not represent a common occurrence, it is typical enough to provide the basis for a closer look at the whole phenomenon of error in medicine.

To start with, we can dismiss some excuses. The case was not so difficult or unusual that it presented new technical problems. Although it ultimately became extremely complicated, that occurred as a result of the errors and was not their cause. Carelessness did not cause the mistakes except perhaps for the missing pre-operative laboratory report. Technical competence, training, and experience were more than adequate to the challenge, as were the technological resources of the institution. Indeed, there are reasons for believing that if the patient had not been in a teaching hospital that was so superbly equipped, the matter might have ended better.

Of much greater importance to an understanding of error in medicine is a look at what would have been the best basis for a malpractice action. Clearly, the continued administration of morphine to this patient, after it was apparent that it greatly impaired his consciousness and respiratory function, was wrong and indefensible. But when the case was over and the family had won their suit, what would the physicians have learned from the trial? Not to give morphine in such circumstances? Any second-year medical student learns that when he or one of his friends in the pharmacology laboratory kills a cat with too much morphine. Although the morphine was the agent of the mistake, the error originated in the conflict between the surgical resident and the internist and the subsequent failure of both of them to protect the patient from their dispute. That dispute would not show up in court unless it was used by the plaintiff's attorney to get one of them to testify against the other.

The function of malpractice law is not to teach physicians what not to do but rather to compensate patients injured by wrong action. However, it is inevitable that something as influential as malpractice law should start to become the teacher rather than the student of an understanding of medicine and medical errors.

One of the things it has taught is that the primary concern of malpractice is with technical mistakes. While certain ethical errors, such as the abandonment of a patient, are grounds for suit, the overwhelming attention is paid to technical errors. There may be good, even inevitable, reasons for that single-mindedness, but an understanding of error that dwells on the technical is simply inadequate.

Errors in medicine are not only technical, but also arise from the moral sphere, social or interpersonal interaction, and from problems of thought. It is in the nature of so complex an activity as medicine that these all interact, but in this case, as an example, each can be seen for its separate effect.

The failure of the internist to come to the hospital on the crucial Sunday was a moral error. So, too, was the failure of the surgeon to remain closely associated with the case after the operation. Similarly, when the resident did not call the internist after the respiratory arrest, he was in error because he was both acting beyond his ability and failing to act in a way that would have been an acknowledgment of his technical error. As noted earlier, errors in social interaction between attending physician and house officer are probably what started the case on its fatal course. Later there were conflicts between house officers of different specialties, common enough, but damaging nonetheless. There were also errors in thought and reasoning. The choice of operation in the first place may have been dubious, and the decision to start peritoneal dialysis certainly was. It may be argued that those were technical errors, but I think not—certainly not by malpractice standards. Medical decision-making is based primarily on the estimation of alternative probabilities. Doctors become very good at that sort of thing. Recently, writers on decision-making in medicine, however, have pointed out that doctors' intuitive methods may lead them far astray, particularly where small probability statistics are involved.[1]

All these kinds of error were probably as crucial in this case as the actual morphine administration. Yet, one might argue that their recitation merely shows that medicine is a human activity and is thus subject to human weakness. That being the instance, such a recital is hardly more illuminating that the opposite single-mindedness of malpractice law.

I believe I can show that these human foibles do not occur at random, and can be systematically understood if we are able to see a "case" in medicine as much larger than a case of, for example, carcinoma of the bladder. That is not merely to say that a patient is a person, but rather to try and find, at least in terms of medical error, what can be seen as an individual entity in medicine. Something individual in the same sense that a person is an individual—discrete and comprehensible in himself, even though subject to outside influence. An individual in the same way that Gorovitz and MacIntyre apply the term to a salt marsh or a hurricane.

Before going further, it is necessary to define better what

usually seems to be meant by error in discussions of error in medicine. Here I mean not to give clarity to the word in the sense of a dictionary definition, but rather to show the special meaning that it seems to have acquired in relation to the behavior of physicians. It does not seem to me that error usually means simply inadvertent action based on ignorance, false beliefs, or notions—inadvertence that applies equally to an action committed or uncommitted. Error in that sense is not something the physician does so much as something that happens to the physician— and through him as agent, something that happens to the patient. That sense of error is morally neutral, and I believe that is not what we commonly mean when we speak of physicians' errors. For one thing, such neutral errors are generally not known to us as mistakes at the time they occur or even soon after. They are revealed by the evolution of knowledge. For example, in years past, keeping patients in bed for long periods after surgery was an error that led to a high incidence of thrombophlebitis and pulmonary emboli. When such an embolus occurred, it was not called error, it was called chance. Generally speaking, that class of mistakes which seem morally neutral—which are conceived as happening to rather than being done to the patients—are perceived as chance events even though they may be causally related to the action of the physician. If, years later, the doctor becomes aware that his action caused the mistake, he may believe that he, as well as the patient, suffered at the hands of fate.

Nor is it usually considered error when, in therapeutic research, patients are randomly assigned to treatment groups and some, therefore, suffer or do less well than others. To preserve that sense of freedom from error, the physician must feel sure that chance alone is operating in the assignment of patients to the treatment groups. In these situations, the physician relinquishes his more comfortable role as the agent of choice, giving over to chance that agency. Should it turn out, as is usually the case, that one group of patients does less well, the doctor may feel badly for the less fortunate patients, but he will not feel that he erred.

I believe that what is commonly meant when people speak of doctors making errors has three requirements. First, the physician is held to be responsible for his choice of action by himself, his patient, or the group. Next, to consider that an error has been committed, the physician, patient, or group must believe that a causal relationship exists between the doctor's action and the injury. Finally, there must be an injury or the awareness of near injury. If something good happens as a result of a mistake, it would generally not be called an error, but, rather, serendipity.

Thus, error, in its peculiarly medical expression, requires a sense of responsibility, an awareness of causal relationship, and injury. What is interesting about each of these terms is that they have both an objective and subjective expression. Most discussions of error in medicine, particularly those centering around malpractice, implicitly or explicitly accept these requirements for error, but deal only with the objective aspects. There seems not to be an awareness that the objective nature of responsibility, causality, and injury (at least in their relationship to medical error) are the societal expression of individual subjective senses of responsibility, causality, and injury. For that reason, these factors in their objective expression are relative to the value structure of the group in which they occur. They are also relative to the group's understanding of the nature and cure of illness and of the function of physicians.

It may be argued that there is nothing relative about the injury suffered by the patient presented here. He was given morphine which led to respiratory arrest and ultimately to his death. But if the highest call on the physician was the relief of pain—indeed in certain terminal illnesses that is believed to be true—then the injury would not have come about through error, but rather as an unavoidable consequence of mercy. So much of what happened to this patient represented not the ineluctable operation of nature, but was the consequence of more or less informed current beliefs about causality in disease, infection, thrombosis, and so forth. The very fact of operating on a ninety-year-old man represents a change from a generation ago in beliefs of what is appropriate to the aged.

The subjective nature of the word *injury* is pointed up by the behavior of modern patients who act as though anything but a perfect outcome from the treatment of curable disease represents injury. If, after a fractured leg has healed, the patient does not walk perfectly, he may well feel and act toward his physician as though he has been injured—not by fate, but by the physician!

Here, as in other areas of medicine, one finds a pervasive and perhaps increasing belief that fate can be controlled or denied. Such a belief is manifested in proposals to create systems of compensation for adverse medical outcome resulting from medical treatment, whether or not caused by negligence. Such proposals suggest that, since the function of modern medical care is to return the patient to health, when that does not happen, despite reasonable expectations based on the existing state of knowledge, then the patient has been injured and compensation is justified.

Quite apart from whether such suggestions are good or bad or will help alleviate the problems of malpractice insurance, they point to something interesting. It might have been suggested earlier that I was wrong in asserting that definitions of responsibility, causality, and injury were relative to the value structure of the group; rather than that, it could be asserted that they are simply relative to our state of knowledge. What was not an injury previously, now becomes an injury, causally related to the action of a responsible physician, because knowledge has advanced to reveal the proper action. While the result of the advance of knowledge is undeniably true, the newer "no fault" malpractice proposals suggest that, in addition to advance in knowledge, there has also been a change in the group's belief—one should be compensated for injury arising *not only* from the negligence of physicians, but also from the action of fate. I am not necessarily opposed to such a belief, but I think the belief and its ramifications are awe-inspiring.

Thus, thinking about injury has changed, and so, too, has thinking about causality—the changes are related. As always, everything is seen to have a cause, but now cause is conceived to be within the control of man. Chance and fate are ruled out as legitimate causes. Injury implies injury *by someone*. And, curiously, when society compensates an individual for the action of fate, that too is an attempt to deny fate. When I buy fire insurance for my house, I do so in recognition that things happen, and that causal chains are not always controllable. But when society begins to compensate its members for injuries arising from chance, the net effect is to deny the power of chance. The next case shows how chance itself is removed from the causal chain.

During an operation to remove an intervertebral disc that was pressing on a lumbar nerve root, the instrument that was being used by the surgeon broke, and a piece dropped into the wound and could not be recovered. The operation was concluded with the instrument fragment still in the disc space. In time, it migrated spontaneously to a more accessible location, and a second operation was done to recover the broken piece. The patient recovered completely. In the trial of the malpractice suit that followed, the history of that instrument from its manufacture to the time of operation was exhaustively reviewed. No responsible party could be shown, and the jury found for the defendants (the surgeon, hospital, and instrument maker). On appeal to a higher court, the case was returned for retrial. Since it was clear that the instrument should not have broken, the jury must find the responsible party(s) and apportion damages. Such a finding by the higher court naturally causes apprehension among physicians and their insurers. In newer proposed systems of malpractice compensation, such cases would fall under the rubric of medical accident—to be compensated on a no-fault basis. It seems equally reasonable, however, to compensate the patient for getting the disc disease in the first place. That, too, was an accident of fate. Or to compensate any patient for any illness. Indeed, in the amendment to the Social Security Law, which extends Medicare benefits to patients with end stage renal disease regardless of their age, we have seen the extension of just that thought.

Another facet of the problem of error in medicine was revealed in the recent series of articles in the *New York Times* on poor practice in American medicine. In discussions of unnecessary surgery and unnecessary prescriptions—both of which are clearly quite common—there seems to be an unspoken basis for the presentation. It is assumed apparently that patients get sick from diseases from which they can be cured. If they are not cured, or if they are given treatments, medical or surgical, which are unnecessary or do them harm, then error has been committed. Such error, the assumption seems to be, is technical in nature and thus always knowable. Therefore, it must always arise from venality or ignorance on the part of physicians. There is no question that there are venal physicians who do wrong acts solely for monetary or other non-medical reasons. There is also no question that there are ignorant, uninformed, or stupid physicians who do wrong things simply because they do not know better when they should know better.

It is my contention that those two sources of error—venality and ignorance—are the least important both numerically and conceptually. There are and always have been venal physicians, and they should be revealed. There are and there always have been physicians who should be retrained. However, I believe the greatest source of error lies in the inherent belief and value structure of medicine, equally shared, as must be the case, by both physicians and patients. Where the belief exists that fate in its expression as illness can be denied or overcome, and where cure is the expectation, there exists a force to act. Medicine is based on a belief in the efficacy of intervention. The focus of the force to intervene is the disease. It is difficult but necessary to point out the difference between disease as entity and disease as symbol. It is clear that the symbolic utility of disease as the cause of human ills is dependent on its concrete utility in individual cases. That is to say that the surgical (or medical) removal of disease must succeed often enough in removing that state of dysfunction called illness to maintain the symbolic importance of disease.

But then, what is meant by disease as a symbol? Diseases such as fibroids of the uterus or tumors of the thyroid gland may be the cause of considerable illness and disability. But not all fibroids of the uterus or tumors of the thyroid cause illness, and it is difficult sometimes to distinguish between those that are or will be the cause of disability and those that will not. For example, tumors of the thyroid are quite common and physicians go to great lengths to try and decide which are at risk of becoming malignant and thus should be removed. Many physicians believe that perhaps all solid tumors of the thyroid should be operated upon. However, oddly, death from cancer of the thyroid is really quite rare. The disparity between the commonness of thyroid tumors and their surgical removal and the rarity of death from thyroid cancer requires some thought. The solid tumor becomes not only the thing itself, but a symbol for the threat of cancer. We strike at the enemy by striking at its symbolic representation. One might argue that all I have shown is that it is difficult to decide which thyroid nodule will become cancerous and calling it a symbol is just fanciness. I think not. Why do we not reason backwards from the very small frequency of thyroid cancer rather than forwards from the large number of thyroid nodules. I think because each thyroid tumor is symbolic of the threat of cancer. The actual fact of cancer, very low in frequency, is not the prime mover, but rather the threat of cancer.

In simple terms, the object of removing disease is to make or keep someone healthy. When we see disease consistently removed or treated with apparently little, or at least obscure relation, to ultimate health (despite good intentions), we may suspect that the real has been replaced by symbol.

Symbols attain their importance as representatives of reality by conferring meaning on reality even when that reality may not be the best concrete expression of the symbol. The symbol remains constant and dependable when reality is not all that constant and dependable. We live in a surgical age in medicine, based on a belief in efficacy of the extirpation of disease. It is essential to remember that for the symbol to retain its force, both patient and doctor must believe in it. It is from this symbolic meaning of disease and surgery that most error in medicine derives. Patients who have unnecessary hysterectomies are not usually dragged kicking and screaming to the operating room. Both they and their surgeons believe in the importance of the operation. The surgeon believes the organ is diseased, and the patient believes that when the diseased piece is removed, she will feel better. But more, it is the surgeon's definition of disease that may confer reality on her feelings. A force exists for the presence of the operation. To eliminate that source of unnecessary surgery, it is almost necessary to eliminate surgery. Put another way, the proven efficacy of surgery has as its inevitable accompaniment unnecessary surgery. Some years ago, it was believed that polyps of the colon should be removed because of the risk of malignant transformation. Such polypectomies often necessitated major abdominal surgery. Evidence was then presented that showed malignant change in such polyps to be quite rare. After considerable debate in the literature, many physicians ultimately agreed and abdominal surgery for such polyps stopped being correct practice. Recently, new instrumentation (the flexible fiber-optic colonoscope) has made it possible to remove those polyps without abdominal surgery and with small risk or discomfort to the patient. Not non-existent risk, but small risk. Now polypectomy has again become common. It is very difficult for physicians and patients to leave tumors alone. It is this relationship of disease as entity to disease as symbol that becomes very difficult to define. Yet, in examining poor practice, the symbolic meaning of disease and the related force to act are forgotten, and each individual operation or combined statistics are treated as only the disease they represent.

Our beliefs in medicine as an attempt to control nature and deny fate, and our confusion of disease as entity with disease as symbol, confound attempts to understand error in medicine. These problems also underlie the persistence with which we view error in medicine primarily as technical. Understanding this or even accepting it does not, however, point to any useful alternative. It is necessary, now, to show why an individual instance of a disease is not a large enough whole in itself to be the basis for an adequate examination of error in medicine.

Appendicitis is a disease whose simplicity makes it a useful example. It is common, usually easy to diagnose and operate upon, and involves inflammation of a vestigial appendix which was thought (probably incorrectly) to be of no use to anyone except surgeons. When a patient fails to recover from appendicitis, it would be common for many, including some physicians, to equate the failure with error. Equating failure with error here, and in so many other instances, implies that we know enough of the nature of disease so that the failure to cure the patient does not tell us about appendicitis but about doctors. In this view, appendicitis becomes the constant against which to measure the performance of physicians. What makes appendicitis the constant in this equation is not the thing represented by the word *appendicitis*, but rather our knowledge of it. We act as though our knowledge truly contains the thing and contains it so completely that it can act as a benchmark for the performance. Indeed, mechanisms are currently being developed to measure quality of medical care that depend precisely on that assumption. In these programs, the actions of medical personnel, as shown by hospital or office records, in regard to certain specified diseases such as heart attacks, kidney infections, and others, will be assessed to see if certain standards have been met. These measurements of quality have a certain galenical cast and may well have a galenical outcome—strictly specified "correct" treatments initially used as measures that ultimately become rules for treatment.

However, any experienced clinician is aware that both the diagnosis and treatment of appendicitis can be difficult. In the aged, the pregnant, or otherwise sick, or when underlying the case there is an uncommon microbe, parasite, or other unusual situation, things may go very badly. Indeed, on close examination, our knowledge of appendicitis is imperfect. What most of us call appendicitis—abdominal pain, tenderness, certain laboratory findings, and so forth—is not appendicitis at all. It is a symptom complex most often associated with inflammation of the appendix and useful in its diagnosis. We have no idea how often the appendix becomes inflamed and then subsides without treatment, presenting none of the features known as appendicitis. For all we know, that is a common occurrence, just as it turned out that poliomyelitis infection occurred ninety-nine times more commonly than paralytic polio. In this country, chronic appendicitis is neither an honorable nor acceptable diagnosis, whereas in Britain it is. We do not even know why appendicitis has become as uncommon as it has in a decade or two. So our knowledge of this banal little disease is very far from complete.

To act in regard to this disease, or perhaps any disease, as though our knowledge contained the thing itself is hubris. What our knowledge does contain is enough information to allow the usually successful diagnosis and sometimes successful treatment. So we must add these peculiarities of disease knowledge to the other deficiencies that arise from trying to equate categorizations of disease with true natural categories or even true, free-standing individual entities. Disease definitions, as undeniably useful as they are and have been, are essentially artificial. They represent man's inevitable drive to bring order to his perceptions by forming those perceptions into categories.

We have thus seen many things that compound our attempts to understand error in medicine. The first is the very way we have come to use the word error in a morally charged manner. We often equate error with failure, inadvertent ignorance, mistaken beliefs, wrong perceptions arising from our view of the world of

disease and the sick. We make equal these morally neutral phenomena with those where the physician is held responsible for an
action causally connected to an injury, real or supposed, suffered
by a patient. Earlier, I pointed out that when a patient suffers at
the hands of chance, the physician, on discovering this, may feel
badly for the patient or even for himself if he was the agent
through which chance operated. In other words, the physician
stands in subjective relationship to his patient such that, even
though mistakes beyond his control have occurred, he may feel
shame, guilt, sadness, or anger. While the rest of us may comfort
him by pointing out that he is not to blame, his feelings are not
inexplicable to us. It is in the nature of the relationship of the
physician to his sick patient that for the brief period of their
bond, the fate of the patient is part of the fate of the physician.
Worse for the one, perhaps, but part, nonetheless, of the other. Is
it any wonder, then, that physicians and patients (and thus, all of
us) should in so many ways support the illusion that fate is
within our control? But it is just those illusions that make it so
difficult to understand error. There is yet another problem that
prevents a more complete understanding of medical error in its
moral, social, and thinking spheres. That problem comes from
choosing this or that individual instance of disease as the conventional framework of reference from which to examine error in
medicine. Such a limited frame of reference is inadequate. For
one thing, diseases as we know them could conceivably be seen
as entities, but they are not individuals in the Gorovitz-MacIntyre
sense that salt marshes are, free standing and unique. Individuals
in the sense of salt marshes or hurricanes are acted on by outside
forces and act on their surroundings, but they are understandable
as wholes in themselves. Comprehensible as wholes, that is, with
the addition of one more element with which science deals
poorly—time. The relationships within and around individuals are
only understood as occurring through time.

Now if we return to our original case, what dimensions of it
will stand up to definition as an individual? Not merely the man
himself, because by himself, we do not know why he is in the
hospital. Not as "a case of cancer of the bladder," for that does
not tell us who he is, his age and the other conditions he had,
such as the eccentricity to morphine, that helped set the stage for

error. It is not until we have added to those the hospital and the set of physicians and the time in which the case occurred that we have the individual entity—free standing and unique.

To put it more simply, one cannot comprehend medicine by looking at disease entities alone. Each case, whether error is present or not, is like a stage play. A setting, an audience, a disease whose story is told, and a set of actors. Only by examining that piece of theatre—medicine's individual—can one gain understanding of error—or even of cure or care.

NOTE

1. William B. Schwartz, et al., "Decision Analysis and Clinical Judgment," *American Journal of Medicine*, 55 (October 1973), pp. 459-72.

Commentary

Errors in Medicine: Let Me Count Some Ways

H. Tristram Engelhardt, Jr.

ERIC CASSELL PROVIDES US WITH A CASE EXAMPLE, drawn from clinical practice, of the origin of error in medicine. This presentation is rich in issues and concerns that transcend medicine and have a bearing on our understanding of error in science and in human conduct generally. What I will offer here is an organization of the issues raised in his paper. I will do this around five sets of issues that Cassell interweaves throughout his paper: (1) the question of error; (2) the question of compensation through malpractice action; (3) the alluring seduction of false conceptions that, according to Cassell, misguide the practice of appreciation of medicine; (4) the role of ontological or disease-entity conceptions of medicine in the understanding of error in medicine; and (5) the Gorovitz-MacIntyre principle of the origin of error in the study of individuals.

I. Error

Eric Cassell holds that, in ordinary considerations of physicians, a physician is said to be in error if and only if (1) someone (the physician, his patient, or some other person) holds the physician to be "responsible" for his choice of action in treating a patient; (2) there is a causal relationship between the physician's action and the injury; (3) there is an injury or the awareness of a near injury.[1] Also, Cassell does not draw a distinction between inflicting injury which involves both damages and violation of someone's rights, and those damages in which no rights have been violated. A distinction of this kind would be useful in sorting out the many senses of error that Cassell catalogues.

It is worth distinguishing the questions that Cassell raises with regard to error into three categories: (A) he often asks who is responsible for the errors that occur in medical practice; (B) he is also interested in distinguishing among the different kinds of errors; (C) he points out that one should not equate failures with errors, or breaches of trust with commissions of error.

The question of who is responsible for the errors that occur in medicine is not only a matter of legal interest, but also bears on our understanding of the nature of medicine, its internal social structure, as well as our assessment of the scope of the physician's powers and, therefore, his accountability. Eric Cassell examines three possible answers to the question of who bears responsibility for medical error. The first and most obvious is the physician. It will suffice at this juncture to indicate that Dr. Cassell's paper lists errors of judgment, carelessness, over-zealousness, and culpable ignorance, to name a few, as origins of physician error. Usually these errors are portrayed as having a single, central actor who bears responsibility and accountability for the errors of his or her actions.

Of course, there is a second and more involved model that Eric Cassell employs in his account of the dispute between the urology resident and the internist. In Cassell's portrayal, the urology resident is in error and the internist is judging correctly. But, of course, it need not be so. In fact, it need not be the case that either one is wholly right or wholly wrong. That example, in short, raises questions of team responsibility and team error. It raises political issues, too—namely, how do individuals with conflicting judgments within a team resolve those conflicts in favor of one course of treatment.

The third type of case has no bearer of responsibility; there are many instances in which error occurs in the sense of the best not happening, but where no one can be held responsible. In a sense, to use the word "error" here is deceptive, as Cassell indicates. No one has made a mistake; no one's rights were invaded. Bad things simply happened. The best choice of treatment fails to be pursued because of our present state of imperfect knowledge, because of the ingredient fallibility of all agents, or because of what could be called the Gorovitz-MacIntyre principle (i.e., that individuals are knowable only up to a point, and that, therefore, the most appropriate treatment for them is knowable only up to a point). I do not believe that Dr. Cassell understands the Gorovitz-MacIntyre principle, and I will return to that issue in section five of this commentary.

Cassell's catalogue of error is quite diverse. I am able to group the examples and remarks he makes under eight headings: (1) technical errors—failure to employ recognized therapy (perhaps what is meant here is failure through lack of skill); (2) errors of judgment (i.e., a vincible failure to see clearly enough the factors to be weighed in deciding upon a course of treatment); (3) errors because of carelessness; (4) errors because of moral failings, such as a choice of an improper course of treatment out of venality or greed (e.g., unnecessary operations); (5) over-zealousness with regard to the practice of one's own art (e.g., an artist enjoys the performance of his art for its own sake—and that includes surgery); (6) error owing to the failure to follow good procedures such as entering into a hospital chart the reasons for and against a course of behavior, so as to make the general character of choices among modes of therapy more explicitly rational; (7) culpable ignorance; (8) subjectively judged error (the issue of the administration of the morphine could, albeit somewhat forced, be placed under this rubric: if one held that it was more important to suppress pain than prolong life, then use of the morphine, as Cassell indicates, is not an error. On the other hand, if one gives a greater value to extension of life, even if it involves a certain period of pain, the use of the morphine with its attendant risks raises the issue of whether an error was made). It is important to notice that the list of errors ranges from non-culpable to culpable error. Moreover, Dr. Cassell indicates important distinctions to be made among the varieties of culpable and non-culpable error.

A third general suggestion in Eric Cassell's paper is that we attend carefully to the meaning and use of the word and concept "error." He suggests that it is wrong to equate failure with error.

That is, it makes sense to say that the physician failed to cure the patient's cancer, even though the physician made no errors in treatment. Medicine in general and physicians in particular are not omnipotent. To fail is not to err. Moreover, one must distinguish error from breaches of trust or what Cassell terms "moral error." The failure of the surgeon to follow the course of recovery of the patient, the failure of the physician to come when called that Sunday night, are, if the physician is culpable, breaches of trust. On the other hand, all resources are finite, including the resources of physicians and surgeons, and one would want to know as well whether providing such follow-up or failing to come that Sunday evening was a reasonable or unreasonable expectation, given other concurrent commitments and the justifiable use by physicians and surgeons of their own time. This does not involve an analysis of error as much as it does an analysis of the nature and quality of trust that can exist between physicians and their patients.

In general, it would seem that this catalogue of errors can be reduced to those in which the damages the patient received are owing to: (1) intellectual errors—failures of the physician to judge clearly, or to act perceptively in the treatment of the patient because of his or her limited analytical ability: what I have in mind here are those cases of non-culpability where a physician finds him or herself in a position where the demands exceed skills; (2) errors owing to culpable ignorance or false arrogation of skills—those cases in which the physician could have, but did not, know better, or in which he could have referred the patient to a more skilled physician and therefore avoided the injury; (3) errors owing to the breach of the patient's trust in the physician. Here the breach is not that of failing to have the knowledge, skill, or intelligence that a patient could reasonably presume that a physician would have on the basis of the usual quality of care in the patient's community, but failures to be attentive or present when the patient has a right to presume that the physician would provide care; (4) that error which is simply owing to chance, or to the fact that patients as individuals are in the end never fully knowable and therefore not able to be treated without error (a set of errors that Cassell does not address).

II. Compensation

As this display of senses of error or an examination of the dictionary definition of error shows, the word has a broad set of meanings, including belief in what is untrue, violation of duty, deviating from a right course, and making a mistake. It is so diverse, though, that we would profit both in understanding error in medicine, and some basic ethical issues in science and medicine, by a more precise appreciation of the kinds and nature of errors that occur in science, medicine, and technology generally. Such distinctions would be particularly helpful for a better understanding of the practice of making compensation for errors in medical practice.

Eric Cassell suggests a number of different bases upon which decisions to give compensation may be made. The first and classical basis is culpable negligence, when compensation is made to recover damages and make the injured person whole. Such compensation is also given to dissuade future negligent actions (not to mention compensation made in virtue of criminal actions such as battery). Secondly, some of the issues to which Eric Cassell alludes suggest that courts are increasingly making awards on the basis of an informal principle of strict liability. That is, awards are being made not only because of culpable negligence, but also in instances of non-culpable negligence.

One can supply two general motives for such a practice. The first is to provide a covert form of insurance. As such, payment for injury is best not considered compensation (indemnification), but better understood as a form of recovery through an insurance policy for patients, paid for by physicians and ultimately by patients through higher medical fees. In such awards, no one is at fault, but society has acted covertly to provide individuals with a security against certain forms of damage. Secondly, one may also advocate recovery on the basis of strict liability in order to motivate greater interest in care and in the avoidance of error. Also, as Eric Cassell indicates, some compensation appears to be given on the false assumption that in every case of error someone must be to blame.

III. The Informal Fallacies of Error

This leads me to the list, which Eric Cassell's paper provides, of false but seductive ideas, informal fallacies concerning the understanding of error. More or less arbitrarily, I have reduced his remarks on this issue to five points: (1) there is the erroneous belief that people have only diseases that can be cured, and if a disease is not cured, or a deformity corrected, someone is to blame. This might be termed the fallacy of medical omnipotence. It is probably a lingering vestige of an older and more embracing fallacy of technological omnipotence.

(2) There is a general human inclination to hold that action is better than inaction. Thus, for example, the mere mention of medical nihilism is likely to suggest immorality. One should remember, though, that this human drive not only leads to aggressive surgery, but has also played a role since the very beginnings of medicine in such practices as bleeding, purging, blistering, etc. In this regard, one should recall the remarks of Hippocrates in *Epidemics*, "Declare the past, diagnose the present, foretell the future [but] help, or at least do no harm."[2]

(3) There is also the allure of practicing one's art for its own sake, even though it exists primarily as a service. This has been mentioned above when referring to the fact that it is quite understandable that surgeons would enjoy practicing surgery apart from any issue of being successful or not (i.e., in the sense of the patient surviving or not). The remark made in caricature, "the operation was a success, but the patient died," highlights this. Surgery, and medicine generally, is a pleasure to practice as an intellectual and technical enterprise, apart from any of the services it exists to deliver. The physician and surgeon can then be drawn to practice their art from this consideration of intrinsic reward, rather than with regard to the services to others that medicine and surgery offer.

(4) Again, one must distinguish failure from error. This is very much similar to the first point made, but is worth repeating separately. It is one thing to err and another thing not to be able to do anything but fail. Humans are often in the latter position. If one does not distinguish failure from error, one can then be sent

on impossible tasks of finding the culprits responsible for failure where no error was made (i.e., circumstances where no one can be reasonably said to be culpable for the failure). In short, one must learn that terrible things happen, even in medicine, for which no compensation can be extracted on the grounds of another's culpable error.

(5) Finally, one must, as Eric Cassell suggests, guard against an overestimation of our knowledge. This is in part a reiteration of the warning against the fallacy of medical omnipotence. But even given a recognition of the finitude of medical knowledge, one tends to overestimate its scope. Such an overestimation can lead to unwarranted disappointments and unjustified allegations of moral error.

IV. Disease Entities

Under the rubric of the symbolic meaning of disease, Cassell argues that diseases are viewed as both entities and symbols.[3] As a symbol, disease represents "a force to act." This point is, to say the least, made cryptically. I suspect he means that disease reminds us of our human finitude which we often wish to repudiate, if not at least in part overcome. As such, the diagnosis of disease elicits something close to a moral imperative to treat, to act. Cassell obliquely identifies a therapeutic imperative. That is, to say that someone is diseased is to say that he or she is in a state that ought to be treated. To characterize someone as diseased is not simply descriptive, it is normative—in fact, imperative. Though he does not say so clearly, I take it that Cassell thinks that this therapeutic imperative can be particularly misguided when it is combined with a view of diseases as things, entities. Thus, if to say someone has a disease is to urge treatment, and if diseases are things that can be best treated by being removed, then surgeons should cut them out, remove the "piece of disease."

Against this, Eric Cassell argues that diseases are not things at all, that what we call diseases are useful collections of phenomena constructed for particular purposes. In other words, he stands on the side of the functional or physiological theorists of disease against the ontological theorists of disease, who have held that diseases are things in the sense of actual entities or enduring constellations of phenomena which can be known and distinguished. Our knowledge of disease, according to Cassell, never contains the disease itself.[4] Even such a well-known phenomenon as appendicitis varies in its expression and is characterized differently depending upon the purposes and presuppositions of particular national groups of physicians (e.g., chronic appendicitis is a much more acceptable diagnosis in Britain than in the United States).[5] "Disease definitions, as undeniably useful as they are and have been, are essentially artificial. They represent man's inevitable drive to bring order to his perceptions by forming those perceptions into categories."[6] In short, Eric Cassell is, with respect to theories of disease, a nomenalist.

I take it that Dr. Cassell is warning us that we can err by acting on the basis of connotations (i.e., the symbolic function of disease) rather than the denotations of our concepts, or when we reify the concepts that we use (i.e., transform an essentially plastic and relational concept of disease into a rigid concept of disease entities). Independently of how one wishes to argue concerning issues of nomenalism in general, it is the case that "disease" does not name entities in the world as "cat" names cats, or "triangle," triangles. The reasons behind these differences are complex and include the fact that disease descriptions are different from disease explanations. Moreover, states of affairs count as diseases for various reasons, and disease explanations gather illness phenomena together on the basis of human goals, as much as on the basis of constraints imposed by an external reality.

V. The Gorovitz-MacIntyre Principle

Eric Cassell completes his critique of disease-entity accounts of illness with a critique of the argument by Gorovitz and MacIntyre that "precisely because our understanding and expectations of particulars cannot be fully spelled out merely in terms of lawlike generalizations and initial conditions, the best possible judgment

may always turn out to be erroneous, and erroneous not merely
because our science has not yet progressed far enough or because
the scientist has been either willful or negligent, but because of
the necessary fallibility of our knowledge of particulars."[7] In fact,
not only does Eric Cassell deny that disease entities are "individuals in the Gorovitz-MacIntyre sense,"[8] a point on which he is
correct, but he also seems to deny that patients are individuals in
that sense.

Now I don't know of anyone, especially Gorovitz and Mac-
Intyre, who holds that disease entities are individuals in the sense
that Gorovitz and MacIntyre speak of individuals (an exception
may have been Paracelsus). As a result, I am not at all clear
against whom Eric Cassell's argument is directed. It is the case
that individuals such as Sydenham and Sauvages held that diseases were entities—but not uniquely individual things, particulars in the Gorovitz-MacIntyre sense. If what Eric Cassell is
attacking are those theories which conceived of diseases as
wholes, as complete entities, then I think his argument succeeds,
but his reference to Gorovitz and MacIntyre is distracting.

On the other hand, if what Eric Cassell is arguing is that
individual patients are not particulars in the Gorovitz-MacIntyre
sense, but rather that the general context of physicians, patients,
and hospitals are such particulars,[9] then the matter is even more
difficult. What would be needed is an argument to show that such
whole contexts are describable as individuals in the way we
naively think patients are. Moreover, it would seem that what
would count for holding that the future of such contexts is not
derivable from abstract rules would hold as well against
being able to predict the behavior of individual patients—which
is the point made by Gorovitz and MacIntyre. In short, if Eric
Cassell wishes to hold that individual patients are not particulars
in the Gorovitz-MacIntyre sense, that their behavior can indeed
be predicted (e.g., which individuals will develop post-vaccinal
encephalitis, etc.—a proposition I do not believe he in fact
wishes to hold), an argument toward that end is needed.

Rather I believe Eric Cassell's point is this: medicine often errs
by focusing on diseases as if they were entities, to the neglect of
patients, and by failing to determine the proper care of patients
through reference to their context of care. The first set of errors

involves (1) a false reification of the concept of disease, (2) a misunderstanding of where the "real" reality lies—that is, the reality lies in the patient, not the disease, and (3) this false reification erroneously misdirects medical attention, often leading to other errors, e.g., unnecessary surgery. A second set of errors arises from failing to realize that the individual patient cannot be understood in isolation from his or her ambience—the role of "patient" is contextual.

VI. Conclusions

As usual, Eric Cassell has provided us with a rich and intriguing set of issues. He has shown that the problem of understanding medicine escapes the confines of medicine itself, and lands us in rather basic analyses of what we should mean by error, disease, and how we are to see generalizations operate in science. It is around these rather abstract considerations, as Eric Cassell has shown, that very practical issues, such as the treatment of patients and the awarding of recovery in malpractice suits, is based, In particular, we are left with the problem of sorting out the meanings and origins of error and how they contrast with concepts of failure and of breaches of trust, so as to highlight the basic ethical issues ingredient in science and technology. We need, in short, to establish the conceptual geography of erring, failing, and breaking trust. Though instances of each are allied one with the other, as the foregoing suggests, many confusions will be avoided by drawing distinctions, even if to some extent stipulative. We have, after all, the impression that there is a significant difference among (1) breaking trust with another and thus injuring him, though no issue of deficient knowledge or skill comes into question; (2) injuring another through culpable ignorance or lack of skill; (3) failing to achieve the goods and ends we may all wish to pursue because of no culpable deficiencies on our part. Finally, the resolution of these questions will require attention to the nexus of disease, patient, physician, health care team and hospital. In fact, it will reach beyond the hospital to such groups as the patient's family, the physician's family, and society.

NOTES

1. Eric Cassell, "Error in Medicine," pp. 300-301.
2. Hippocrates, *Epidemics I*, xi, trans., W. H. S. Jones, *Hippocrates*, (Cambridge: Harvard University Press, 1923), I, p. 165.
3. Cassell, "Error in Medicine," pp. 304-305.
4. Ibid, p. 307
5. Ibid.
6. Ibid.
7. Samuel Gorovitz and Alasdair MacIntyre, "Toward a Theory of Medical Fallibility," in *Science, Ethics and Medicine*, ed. by H. Tristram Engelhardt, Jr. and Daniel Callahan (Hastings-on-Hudson, N.Y.: Hastings Center, 1976), p. 262.
8. Cassell, ibid., p. 308.
9. Ibid., p. 309.

Preface

IN THE APOCRYPHAL Old Testament book of Ecclesiasticus, Jesus, son of Sirach, remarks that "the wisdom of a learned man is the fruit of leisure." (Ecclus. 38:25) Unfortunately, most interdisciplinary work has lacked this recommended leisure, or at least the time to allow issues to digest at leisure. Still, this project, well into its second year, has progressed to the point that some interdisciplinary themes have become apparent. Or, rather, a number of interdisciplinary connections between science and ethics have become clear. These have included: (1) reciprocal borrowings of concepts between science and ethics; (2) common problems concerning the meaning and scope of rational explanations and justifications; (3) special roles played by particular constellations of values in framing the sciences as professions; (4) causal influences on evaluations; and (5) the influence of values on explanations. In addition, there are some apparent dependencies of ethics (if not also science) upon transcendent values. These relations among disciplinary provinces led to the exploration of the conceptual, symbolic, and causal interconnections between the foundations of ethics and the sciences. Given this volume's concern with knowledge, values, and belief, the discussion here has embraced interrelations among science, ethics, and theology.

These explorations have included not only interdisciplinary analyses of common subject areas (e.g., the determination of the place of man in nature) or disputed intellectual territories (e.g., the biological versus the conceptual basis of ethical behavior). It has also led to initial comparisons of methods and criteria for valid reasoning in science and ethics (e.g., the role of values in scientific versus ethical reasoning). Comparative attention to methods is more difficult and will be given special attention in the fourth and last year of these volumes.

This final section of Volume II offers an explicit analysis of interdisciplinarity. Although the discussions in this project have, in general, been interdisciplinary in character, it is only in these last two essays that the concern shifts from method to methodology. That is, this section moves from engaging in an interdisciplinary enterprise to reflecting on the interdisciplinary character of that enterprise. Interdisciplinary method or approach to issues is itself made thematic in the two papers that follow.

Finally, as Corinna Delkeskamp indicates, interdisciplinary undertakings are dialectical in character—they must transcend particular disciplines without obliterating them. Only insofar as interdisciplinary investigations transcend disciplines do they succeed in their bridging functions. But only insofar as the disciplines bridged maintain their integrity, do the bridges lead from somewhere to somewhere. And finally, if this dialectic ceases to be dynamic, it crystallizes into yet another discipline, itself requiring interdisciplinary bridging. One can see how this happens not only in bioethics but also in philosophy, which should (to use a Miltonian play on etymology) be pontifical as bridge building, not pontifical as speaking with authority only for its own discipline.

In reading these essays one must distinguish a logical and psychological dimension of analysis. The logic of interdisciplinarity concerns the logic of interdependence among the concepts and methods of various disciplines. The psychology of interdisciplinarity concerns the heuristic of interdisciplinarity—how one can be brought to see things anew in one's own or in another's discipline, or to see connections between them. While the essay by Corinna Delkeskamp focuses primarily on the logic of interdisciplinarity, Eric Cassell's paper focuses primarily on the psychology of interdisciplinarity.

What follows is an analysis of interdisciplinarity combined with an analytic overview of the last two years of this project. The essays offer a critique of interdisciplinarity and, as well, a synoptic view of the first two volumes in terms of their interdisciplinary character. These two essays offer, as well, insight into the character of the interdisciplinary enterprise in general, complemented by a presentation of some of its more successful maneuvers and methods. In addition to providing some views of the foundations of ethics in relationship to the sciences, we hope to have developed as well a portrayal of the ways of achieving such views.

H.T.E.

Interdisciplinarity: A Critical Appraisal

Corinna Delkeskamp

MY REMARKS ON INTERDISCIPLINARITY will—for clarity's sake—be divided into three parts. The first section will present some general considerations in which the interdisciplinary endeavor is critically examined. In particular, I shall focus on conceptual puzzles involved in the arguments commonly adduced for the meaning and function of this endeavor. In the second section I shall illustrate my conclusions by reference to the essays in the first two volumes of *The Foundation of Ethics and its Relationship to Science.*[1] These essays are part of a project already into its second year. The project itself fosters an interdisciplinary dialogue centered around an attempt to analyze the foundations of ethics and the relationship between ethics and science. It thus provides an opportunity to specify the difficulties attending such a dialogue with reference to a concrete case study. My discussion of the essays contained in these volumes will, moreover, illustrate various degrees of sophistication which have entered into this dialogue. Finally, in the third section, I shall return to my general conclusions regarding interdisciplinarity, exposing their ethical bearing and specifying their philosophical significance as to the particular project under examination. In this way I hope to portray in a concrete fashion how the dialogue between disciplines should be understood and how its difficulties may be overcome.

I. General Critical Considerations

Any contemporary study of interdisciplinarity is hampered by the differing methods of investigation, areas of concern, and mutually incompatible terminologies in the literature available on the subject. Two stipulations from the Centre for Educational Research and Innovation[2] may serve as points of departure. First, *discipline* is defined as "a specific body of teachable knowledge with its own background of education, training procedures, methods and content areas"; second, *interdisciplinarity* is defined as "interaction among two or more different disciplines" ranging from "simple communication of ideas" to "mutual integration of concepts, methodology, procedures, epistemology, terminology, data . . ." Interdisciplinarity in this latter sense is usually seen as a step towards *transdisciplinarity* (i.e., a "common system of axioms for a set of disciplines") as its logical consequences.[3]

In view of these definitions and their implications, this first section will examine four arguments on behalf of interdisciplinary studies.[4] I shall hope to ascertain whether they can justify anything more than the pursuit of such studies as a complement to our traditionally accepted fields of scholarship. In particular I hope to determine whether there are good grounds for pursuing a transdisciplinary unification which would imply the abolishment of our present departmentalized academic learning.

1. The argument from the object of study. Research concerning issues at the boundaries of given disciplines has always required the cooperation of specialists from neighboring fields. Such cooperation is either restricted to providing additional information ("auxiliary" interdisciplinarity) or—at the other extreme—contributes to the development of new "inter-disciplines" between the established fields. A growing trend towards the study of borderline issues can be observed. Hence, theoretical frameworks should be designed to justify conceptually the resulting cooperation by a common epistemology, method, or purpose. In view of such a conceptual unity, assumed to be underlying the manifest diversity of disciplines, it is tempting to denounce the division of scholarly work into specialized departments as a state of alienation, and to infer that truth and salvation can be expected only from an eventual reunion.

This conclusion follows only if a claim for reconstructive intelligibility is confused with a claim for conceptual constitution—if what was achieved by the former is taken as credit for the latter. What started as a stipulative framework in terms of which the interdisciplinary endeavors already existing receive a unifying interpretation is confusedly taken as a definition for the very essence of these endeavors and is used to prove the need to pursue them exclusively. Historically speaking, interdisciplinary cooperation has been fruitful ever since at least the early nineteenth century, or since that very time in which an increasing differentiation of academic learning and crystallization of disciplinary methods and subject matters occurred. This cooperation was not impeded by progressing specializations, but derived from them the very concepts it would subsequently modify. Consider the conclusion advanced by Briggs and Michaud:[5]

> . . . change in the pursuit of intellectual enquiry itself and in the modes of intellectual discourse have rendered obsolete the organization of universities into vertical structures corresponding to the idea of "subjects" or "disciplines" and "faculties" or "departments".

This endorses a denial of those very presuppositions from which the unifying frameworks derive their stability and relevance.[6]

2. *The argument from social concerns.* Certain urgent societal issues are so complex that their solution requires not only communication among experts from various fields, but coordinated effort to integrate their approaches. This task can be effectively carried out only if the educational system is subjected to a thorough restructuring. The inconvenience involved in such a reorganization, it is assumed, will be amply compensated by a more successful application of the knowledge thus unified.[7] This assumption, however, itself stands in need of justification. The quest for unification of methods rests on a philosophical conviction that a subject matter, because it transcends the boundaries of any given discipline, requires a method which similarly transcends any particular discipline. Although methodological considerations aiming at philosophical consistency are to be cherished for their heuristic value, it does not follow that their pursuit will always pay off in a successful application. A poor methodology

(as distinguished from poor method) sometimes admits of useful results, while immaculate methodological theorizing may prove— in practice—sterile.

Furthermore, the adaptation of academic structures exclusively to societal needs, as suggested in such arguments, would reduce the function of scholarly learning to solving predetermined social problems.[8] Social practice would become a function of the results of academic research, while research would in turn degenerate into a function of immediate societal needs. In the account of Eric Jantsch[9] a supra-disciplinary systems-theory is developed. Its application is designed to guarantee the prevalence of one particular, ideologically determined definition of "useful" scholarship throughout the academic world. Morgan[10] is correct in observing that the established disciplines are unable to deal with the great human problems confronting us. But in implying that we should abandon disciplines altogether, he disregards the possibility that a relatively independent academic enterprise might uncover empirical data and evaluative categories on its own. He denies, thus, that such an endeavor could give reasoned voice to societal problems not previously addressed.

3. The existential argument. The case for interdisciplinarity rests on a further belief that human life in modern society is fragmented into unconnected segments of activities. It appears alienated from a primordial wholeness to which it must be restored. For the subject matter of academic learning this implies that the division between what concerns the investigator as a human being and what concerns him professionally must be overcome. Man should finally be made the proper study of man. The various disciplines, which are, in the present university system, abandoned to issues irrelevant to humanity, should be subsumed under anthropology or the life sciences.[11] It seems as if an unhappily phrenologized university should no longer be allowed the use of its several organs to pursue the disparate activities of quasi-sensing, remembering, analyzing, associating, imagining, and willing, but must be granted a divinely instantaneous intuition (which is *totum in toto* and *totum in qualibet parte*, like a scholastic soul that has swallowed its body).

On the level of teaching, vocational considerations must take precedence over research. Social practice, presumed the proper focus of man's humanity, must be made to encompass all scholarly activities. These activities can then be subsumed under the general headings of "communicative interaction," "realization of purpose," and "optimization of benefits by minimizing the costs." Advanced in support of interdisciplinary restructuring, this quest for "wholeness" is construed on the analogy of a claim for natural rights—it points to an obligation of the community. Understood as a social need, this quest for wholeness must be collectively satisfied. It can be so satisfied only by reducing the complexity of human externalization. Yet it is this complexity which would have warranted the relevance of such wholeness, if its realization had been conceived as a personal task.[12]

4. The ethical argument. The existential concern is complemented by an interpretation of the ethical dimension of disciplinary and interdisciplinary engagements. Dissatisfaction with the established university structure arises partially from a disenchantment with the contrast between ideal and actual academic humanism. The accomplished (and tenured) experts in special fields are denounced as creatures of settled habits, lacking in information, subject to structural inertia, moved by a secret anxiety about the morrow and by a fear of the unknown (Briggs and Michaud, p. 192 f).

> Modern thinking typically carries the seal of a 'field' of 'discipline.' The scholar sees himself committed to the study of physics, biology, psychology, or literature. His work is governed by a sense of responsibility to his profession. The primary commitment of a person engaged in human studies, on the contrary, is not to a field, but to comprehension of man's humaneness and his situation in our time. The person's chief responsibility is not to a profession but to all those who would turn to him for help in their own effort to seek understanding of human life and its problems. (Morgan, p. 263)

This "human discipline" is the discipline "of an independent and responsible thinker," who has "no fixed criteria," who "does his utmost to respect the reality he confronts," "to be attentive to other person's ideas" and is prepared to "faithfully communicate his understanding." (p. 265)[13]

In juxtaposing a commitment to a discipline with a commitment to man's humaneness, Morgan separates humaneness from man's intellectual history. That history, after all, is embodied in the multiplicity of aspects, methods and goals constituting the present fields. In this sense, the definition of "discipline" offered by CERI (cf. p. 2) and accepted by many writers on the subject must be considered incomplete.[14] Areas of scholarship must be granted their own histories; these are indispensable for understanding the present set of norms which characterize these disciplines. They also provide an arsenal of concepts and presuppositions through which criticism and intelligent change may occur. A clear assessment of this historical dimension is significant in two respects. First, this assessment is a condition for securing the *good* effects of those "humanistic intentions," which have been used to repudiate the relevance of that dimension. No "feeling of responsibility" and no amount of "utmost effort" can compensate for a lack of historical perspective. For perspective alone allows one to check one's benevolent designs against the fate of previous analogous endeavors, and to compensate for the blinding effects of present ideologies by comparing them with their predecessors. Second, only a thoughtful choice among the values of the past and a reflective modification of established categories can enable us to acknowledge what we wish to overcome, and to show our gratitude toward our academic teachers through pertinent criticism. The commitment to established disciplines is a commitment to the preservation and transformation of tradition. Thus, it balances the concern with the human condition of the present and future (which underlies the argument for interdisciplinarity) by a concern with the humanity of the past.[15]

It may indeed be one of the functions of professional and academic jargon to forge obstacles for an outsider. But the specific terminologies have been defined and refined in the process of specifying a subject matter and body of knowledge. The hermetic character of a terminology is thus a necessary condition for the disclosure of more-than-common-sensical differentiations in need of study. The difficulty of communicating beyond the barriers of the field is a natural consequence for there being something worthy to communicate.[16]

The case for interdisciplinarity is, as a result, much weaker than is generally supposed. The arguments usually forwarded for interdisciplinary studies at most justify those studies as a desirable complement to our traditional scholarly pursuits. The arguments, though, are not strong enough to establish the need for abolishing these various traditional fields and replacing them with a single unified transdisciplinary framework.

II. Diacritical Examination of a Special Case

In order to illustrate the consequences which follow from my conclusions of the first section, I shall now turn to an example of interdisciplinary studies *in vivo*—the first two volumes of the series *The Foundation of Ethics and Its Relationship to Science*. Here I shall attempt to map the conceptual bases upon which a "disciplined" interdisciplinarity, or interdisciplinarity as a complement to disciplinary studies can be justified.[17] To begin with, I shall summarize the particular difficulties which have arisen for the chosen example and which have presented obstacles to the interdisciplinary dialogue. As a result, three questions will be posed concerning the possibility and the relevance of such a dialogue. As a condition for answering these questions, I shall examine the essays published in the two volumes. These essays will be scrutinized as to the various understandings of interdisciplinarity which implicitly characterize their methods. I shall arrange these essays in such a way that their discussion can ascend from the less to the more adequate notions of interdisciplinarity betrayed by them.

Most examinations of interdisciplinarity either aspire to overarching theoretical schemes for unification or else focus on experimental educational programs.[18] In contrast, I shall analyze the results of interdisciplinary discussions addressed to a societal problem described in Daniel Callahan's introductory report on "The Emergence of Bioethics" (Vol. I). Such discussion takes place in what Callahan calls the "field" of Bioethics (or, for that matter, the more encompassing consideration of the relation of ethics and science), and it encounters two immediate obstacles to fruitful study. The first arises if "Bioethics" is subsumed under one of the already existing disciplines, as a special area to which its method can be applied. As a result, the participants disagree which of those disciplines is best qualified for such a function, and which other ones should be reduced to providing merely auxiliary information. The second obstacle arises, if "Bioethics" is considered an interdisciplinary discipline in its own right. As a result, this new discipline has been challenged to justify its independent status according to both the standards of academic fields in general and the political influence this supposed field has been acquiring in particular.

These obstacles arise from different attempts to avoid the pitfalls of interdisciplinary communication. In the first case, the interdisciplinary enterprise is surrendered to one of the existing disciplines; in the second case, it is transformed into yet another department of study. Part of the difficulty in establishing a balanced cooperation for the particular project here discussed seems to derive from the peculiar combination of disciplines involved. The majority of claims about interdisciplinarity have concerned the social and the natural sciences.[19] The essays in the two volumes, however, focus on values and reason, knowing and caring, progress and responsibility. They involve the sciences—here including medicine—and the humanities—here, in particular, moral philosophy. We are, thus, led to consider a third obstacle to interdisciplinary study, peculiar to our chosen example. While philosophy allows one to address explicitly the ethical implications of scientific knowledge as applied to society, the participation of philosophy as a discipline different in kind seems to suggest an inequality in the interdisciplinary cooperation.

These three obstacles lead to three questions concerning our project of arguing for a complementarity of disciplinary and interdisciplinary studies: (1) Since the *practical* advantages or disadvantages attending various methods of multidisciplinary cooperation are difficult to ascertain (particularly in the case of our chosen example), we should ask what the *conceptual* advantages or disadvantages of these methods are for the participating disciplines? Granting that every interdisciplinary project is as good as its (disciplinary) input, can we understand intra-disciplinary work in such a way that the quality of this input in turn is understood to depend on some interdisciplinary inspiration? (2) Can the problem of communication across the academic fields be solved in some way other[20] than imposing the language of one such field

on all the others, or by generating a new disciplinary language
for another inter-discipline?[21] (3) Is there a way in which philosophy can enter into a truly interdisciplinary engagement? And how
does this way relate to any ethical meaning imputed to "interdisciplinarity"? In order to answer these questions it will be
necessary to investigate the various understandings of how disciplines relate to one another, which are implicitly exemplified in
the essays to be examined. By discussing these several kinds of
interdisciplinary efforts I shall hope to isolate general characteristics which determine the value of the interdisciplinary enterprise
when rightly understood.

Bernard Towers, in his essay "Toward an Evolutionary Ethics"
(Vol. II), has interpreted the title of the published series as
suggesting a priority for the metaphysical basis of an ethical
theory which must subsequently be "applied" to the sciences and
to medicine. He maintains that this understanding of the interdisciplinary task should be reversed. A properly evolutionary
biology, in that it delineates the development of those "increasingly complex nervous systems without which conscious
awareness and ultimately ethical decision-making would not have
been possible," should provide the scientific foundation for sensible philosophizing.

In a very different spirit Michael Scriven, in "The Science of
Ethics" (Vol. 1) has made a similar claim: Ethics is the "em-
press" of the sciences, and controls all their applications. Yet she
is qualified for this office only because she herself has been
established on a scientific basis. While for Professor Towers the
paradigmatic science is determined by biological evolution, Professor Scriven defines it in terms of game theory. In both cases
philosophical ethics is grounded on a supposition not philosophically reflected upon, namely that the survival of species or
individual, respectively, is the most fundamental value.

John Ladd, on the other hand, endeavors to disprove what he
takes to be a claim on behalf of scientists' professional commitments. If the search for truth is man's noblest enterprise and the
values realized in scientific activity are superior in rank to other
values, the scientist may claim that no genuine value-conflict can
arise out of the pursuit of scientific goals. In his essay "Are
Science and Ethics Compatible?" (Vol. I), Ladd addresses the

issue of such commitments versus the scientist's social responsibility. He solves it by arguing that claims concerning values
have to be rationally defended. He shows the proofs which can
be offered for the existence of "scientific values" to be inconclu-
sive. Hence there exists no ground for an ethical commitment to
science. His position seems to imply that since the ethical value
of scholarly pursuits as such cannot be proven, some moral
authority outside of science must be appealed to whenever conflicting societal values to be realized by scientific activity require
a decision.

And again in a very different spirit, Lester King, in "Values in
Medicine" (Vol. I), has made what amounts to a similar claim.
There are genuine value issues implied in the scientific, practical
and social aspects of medicine. These aspects, as they constitute
different value systems, give rise to ethical conflicts. Such conflicts, especially as they may arise from the physician's commitment to the well-being of his patient and from his scientific
interest in an unusual "case," are exposed in greater detail in
Stephen Toulmin's "The Meaning of Professionalism" (Vol. II).
Yet, unlike Toulmin, Professor King relies on the philosopher to
provide "an ethical theory," which, it is hoped, will solve the
problem.

It cannot be our task in the present inquiry to quarrel about the
philosophical difficulties involved in these suggestions. Obviously
the "facts" chosen by Towers and Scriven presuppose some decision concerning relevance. The derivation of an "ought" from an
"is," even if we disregard the logical pains involved in the
operation, requires (in all non-trivial cases) that the particular
determination of what "is" in the premise be justified by reasoning. It is the acceptability of that reasoning on which the persuasive power of the conclusion will depend. The assumption in
both papers, moreover, that survival is the greatest good, is
powerfully repudiated by Professor MacIntyre's deathbound dignity (Vol. II).[22]

Professor Ladd's paper, to continue this review, contains some
problematic metaphysical assumptions. His argument seems to
reflect an earlier systematic account of the interdisciplinary affairs, namely Kant's *Streit der Fakultäten*. In this quarrel conducted between the three higher faculties—theology, juris-

prudence, medicine—and philosophy, as the lower faculty, the struggle is to win the favor of the public. For the analogy to work in a contemporary American setting we must replace theology by the empirical sciences, which sciences Kant had still reserved for the philosophical faculty (since their object is the truth). Then for Ladd, just as for Kant, it is the task of philosophy exclusively to examine the teachings of the other disciplines and to judge them in view of what is true and what promotes the well-being of the public. Its jurisdiction over truth derives from philosophy's unique academic freedom. Its competence concerning the public good derives from an appeal to the only source of public happiness, the liberty of rational beings. For Kant the quarrel between philosophy and the other faculties arises only when they transgress the proper limits of their competence and arrogate the determination of public well-being to their own specialized ideologies. John Ladd, by contrast, is much less tolerant. His *onus probandi* rule (cf. p. 11f.) does not even grant the sciences their own professional ethos. But then his rule supposes either that something exists as a matter of fact only if reasons can be given for it (which is false), or that something exists as relevant for philosophy only under this condition. In the latter case Professor Pellegrino's testimony[23] to the real efficacy of a scientific ethos in the minds of scientists reduces the relevance of a philosophizing in which being is recognized only insofar as there are arguments for it.

One readily perceives that there is something inappropriately "beckmesserian" about philosophical quibbling with attempts to establish an interdisciplinary discourse. The fact, however, that these attempts lay themselves open to such "professional" attacks must either imply that interdisciplinary endeavors are, in principle, not up to disciplinary standards or that present endeavors could be improved upon.

In order to clearly distinguish the several senses in which the interdisciplinary dialogue can be understood, let us turn to one of the earliest documents of such an encounter: The Platonic *Symposium*. In this work, just as in the example studied here, representatives from various disciplines are engaged in examining the interrelations between society, ethics, and the life sciences. There, just as here, the manner in which that subject matter is defined in the various speeches, acquires a symbolic significance for the manner in which the participants envisage their interdisciplinary interaction among one another. We shall merely have to replace the task of praising *Eros*—which provides the occasion for the Platonic dialogue—by the problem of how to define Bioethics, and see how far the analogy will carry us. Bioethics (our more particular example of the interplay of ethics and science), then, will appear as the child of the biomedical sciences and of ethics (or, more generously, of philosophy). It is, like the Eros in Diotima's account, a product of poverty (as philosophy claims to "know nothing") and of (scientific) contrivance, who is the son of invention.[24] But whether the drunkenness of contrivance, by which poverty sought to "enrich" herself, came from divine inspiration or just from an intoxication with the spirits of the time must now be investigated. Let us first review the essays mentioned above and see how the Platonic categories can be applied to them.

In Michael Scriven's account, that (interdisciplinary) child accuses his parents of incestuous relations, for ethics (as the mother) conceived by science her own son—a state of affairs complicated by the fact that ethics is equally said to have descended from that son, who is therefore her father as well. A similar inbreeding is suggested in Bernard Towers's theory, but here it was the father (science) who abused his daughter (ethics) to beget the interdisciplinary result. By contrast, John Ladd appears to view the child as engaged in disproving its father's claim to have effected it alone by a sort of "androgenesis," and that science and ethics, being "logically incompatible," are a fortiori distinct and thus his natural parents. Finally, in the case of Lester King, the child is busy properly administrating the mother's assets in values, as they are constantly in danger of being squandered by the trouble-ridden biomedical father.

In each of these cases the fairly scandalous background stories can be thought to account for the ensuing interdisciplinary battle of arguments: No universal agreement will credit a position in which the independent standing of one of the participating disciplines is denied. But perhaps it is a mistake to limit the purpose of disciplinary communion to the begetting of children. The higher erotic activities, after all, aim toward "procreating beautiful speeches."[25] The preceding moralistic considerations could, then, be replaced by a methodological account. The positions quoted above each subsume the liabilities of one discipline under those of the other. They thus repudiate the very conditions which would make interdisciplinary reflection possible. To use a further platonic suggestion—should not interdisciplinarity be, instead, an intermediate spirit,[26] a messenger to convey and interpret addresses from one field to the other, bridging the gap between them and preventing the universe of learning from "falling apart"?

Stephen Toulmin's deliberations on "Ethics and Social Functioning: The Organic Theory Reconsidered" (Vol. I) deal with an "interplay" between biology, medicine, and human values. On the one hand, medical practice and biological theory furnish values upon which ethical thought may reflect. Toulmin emphasizes the problematic aspect of this relation when he discusses the political use of outdated biological models: It is by reference to such models that conservative views of social values acquire a pseudo-scientific rationality. On the other hand, we learn from the history of physiology that basic concepts of this field in turn depend on external value judgments. This historical account may be used to illustrate, as a point in method, how to expose value assumptions which are unconsciously taken for granted within the scientific thought of a given time and which, therefore, encourage the apologetic use of such thought in political discourse. On a methodological level, these hidden value implications can be taken to provide a common ground on which ethics and biology may conduct a more properly interdisciplinary dialogue in which each discipline can scrutinize its dependence on the other. (As a practical consequence, a more enlightened usage of biological imagery in political arguments may ensue.)

In a discussion of cognitive categories rather than of value implications, Marx Wartofsky examines a similar interplay between philosophical epistemology and its relation to the medical intertwining of theory and praxis. In "The Mind's Eye and the Hand's Brain: Toward an Historical Epistemology of Medicine" (Vol. I), he, as well, has given an historical account, but now of the influence epistemological frameworks within disciplines exert on one another. And again through this account a methodological condition is provided for philosophy and medicine to reinterpret their respective conceptual schemes with regard to one another.

Both cases present "more properly" interdisciplinary dialogues because judgments are no longer pronounced by one discipline over the other. Rather, once the disciplines discover their common conceptual roots, each comes to review its own categories. Moreover, both accounts piously follow the conditions laid down for the Platonic messenger-spirit:[27] conveying prayers (for enlightenment) and sacrifices (of mutual self-criticism) from the earth (defined by biology and political thought in Toulmin's, or by medicine and philosophy in Wartofsky's case) to the heaven of historical contemplation, from whence he returns with the corresponding commands and rewards.

But neither of them presents the required dialogue in "quite" the proper way as appears from a methodological deformity in the procreated speeches. Indeed, biology and medicine are encouraged to become philosophical, philosophy is asked to consider its medical roots, and politics is enjoined to be more serious about the biological facts underlying its metaphors. However, in each of these cases such interdisciplinary therapy is prescribed by a discipline whose qualifications are not in turn critically examined—history. Yet a historical perspective is itself a historical phenomenon, and the presuppositions of any form of historicism involve philosophical assumptions which must be subjected to philosophical analysis. Thus, on the methodological level—just as before on the level of method itself (where disciplines were simply subsumed under one another)—one discipline is granted a prerogative over the others, or critical reflection among disciplines is demanded from an uncritical and unreflected position. (This same diagnosis holds for Jack Bemporad's "Morality and Religion" [Vol. II] where a theological perspective is recommended as a common ground—of unquestionable authority—for ethics and science to become transparent to one another.)

It is necessary, therefore, to proceed to yet another stage of the Platonic presentation. Indeed, the lover, as he ascended in the mysteries of contemplation, has learned to direct his prayers and supplications to a beloved only insofar as he has recognized in him beauty—absolute, separate, simple, everlasting,[28] and, hence, divine (up to this stage the deification of history—or theology—in the last three examples seems unobjectionable). But immediately after this Socratic interpretation, Alcibiades' intoxicated description of Socrates portrays a reversion to the roles of lover and beloved, where messages of prayers and commands between them can be thought to be returned on equal terms. Thus, the interdisciplinary inspiration must affect every one of the parties involved if methodological consistency of the resulting speeches is to be warranted. While such an inspiration is lacking in the previous essays, it can be shown to move the authors I shall consider next.

An interesting intermediate position is presented in Gunther Stent's paper on "The Poverty of Scientism" (Vol. II). He establishes a fundamental difference between the sciences and the humanities. Propositions of the former can be validated but are irrelevant to the exploration or even realization of societal values. Propositions of the latter cannot be validated but address the humanely important issues. Such rigid separation of what is scientifically "true" from what is valued for social practice may lead us to conclude that Stent repudiates the relevance of interdisciplinary cooperation. Yet with his structuralistic interpretation of biology, Stent provides an "intermediate" field between the truth-finding sciences and the value-finding humanities. He applies this interpretation first to Kant's epistemology. Kant's answer to the question of how science is possible is given in terms of a categorial reconstruction. Thus the discovery of deep structures which the mind has phylogenetically acquired can be taken as scientific corroboration of Kant's quasi-categorial grammar for framing empirical judgments. Second, this interpretation of biology is used to corroborate in a similar way Kant's answer to the question of how morality is possible. Stent assumes a corresponding "moral deep structure" which allows for the several moral imperatives on the surface level to partake in a common principle.[29]

Yet, whereas Kant takes pains to explain the validity of moral judgments by reference to the rational principle in human beings, Stent finds the rational and the moral deep structures not only different from but incompatible with one another. The resulting theory is no longer philosophical but scientific (in a speculative sense of the term). It is no longer a conceptual framework designed to show the validity of scientific knowledge and moral obligation and to interpret empirical findings about the knowing and moralizing subject. Instead, it is a theoretical account designed to accommodate empirical findings according to standards of scientific knowledge derived from what is assumed to be evolutionary, i.e., empirical facts. What was stipulated as value in Kant is now stipulated as a fact. Yet value questions reappear in a final ethical twist to Stent's argument: Given the fact that one particular kind of rational deep structure has been favored by evolution, should we welcome the rationale of that evolution and endeavor to complete the task accordingly? Should genetic engineering be directed towards setting our moral grammar "straight"? Or should we try to make "ethical" sense of our paradoxical condition?

What is—in view of the interdisciplinary enterprise—interesting in Stent's essay is the manner in which the sciences and the humanities, while remaining fundamentally distinct (biology is still a science, only its structuralistic interpretation links it with linguistics and psychology), are made to relate internally to one another. The biological concern for the evolution of the human species is used to integrate in scientific terms those very facts which can be taken to account for the possibility of the humanities. Conversely, an ethical evaluation of the possible consequences flowing from such a universalized science is called for. Thus a sense of interdisciplinarity can be conceived that involves not merely an external application of the peculiar categories of one party to the method or subject matter of the other. It rests, instead, on a systematic conceptual justification of the liability of both the sciences and humanities to consider one another's issues as their own and to reflect upon their own in terms of one another.

Similar conditions for the possibility of an interdisciplinary discourse are exposed in Lappé's essay on "The Non-Neutrality of Hypothesis-Formulation" (Vol. I). He opposes two common assumptions: one, that "scientific scrutiny and criticism are essential to the process of justification, not that of discovery" (p. 96), and the other, that social concerns pertain only when the practical application of scientific findings is at stake. Lappé holds that in the very activity of formulating hypotheses and choosing which to test, the possibility of epistemological mistakes (where the immanent standards of the craft are violated) combines with the influence of the prevailing world view (encompassing judgments concerning societal values). These determine in advance what later is claimed as purely scientific knowledge.

Thus, Lappé considers even scientific hypotheses to be the result of an activity which is relevant in societal terms. Yet his account differs from a simple subsumption of such purely scientific activity under the categories of the social sciences. An internal analysis of the presuppositions and implications of scientific activities has itself furnished the facts to which sociological categories can, as a consequence, be properly applied. An external imposition is replaced by an internal disclosure. As a result, the social sciences are confronted with a body of observations which would not have surfaced in a purely sociological analysis. Furthermore, at the heart of what has been considered a purely scientific concern, an intriguing possibility has been exposed. Scientists, in their scientific criticism of hypotheses, may reap advantage from considering the sometimes blinding effects of underlying value prejudices.

This extension of the scope within which an investigator can reconsider his science in terms of the humanities, was possible because Lappé used the concepts of a philosophical hermeneutics to criticize some basic tenets of the scientific understanding of science. But his appropriation of a philosophical method for modifying a scientific prejudice raises a corresponding challenge for philosophy. Once hypotheses have been classified by the proper experts themselves as, for example, "socially invidious," it becomes incumbent upon philosophy to reconsider the grounds on which those "social and moral norms" are established, and to examine whether they depend on such purported "facts" as might be disproven by the hypothesis in question. While scientists thus come to envisage the "moral costs" of testing or not testing given assumptions, moralists will have to scrutinize whether the "conceptual costs" of considering such "moral costs" are really balanced by the dignity of the moral values at stake.

An interesting extension of such an understanding is presented by the studies of Eric Cassell. His quest for a "disciplined applied moral philosophy" in "Moral Thought in Clinical Practice" (Vol. I) is not really directed toward an extension of philosophy's competence. It implies a more radical necessity for philosophy to reconsider those concepts which, when applied to the clinician's practice, fail adequately to account for his concerns. Professor Cassell argues that the abstract nature of philosophical considerations favors a one-sided attention to the extreme or tragic cases and thus neglects the daily and seemingly trivial but more urgent ethical issues. Yet Cassell overestimates what philsophy can do when he demands of it guidance in dealing with individual cases. Rather, a specification of the general principles of ethics, established by clinicians themselves, is needed for the practice of medicine in order to fill the gaps left by philosophy. Only after such a "particularizing code" has been formulated by medical practitioners and has provided a new subject to which the concepts of moral philosophy are applicable, will the concept of individuality itself (and its logical relations to other philosophical universals), as constitutive of such a code, have to be developed within philosophy.[30]

Thus Samuel Gorovitz and Alasdair MacIntyre undertake in "Toward a Theory of Medical Fallibility" (Vol. I) to specify philosophically a notion of particularity. In their effort to establish a knowledge of particulars alongside that of universals, they argue for a philosophical readjustment of the concept of knowledge such that it can account for both general and particular subject matters. They recognize that the previous philosophical understanding of knowledge as essentially universal, when applied to the sciences and to medicine, has failed to do justice to the problems inherent in those fields.[31]

The essays by Cassell and MacIntyre-Gorovitz, while dealing with ethical and epistemological issues respectively, do so in a manner which argues for the possibility as well as for the need of interdisciplinary communication. This communication is characterized by the discovery that categories used in one discipline (i.e., medicine) depend on categories developed in the other (i.e., philosophy). Hence any insufficiency attending their derivative use (in medicine) implies a challenge for medicine to specify the required modifications, and for philosophy to effect corresponding adjustments in its own categorical system. In a similar vein, H. Tristram Engelhardt's "Human Well-Being and Medicine"

(Vol. I) has drawn attention to the vagueness attending both the philosophical and the medical understanding of what are properly human functions and goals. He has argued the need for more concrete definitions of the concepts of well-being, health, and disease within these disciplines. Such definitions, however, can only be reached on the ground of a consideration of categories taken over from one field into the other. The interdisciplinary dialogue, thus understood, leads not merely to a mutual consideration of one another's issues, but occasions a critical revision of conceptual assumptions within each discipline.

III. Metacritical Conclusions

Given this review of the interdisciplinary endeavor at hand, it is now possible to return to our three questions concerning the possibility and relevance of such an endeavor. In order to specify an answer to these questions, I shall first—as a result of the foregoing discussion—envisage an idealized version of the several phases which an adequately interdisciplinary entertainment requires.

The first phase is one of exposition or of "external" criticism. At this stage, experts from various fields learn about how their own professions are being viewed in terms of the other disciplines. Conversely, each expert externally applies the categories of his own field to each of the other fields and exposes his own knowledge to the distorting impact of a translation into a foreign variety of knowledge. The second phase is one of solitary confinement, or of "internal" criticism: Each specialist, on the grounds of his professional acquaintance with his own field, seeks to uncover areas to which those foreign concepts could be internally applied—areas which provide those concepts with appropriate material. In the third phase, finally, each participant is presented with modified self-interpretations of the other disciplines, resulting from the application of terms he had originally used (as an outsider), but now to more adequately determined materials. Such previously unsuspected ranges of application, however, require in turn an adjustment in one's own understanding of these terms in order to accommodate the novel facts. This phase may be considered one of reflective criticism, and will obviously result in modified external criticism, thus requiring new meditative monologues, and so on, until all participants and funds are exhausted.[32]

The essays in the series, *The Foundation of Ethics and Its Relationship to the Sciences*, are, thus, both results of previous, and conditions for further, more fruitful interdisciplinary study. They are *results* in that they betray questions and problems within a given discipline which presuppose an exposure to the concepts and methods of other disciplines. As a consequence, when scientists themselves are motivated to exhibit the ethical implications of scientific activities, the philosophical considera- tion of these implications may result in more than just a confir- mation of what is already known, or in more than a simple reassertion of philosophical positions. These essays indicate a *need* for further such cooperation in order to stimulate the re- quired realignment, wherever the concepts originating in one field fail in another. Furthermore, if the reflection on ethical implica- tions of scholarly activity has been introduced into some scientific fields, then a philosophical account of such reflection will require that an analogous consideration be inaugurated for the ethical implications of philosophical activities. This will result in a cor- responding revision of philosophy's understanding of itself. Once, for example, the dichotomy of internal and external criteria for evaluating science breaks down—as is suggested in the essay by MacIntyre and Gorovitz—it becomes equally necessary to re- evaluate the corresponding philosophical distinction between mo- rality as an intrinsic and prudence as an extrinsic virtue—an endeavor which the study by Burrell and Hauerwas[33] seems to undertake. The interdisciplinary implications of an exchange be- tween specialists from various disciplines can then be measured by the change in self-understanding achieved.[34]

The question about how interdisciplinary communication is possible can now be answered. Such communication is possible by an alternation between "everyday language" and the "technical language" of the various disciplines in oscillating phases of inter- action and reflection. Yet the "everyday language," by which an expert communicates with a non-expert, differs from that em- ployed by the non-expert. The specific nosology and syntax governing the language of his discipline operates as a screen, imposing certain restrictions on and necessitating a certain stretching of the ordinary usage. Just as a Russian will teach us Russian by the very manner in which he violates and improvises upon the rules of English grammar, so the expert from one field using ordinary language to address issues within another field will teach the specialist of the latter the rules of the former. Correspondingly, even though the idiom of a certain discipline is maintained, its referents will—in the second phase—be subjected to the scrutiny of foreign categories and its concepts will—in the third phase—be confronted with issues previously overlooked. This terminology will, therefore, suffer an extension or shifting in the meanings of its terms, or in the formation rules of its propositions. The miracle of "mutual understanding" can be thought to manifest itself slowly in the process of each participating discipline as it is modified by its own adherents in such a manner as to provide the other disciplines with matters ready for their conceptual digestion.

The dichotomy between specialists and interdisciplinary dilettantes could then be replaced by a multiplicity of degrees to which such specialists may practice their interdisciplinary engagement. Instead of creating yet other "fields" calling for further inter-interdisciplinary mediations, a gradual proliferation of "foreign" perspectives in the studies of the field itself would slowly transform its "provincialism" into an enlightened "cosmopolitan" orientation.

The question concerning the desirability of interdisciplinary cooperation for the participating disciplines themselves can now be decided as well: The resulting non-trivial extension in the range of application of categories within a discipline is desirable to the degree that such extension calls for conceptual differentiation and, thus, for a growth in reflective self-understanding. In this sense the increasing transparency of disciplines to one another can be expected to contribute to better disciplinary work.

It must be noted, however, that the criterion for "better" disciplinary work is primarily philosophical; conceptual differentiation and reflective criticism of implicitly functioning presuppositions are the mark of philosophical thoughtfulness. Would not our argument for interdisciplinarity therefore suffer from an inherent contradiction? For philosophy enters not only on the level of disciplines into the actual business, but seems, according to its own provincial preferences, to legislate the manner in which that business ought to be conducted and to determine its goal.

It is at this point that the special status of philosophy as a discipline must be considered, and that the "spirit" of that discipline must be appealed to. It is inherent in a truely philosophical understanding of philosophical thought that the validity of such thought be critically relativized. Philosophers are not presented with data; they invent them. Hence, philosophers are aware that their concepts are not immediately "applicable" to issues outside of their theoretical context. They may indulge in seemingly unrestrained speculation when devising these frameworks, but they are skeptical as to the practical relevance of such rational dreams. This skepticism (constitutive of the philosophical mind as a "Timaean" knowledge that necessity yields to the soul's persuasion only with some reluctance)[35] is designed to balance the equally constitutive philosophical arrogance betrayed in the claim that philosophizing is at least one of the exemplary ways of being truly human and that some quasi-philosophical reflexivity would benefit other disciplines by humanizing them.

As a result of this balancing counterpoise, a practical "repulsion" is found to answer to the theoretical "attraction." This repulsion consists in the prudent refusal to accede to the imprudent request from representatives of the other disciplines that philosophy should provide them with moral guidelines, exculpating them from the burdens of their own responsibilities. On the grounds of a philosophical reflection concerning the limits of philosophical competence, the task of developing ethical codes is returned to each of the professions themselves. For only the experts of a given field can judge correctly (once they have been exposed to the philosophical manner of asking moral questions) where the need for moral guidance arises and what concrete determinants of professional activity must be considered for its realistic formulation and its practical enforcement. If conceptual criticism, as extended by one discipline over the others, has been found inconsistent with the interdisciplinary endeavor itself, then this same reasoning applies to moral criticism. Only if the sciences and the medical profession are called upon to develop their own moral codes on matters of their immediate competence, and to determine their own hierarchies of values as they reflect the bearing of those disciplines on other fields and on the society in general, can their ethical problems be discussed without categories held dear by one discipline being imposed on the work of another. Only when such responsibility is entrusted to specialized rules of the guild[36] is that autonomy of disciplines recognized which makes an interdisciplinary discussion possible.

If, therefore, the "field" of bioethics is considered more like a magnetic field in which currents of thought are being redirected and particles of ideas are acquiring a new order, then even the Pandora's box of political influence (about which Dr. Callahan's report expresses prudent concern) can be returned unopened. With the development of professional "guides to action," or with the problem of allocating responsibilities entrusted to the professions themselves, the competence of outsiders to consult would be restricted to occupying the left bench of a Kantian parliament. They are granted the voice of criticism, but not the power of legislation. No hybrid bioethical hermaphrodite would call for a second Zeus to split it.[37] With regard to such outside scrutiny, each profession would endeavor to be sufficiently rigid in determining its liabilities in order to avoid the need for a government agency to impose what it has failed to choose—and thus to preserve the integrity of its reputation. It would be this very interest in preserving its autonomy which would motivate each field to seek the interdisciplinary opportunity of integrating the other concepts into its own justifications.

The desirability of such a procedure rests in a pernicious inconsistency within the only alternative so far in view. If we want doctors to treat their patients as persons, that is, to take seriously their dignity as autonomous and responsible rational beings, then it is odd to deny doctors a similar autonomy and responsibility by *forcing them* to treat patients as persons. Bureaucratized morality or humanity, ordered from above, has always defeated its own goals. What should have arisen from the individual's self-determination is ruined when it is demanded from without.

We are now in a position to answer the final question: Is there a sense in which philosophy makes a difference as a participant in the interdisciplinary encounter? Indeed, the peculiarity of an interdisciplinary discussion which includes philosophy among the participating fields consists in the fact that those very (philosophical) principles, on which any commendable interdisciplinarity has been claimed to proceed, now enter into the interdisciplinary discourse itself. Hence, such a discourse not only occasions each specialist to reflect upon his own discipline in terms of others, but to reflect on this process of reflection as well. That is, interdisciplinarity becomes "self-conscious."

This self-consciousness also extends to the ethical implications of such an undertaking. The ethical question Gunther Stent posed at the end of his essay concerned the desirability of drawing a line between rational and moral thought. This question, thus, pertains not only to the condition for future ethics (whether it should be subsumed under the sciences). As a meta-interdisciplinary question it bears as well upon the condition for future interdisciplinary discussion between the sciences and the humanities. It is to be expected, then, that such discussion itself presents an occasion for ethical behavior. If, as a result of such interdisciplinary discussion, we demand some ethical considerations within the sciences or some respect of others in medical practice, it seems appropriate philosophically that the interdisciplinary discourse, while theoretically grounding such a demand, should itself exemplify its realization.

The ethical significance of human communication has most clearly been described in the metaphysics of Levinas[38] as the disposition to accept the other not only on his own terms as "other," but also as teacher in the eyes of whom one is judged. It is just such a disposition which has been found to underlie the interdisciplinary endeavor. Such exemplification on the methodical level of what the subject level is about gives rise to that internal coherence which at least some philosophers are inclined to take as a signature of truth.

NOTES

I would like to thank Vincent Kawalowski for his help in finding bibliographical material on the subject of interdisciplinarity. I am especially grateful to H. Tristram Engelhardt, Jr. for criticism that fostered both discipline and inspiration, and to Edmund Erde for his painstaking effort in making my language games less private. John Moskop has given helpful criticism of the final version.

1. D. Callahan and H. T. Engelhardt, Jr. eds. (Hastings-on-Hudson: Institute of Society, Ethics and the Life Sciences, 1976).
2. *Interdisciplinarity: Problems of Teaching and Research in Universities* (Paris: Organization for Economic Co-operation and Development, 1972), p. 25. Hereafter cited as OECD.
3. Joseph Kockelmans, *Interdisciplinarity, New Experience in Higher Education* (manuscript to appear in December 1976, The Pennsylvania State University Press), provides a comprehensive discussion of various interdisciplinary theories, of the historical roots of the present disciplines, and of the interdisciplinary endeavor itself. He distinguishes "multidisciplinarity," which concerns the educational aspect of a *studium generale*, and "pluridisciplinarity," as descriptive of the various utilizations of one field of scholarship for the purposes of another. Both are different from interdisciplinarity in that no real reciprocity takes place.
4. The categories used for ordering those motivations have been extracted from what usually is presented as a muddle of very divergent concerns. Thus, the holistic nature of interdisciplinary studies has, even in the otherwise carefully reasoned exposition of A. Briggs and D. G. Michaud ("Interdisciplinarity, Problems and Solutions," in *Interdisciplinarity*, OECD, p. 185 ff.), been indiscriminatingly recommended not only for attempts at conceptual (e.g., structuralist), operational (e.g., system theoretical), epistemological (e.g., empiricist), and linguistic (e.g., formalizable in mathematical notation) unifications of sciences. It has, in addition, been suggested for practical issues (i.e., for the solution of problems presented by a constantly changing society, the organizational confusion within the systems of higher education, the ineffective manner in which European universities are run, the trend towards democratization in Western societies, and the ensuing change in student needs, finally, the insufficient integration of university and society, research and vocational training in general). In contrast to this confusion, the "Common Outline for Preparation of Casestudies" (in *Innovation in Higher Education*, issued by the OECD, see E. Böning and K. Roeloffs: *Three German Universities: Aachen, Bochum, Konstanz*, 1970) has at least conceptually separated the question of interdisciplinarity from the general problems encountered by modern universities.

5. See note 4.
6. "To be ready for interdisciplinary research, the disciplines involved must have arrived at a stage of sophistication." (M. B. Luszki, *Interdisciplinary Team Research, Methods and Problems*, no. 3 of the Research Training Series [New York: New York University Press, 1958], p. 11.)
7. When dealing with the problem of organizational change within the university, one really addresses a continuum of proposals. They range from rather harmless administrative decisions of reducing, for example, the needlessly comprehensive "Fakultäten" in the German system into more manageable units of closely related fields (and thus to leave those fields themselves intact), via the creation of various overreaching "Dimensions of Learning" (P. C. McCoy, "Johnston College: An Experimental Model" in *The New Colleges: Toward an Appraisal*, P. L. Dressel ed., Iowa City, The American College testing program and the American Association for Higher Education, 1971), such as an "Environmental Dimension" requiring interdisciplinary studies that "naturally involve a grounding in the fundamental fields of mathematics, physics, chemistry, biology, psychology, political science, sociology and communication" (p. 59), to a complete unification of teaching, methodology and administration. The criticism expressed here concerns only such proposals which would, in theory or in effect, vitiate the academic pursuit of disciplinary studies.
8. It is revealing that Böning and Roeloffs find it necessary to emphasize the traditional self-understanding of the German university: "It may not, for instance, have the same idea as the general public about what the main needs and interests of society are. It considers its essential function to instill the ethos of scholarship and not just to train students professionally" (*Three German Universities*, p. 28).
9. See E. Jantsch, "Towards Interdisciplinarity in Education and Innovation," in *Interdisciplinarity* (OECD, p. 97 ff.).
10. See G. W. Morgan, "Disciplinarity and Interdisciplinarity: Research and Human Studies," in *Interdisciplinarity* (OECD, p. 263 ff.).
11. Cf. G. Gusdorf, "Interdisciplinarité" in *Encyclopedia Universalis* (Paris, 1970, p. 1086 ff.): ". . . un regroupement des saviors doit restituer à l'être humain sa place privilégiée de point de départ et de point d'arrivée de toutes les formes de la connaissance. Affolées par l'emballement de leurs technicités respectives, les sciences de l'homme ont trop souvent oublié qu'elles doivent demeurer des sciences humaines. Et même, les sciences qui n'ont pas l'homme

pour objet, dans la mésure où elles ont pour séjour des hommes, sont aussi des sciences humaines. L'oubli de ce principe fondamental constitue l'une des formes les plus pernicieuses de l'obscurantisme contemporain." It is easy to see how underneath a generally human—and hence harmless—concern for man a very particular anthropological assumption about his nature is utilized ("Le savoir universel n'est pas une mathématique universelle, mais une anthropologie culturelle"), which is really not so harmless in that it pretends to an objective validity, where argument is required. The assumption that man (or human life) ought to exhibit a unity understood in an undialectical sense should at least be defended against the equally possible view that some sort of alienation is what distinguishes human from animal life.

12. Why, in the end, should we resign ourselves to the fragmentation of humanity into male and female, and into various races and cultures? Should not the genetic sciences be employed to breed the ultimate wholesome androgyne of carefully intermediate color and, true to the principles of advanced demonology, capable of serving as *succubus* and *incubus* alternatively? (Martin Del Rio, *Disquisitionum Magicarum Libri Sex*, Mogunt., apud Ioannem Albinum, 1903, lib. II, Q. 15; 1st ed.: Louvain 1599-1600).

13. The disjunction between a heartless technocrat of learning and the humane interdisciplinary fellow-thinker recurs in Briggs and Michaud: "Interdisciplinarity is first and foremost a state of mind requiring each person to have an attitude that combines humility with openmindedness, a willingness to engage in dialogue and, hence, the capacity for assimilation and synthesis. Furthermore, it is a discipline in the ethical sense of the word and demands from the start that the representatives of different sciences accept teamwork and the necessity of searching together for a common language" ("Interdisciplinarity . . ." p. 192). Of course, such a state of mind does not differ from that required for intra-disciplinary work. Yet if, independently of the demands of the respective subject matter, teamwork and search for a common language are raised to the status of moral precepts, then any solitary pursuit of truth would have to be judged as morally deficient—a somewhat harsh verdict, even when pronounced over that habitually solitary attempt at thinking through our ethical intuitions and reasoning out our humanitarian predilections.

14. An exception is H. Heckhausen, "Discipline and Interdisciplinarity," in *Interdisciplinarity*, OECD, p. 83 ff., who lists among the criteria for a discipline "sensitivity to historical change."

15. An admirable example of such revolutionary conservatism is R. McKeon, "Character and the Arts and Disciplines," in *Ethics*, 78, 1968, p. 109 ff.

16. We even have disregarded another grave disadvantage of non-disciplinary learning: to wit, its indistinguishability from demonic (hence forbidden) science, the adepts of which art have been characterized by a leading authority in the field: "neque acquirunt illam scientiam naturaliter, hoc est, per modum disciplinae, & artis, nempe per speculationes, libros, & praeceptiores; sed quadam traditiva, quam qui habent, statim inusitatos illos effectus producunt. . . ." (Candidus Brognolus, *Alexicacon*, Venet., apud Nicolaum Pezzana, 1714.)

17. This attempt to reconcile disciplinary with interdisciplinary studies contradicts J. Piaget's thesis ("The Epistemology of Interdisciplinary Relations," in *Interdisciplinarity*, OECD, p. 127 ff.) that the principle of interdisciplinarity is "contrary to that of natural boundaries separating the various categories of observables from each other" (p. 128). This latter assumption he takes to underlie disciplinary studies. In view of such criticism it is necessary to keep in mind that the present attempt at understanding interdisciplinarity is neither committed to ontological boundary assumptions (but rather to a dialectical view of the interrelation between in part culturally determined methods and their objects), nor to the supposition that the existing disciplines should be endowed with some universal credentials of eternal necessity. The importance of disciplines will be emphasized not in an attempt to justify their particular present manifestations, but in order to delineate, on the basis of the extant samples of the species, a way in which interdisciplinarity can make sense with respect to disciplinary work as such.

18. An exception is Luszki's truly admirable work on case studies in interdisciplinary research on the anthropological, psychological, psychiatric, sociological aspects of problems of mental health. *Interdisciplinary Team Research . . . .*

19. Excepting Francis Bacon, in *The Two Books of the Proficience and Advancement of Learning* (London: Henrie Tomes, 1605), who demands (p. 26) that contemplative and practical philosophy, as Saturn and Jupiter, join efforts in the service of mankind.

20. Another alternative we will be well advised to avoid is Professor G. Frey's hopeless quest for meta- and metameta languages sufficiently diversified to deal with any combinations of one-, two- and three-level sciences, the relevance of which seems happily repudiated by an inexplicable success of interdisciplinary chatting (see "Meth-

odological Problems of Interdisciplinary Discourse," in *Ratio*, 15 [1973], p. 161 ff.).

21. Scrupulous attention to historical precedents obliges us at this point to remind the reader of that truly interdisciplinary machine, which on purely combinatoric principles represents a depository of universal knowledge, designed by the first professor of Speculative Knowledge introduced to the reader in the Grand Academy of Lagado (J. Swift, *Gulliver's Travels*, New York: The Modern Library, 1958, p. 145 ff.). It seems that the device described there has overcome all problems of interdisciplinary communication.

22. See his essay "Can Medicine Dispense with a Theological Perspective on Human Nature?" Vol. II.

23. See E. D. Pellegrino, "Science and Moral Neutrality: Some Notes on Ladd's Method of Logical Negation," 1, 84.

24. Plato, *Symposium,*, 203 b.

25. Ibid., 209 c.

26. Ibid., 202 d.

27. Ibid.

28. Ibid., 211 a.

29. It may be noted that I am here sympathetically circumscribing Stent's more ambitious claim to give a non-normative account of Kant's moral theory.

30. It is this resulting modification in the fundamental concepts of the "other" discipline which distinguishes applied anatomy, applied biochemistry, applied pathology (p. 147) from the inspiration philosophy, psychology, and the medical ideology can derive from their involvement with the clinical field (see note 31). If some aspect of anatomy, biochemistry, or pathology fails in its clinical application, then what is usually required is only some research on the respective topics in those fields—not, however, that critical revision which characterizes the truly interdisciplinary quality of an interaction between disciplines. Such revisions are especially valuable for philosophy, as the interdisciplinary perspective confronts its theoretical constructs with their practical realization. Such a regard—even though alien to philosophy as such—can provide an essential motive for specifying its claims.

31. In a similar way the person to person clinical situation confronts the doctor with practical dilemmas for the evaluation of which the psychological explanatory model fails. Again, it would not be fair to demand of psychology that it should consider its objects of research as subjects of a personal encounter in the sense in which clinical treatment requires such an approach. Rather, an indepen-

dent clinical psychology is needed which allows the use of psychologically inexplicable mechanisms by which to deal with their psychologically explicable counterparts. But then again, for a psychological consideration of that particular application of psychological knowledge, a manner of reviewing its claims to explain is needed to account for a region of theoretically opaque but practically crucial phenomena. When Cassell (in "Error in Medicine," Vol. II) argues that a major source of medical error arises from an incorrect perception of the role of medical technology in its struggle with the contingencies of life, or from an incorrect perspective of "fate in its expression of illness," then this unhappy consequence in the application of medical knowledge so understood suggests a revision of that perception.

32. This concept of interdisciplinarity (requiring the participating disciplines in their particular determination by methods and criteria of acceptable knowledge to enter into the dialogue) is not altogether different from the account of an interdisciplinary team by Luszki: ". . . a group of persons who are trained in the use of different tools and concepts, among whom there is an organized division of labor around a common problem, with each member using his own tools, with continuous intercommunication and reexamination of postulates in terms of the limitations provided by the work of the other members . . . " (Interdisciplinary Team Research . . . , p. 10). A similar dialectic of disciplinary and interdisciplinary aspects is suggested in E. Quinn, *et. al.*, *Interdiscipline, A Reader in Psychology, Sociology and Literature* (New York: The Free Press, 1972), where the preface states that the purpose is: ". . . to point up the interrelatedness of the disciplines of psychology, sociology and literature, and to define each discipline by distinguishing it from others . . . ."

33. See their essay "From System to Story: An Alternative Pattern for Rationality in Ethics," II.

34. A "Philosophy of Medicine" (Cf. H. T. Engelhardt, Jr., "Is There a Philosophy of Medicine?" *Proceedings of the Philosophy of Science Association*, 1977) is said to be possible if a reconsideration of medicine in terms of concepts borrowed from philosophy discloses "hidden" structures of reasoning that lend themselves to philosophical reconstruction. It is said to be especially interesting if this consideration reveals categories not otherwise treated by philosophical inquiry. Such reinterpretations subject the medical understanding of medicine, just as the philosophical understanding of some philosophical concepts, to modifications. Hence "Philosophy of

Medicine" can truly be held to be a result of, as well as a demand
for, further interdisciplinary study. In a like manner "Bioethics" can
be conceived in relational, rather than in substantive terms.

35. Plato, *Timaeus*, 48 a.
36. "Bei diesen freien Vereinen (i.e., of the gardeners, the weavers,
    and the tailors), denen alle Handwerksverbindungen nach und nach
    sich gleichstellten, ersetzte theils das genossenschaftlich Ehrgefühl,
    theils die Rücksicht auf ihren Vortheil durch Erhaltung des Ver-
    trauens die polizeiliche Aufsicht der Obrigkeit, indem sie selbst nun
    daruber wachten, dass niemand schlechte Arbeit verfertigte oder
    verkaufte." (W. E. Wilda, *Das Gildenwesen im Mittelalter*, Neu-
    druck der Ausgabe Halle 1831, Aalen, Scientia Verlag, 1964, p.
    323). As a sample of what such rules looked like in a field more
    related to Bioethics, the item number 19 from the order for the
    Salisbury Barber Surgeons of 1676 is quite instructive: "Women to
    forbeare takeinge Chirurghery on them contrary to Lawe. Item, It is
    further ordered that whereas there are diverse women and others
    within this Cittie altogether unskilfull in the art of Chirurgery who
    doe oftentimes take cures on them to the great danger of the
    patient, It is therefore ordered that from henceforth noe such
    woman or any other shall undertake or inter meddle with any cure
    of Chirurgery for which she or they shall directly or indirectly have
    received or take any money benefitt or other reward, upon paine
    that every one shall for every cure taken in hand or meddled with,
    unless she or they shall first be allowed by this Company, forfeite
    and loose to the use of this Company the sume of tenne shillings."
    (A. C. Haskins, J.P., *The Ancient Trade Guilds and Companies of
    Salisbury*, [Salisbury: Bennet Brothers, 1912]). This quotation is
    illuminating in that it also reminds us of the problematic inherent in
    the guild system: its intolerance against unorthodox competition
    (see T. Szasz, *The Manufacture of Madness* [New York: Harper &
    Row, 1970]).
37. Plato, *Symposium*, 190 c.
38. Emmanuel Levinas, *Totalité et infini: essai sur l'extériorité* (The
    Hague: M. Nijhoff, 1961).

9

How Does Interdisciplinary Work Get Done?

Eric J. Cassell

INTERDISCIPLINARY WORK CAN GET DONE AND very well too—witness the work of this group. From my experience with this and other efforts at the Institute, I would like to make some observations on how it happens. I feel that the personal reference is justified because I believe that successful interdisciplinary work is based primarily on the participants undergoing personal change. Since none of us is all that willing to change beliefs and viewpoints, perhaps we should look at what softens people up enough to allow them to change.

The first essential is a healthy respect for the problem at hand. As a physician, I am quite accustomed to working with experts from other disciplines. Only I call it asking for a consultation, not interdisciplinary work. I do not do this out of largeness of character, but because I am scared of error and afraid of doing harm to a patient. That fear usually overrides pride because doctors soon learn how much damage can follow the failure to admit ignorance. If the first requirement is a healthy respect for the problem at hand, then the problems of ethics in the life sciences lend themselves naturally to interdisciplinary work. One must simply stand in awe of any set of issues which have withstood solution since the beginning of recorded time. Before working in these interdisciplinary groups, I thought that the difficulty was merely that well-established ethical systems or philosophical understandings had not been applied to the issues raised by modern biomedical science and technology. While that may be partly true, to a larger degree it is basic understanding that is lacking. As in other fields, exposure to new challenges has revealed gaps in previous knowledge, insight, and methods of analysis. In other words, it is not merely that we are seeing situations in medicine and the life sciences that are new and unique—to which, for example, Aristotle's *Ethics* have never been applied. Rather, these new things would pose exciting challenges to Aristotle (as only one example) if he were around today. Indeed, I am distressed with my own tradition, Judaism, because I believe Jewish ethicists have not by and large yet understood that we are dealing with situations that are new and unique in the experience of mankind.

If the first requirement for interdisciplinary work is respect for the problem, then I think that the second requirement is a belief that the problem demands solutions. When I call a consultant to see a patient with a puzzling illness, I do not do so solely out of intellectual curiosity. I ask for help because I know that decisions must be made and actions taken. Here again, the similarity to the problem of ethics in medicine and the life sciences is clear. Discovery, invention, and change proceed with consequences good, bad, and who knows what in between. Our disquiet with medicine and science, which for some reason continue to see themselves as "value free," is deepening. There is an urgency here that is pressing despite the fact that the work may go on at this pace for many decades.

These two basic requirements, respect for the problem and an urgency for answers, are necessary, I believe, because of the effect they have on the people who must participate across disciplines. They create a community of interest that, at least for a time, directs the interests and attention of the participants toward the outer need and not so much toward each other and each other's discipline. I know well that attention falters and that side issues may obscure common interest in the challenges, but I also know that the fundamental issues are so compelling that it is necessary only to raise them again to return common direction to the work.

What is being asked of those who do interdisciplinary research is that they leave the fixed intellectual navigating platforms from which each discipline or specialty views the world. For all its importance, I find that no easy thing. A person is defined, in part, by his conceptions, by the paradigmatic structure of values and beliefs about the world that relates each conception to the other. To ask of someone that he be prepared to call that conceptual structure into question is to ask that he be prepared to give up a piece of himself. People do not hold white-knuckle tight to their frames of reference out of pure reason but because to give up a frame of reference is extremely unsettling. The design of settings in which we do interdisciplinary work and the methods by which it is accomplished must take that potential for anxiety into account. It takes time for people to change their views; they are not changing something external to themselves, rather, they are changing themselves. Personal support is also required, and the best support is the sense that one is among friends and equals.

Therefore, to the requirements of respect for the problem and awareness of its urgency I must add more personal necessities for interdisciplinary research. I cannot emphasize strongly enough my belief that in successful interdisciplinary research, those things that promote change in individuals promote the work.

First among these is, I think, respect for the other participants. I lay aside a bit of myself out of the belief, derived from respect, that the view of the other person will support me even though I have not yet had time to test it myself. It is respect for the physician that enables a patient to do something for his health that he does not want to do, or that threatens injury or discomfort. In the setting of transdisciplinary work, respect arises from several diverse (and sometimes related) characteristics. One is sheer intellectual power: I do not see the problem as that man or woman does, but if someone as intelligent as that believes it to be so, I am forced to re-examine my own belief. Another characteristic often related, although not necessarily so, is depth and breadth of scholarship. Someone who knows his field and its literature so completely that it has become a part of him also commands my respect for I love learning itself. The personal integrity of a participant may make us accept what he or she says as something not idly come to or lightly held.

At the first meeting I ever attended at the Institute, when I wanted to play tapes of patients' conversations I found myself in direct conflict with the late Henry K. Beecher, M.D., over the lack of written permission for the recordings.[1] The patients had known their conversations were being recorded, and I did not see the necessity for formal permission. Some sharp words ensued, and I left the session angry. At the meeting the next morning, I apologized somewhat reluctantly, as much out of respect for Beecher as from agreement with his point of view. However, I did start getting written permission after that, and by now, I have taken Dr. Beecher's position on a number of occasions. Change is gradual, but the first willingness really to listen may come out of respect.

I may appreciate what another person has to say but I may not respect his discipline. Interdisciplinary efforts do not go well when the participants do not respect each other's disciplines or their methods. Most of us have prejudices against this or that branch of science, against all physicians or some specialties, against all philosophers or some philosophical schools, or against all theologians or some professed beliefs. No seminar, working group, or conference can survive too many participants with such feelings. On the other hand, there is no such group that does not carry some burden of simple prejudice. The solution for the problem of prejudice is, once again, personal respect and the appreciation of the importance of the goals of the work.

Having discussed these personal issues in transdisciplinary research, it seems necessary to mention some specific things that either promote or hold back the work. The first and foremost specific is language: social and professional communities are communities of language. The extent that any of us share the same conceptions or world view, or can come to know that we do, is the extent to which we share a common language. By language, I mean, of course, not merely the same words, but the same meanings and usage.

The problem of jargon is well known, but the meaning of the

use of jargon is not as obvious. Jargon is often used as a short cut to pack wide meaning into few words. But, similarly, jargon is often used to cover up an absence of precise meaning. By convention, we all agree to use the word to denote the thing. However, we all also agree not to examine further the issue so denoted, knowing we might drown in any attempt at true explication. Perhaps for ordinary conversations we are better off to look no further, but interdisciplinary research is not ordinary conversation.

The use of jargon also symbolizes the fact that the user belongs to a special group. I believe the reason medical students and young physicians, for example, use more jargon than older physicians is the need the young have to feel a part of the group. Nonetheless, for any successful interdisciplinary work, the jargon has to go. When it goes, it is rather like pulling off a wart; it leaves bleeding. Daniel Callahan's dictum seems the best advice: you should always talk to others in the language you use to talk to yourself. (I wonder why we do not talk jargon to our inner selves?)

Problems of language usage, however, go deeper than jargon or technical terms. Both jargon and technical terminology can be translated into ordinary language. Further, people know and request clarification when they hear a word whose meaning they do not understand. The diverse meanings of everyday words may provide an even greater stumbling block. I suspect that the word "pain" has a different meaning to physicians than to non-physicians. Seeing a movie of a woman delivering a child by Cesarian section, under hypnosis and without anesthesia, had a profound effect upon me. I remember thinking that I had to revise my entire understanding of the meaning of pain. But both before and after that movie, I used the same word, pain, to label what had become different understandings. Difficulties in ordinary language are much harder to clarify precisely because we often do not know that the problem exists. Certain concepts can illustrate this confusion. It is quite common still to hear some philosophers talk of the difference between man and the animals. The distinction is most often made in discussing man as a rational being. To most biologists, such dichotomous distinctions seem unnatural since we see life much more in terms of similarities than of differences, as a continuum rather than as a step-like progression. This difference between life scientists and philosophers or theologians is absolutely fundamental. It is not merely something life scientists know, but it is a part of their being that underlies everything they learn and the way they approach the world. And, of course, the reverse is true. Kant is just a name to me, albeit an important one, but it is clear to me that for philosophers, Kant stands for something very much larger than I am able to comprehend.

These last two examples, difficulties arising from diverse meanings of everyday language and differences in a fundamental world view would seem to deny the possibility of successful interdisciplinary research. And yet, success is achieved. How does it occur? Given the conditions of respect I noted above, respect for the problem and its urgency, for the other participants and their disciplines, personal change does take place. This change seems to me to have one fundamental characteristic to which all others are subservient: the change in one's frame of reference. Previously, I saw my work, the knowledge of my profession—its problems, goals, methods, ideas, and ways of thought—as being self-contained and existing alongside other similarly self-contained systems of greater or lesser interest to me. To be sure, these self-contained systems were seen by me as impinging on one another or of having importance one for another, but their distinctness was preserved within me.

Slowly dawning but then suddenly clear, the frame of reference enlarges. For me, it was coming to see medicine as existing within the much larger system of the moral life of mankind. I do not mean merely the realization that there is a world outside of medicine (although that, too, could be a first and vital change in a frame of reference). Rather, I realized that understanding in moral philosophy is fundamental to understanding medicine. With that change, what other participants had to say became not merely something I would have liked to understand in order to broaden my knowledge of the world, but rather something I realize that I *must* understand so that I can bring order back into my comprehension of medicine. The point is, of course, that with the enlargement of the frame of reference, the previous structure of my comprehension of medicine has become uncertain and the new knowledge from other disciplines is not merely useful but necessary to restore stability to the conceptual structure.

For a philosopher or a theologian, a similar change in reference frame might be the developed awareness that the biology of man is an overriding force. I cannot know what it feels like suddenly to become aware of biology, of its ineluctable operation of nature's finitude. I cannot know this because it is a part of me that developed as I developed. But I can guess that the change is as exciting for the philosopher as the reverse is for me.

The process I have described—and above all it is a process—is one of personal change. I know of no other terms that can adequately describe the nature of successful interdisciplinary efforts. Like all personal change, it takes place over time. The process is not smooth, but moves in fits and starts. For an outsider, watching it may prove exasperatingly slow and inefficient. Verbose and argumentative interchange may be more apparent than consensus. But appearances can be misleading because things are happening. Certain circumstances promote the process: obviously, judging from these meetings good food is not necessary, while alcohol seems quite useful. The idea of having papers and commentary read at one meeting and then presented again at a subsequent meeting has proved excellent. At first that seemed to me to be redundant. Why say the same thing a second time? Often, however, the discussion only comes alive at the second presentation, as the other participants begin to understand fully what the writer is saying. Problems of language and point of view are clarified over time.

As in every circus, good ringmasters are essential. Keeping all the tigers in the cage and sitting on their pedestals (each just the proper height) is no easy task. For any success we may enjoy, we are indebted to our trainers, the editors of this volume.

NOTE

1. Dr. Beecher was the author of *Research and the Individual: Human Studies* (Boston: Little, Brown and Co., 1970), a seminal work on the ethical problems of human experimentation.

Index

Abortion, 116, 120
Abraham, 10, 39, 68
Alienation, 122-24
American Bar Association, 256, 258, 263, 268
American Medical Association, 256, 258, 268-69
Anselm, 161
Aristotle, 19, 28, 34, 38-39, 89, 127, 131, 136, 154, 172, 211, 282, 287, 356
Austen, Jane, 50
Austin, J.L., 76
Ayer, A.J., 2

Bacon, Francis, 262
Barth, Karl, 36, 60
Becker, Ernest, 139
Beckett, Samuel, 40
Beecher, Henry K., 359
Beethoven, 182
Bemporad, Jack, 7, 9-10, 337
Bettelheim, Bruno, 253
Biology, as foundation of ethics, 15-16, 226-31, 237-40
Blackmun, Harry A., 71
Boorstin, Daniel J., 212-13
Bradley, Francis H., 30
Briggs, A., 326, 328
Brunner, Emil, 60
Bultmann, R.K., 36
Burger, Warren, 266
Burrell, David, 11-13, 17, 22-23, 116, 153-56, 162-66, 168, 343

Butler, Bishop, 81-82

Callahan, Daniel, 13-14, 330, 346, 359
Calvin, John, 76
Camus, Albert, 164, 167
Cassell, Eric, 19-21, 113, 274, 310-19, 322, 340
Chomsky, Noam, 235, 241, 251
Christian ethics, 45-46, 51-52, 59-61, 62-68, 88-89, 111-12
Churchill, Winston, 179
Cleanthes, 81-82
Cohen, Hermann, 104
Comte, Auguste, 125
Cook, Captain, 30, 35

Dante, 29
Darwin, Charles, 211, 238, 241
Delkeskamp, Corinna, 7-9, 13, 20, 322
Demea, 81
Demos, Raphael, 36
Descartes, René, 1, 229
Disease entities, 316-19

Engelhardt, H. Tristram, 341
Error, medical, 19-20, 295-309, 310-319
Ethics, 1-19
  and Christianity, 45-46, 51-52, 59-61, 62-68, 88-89, 111-12
  and Judaism, 59-60, 62-68
  and evolution, 207-21, 247-53

and professional codes, 18-19, 254-77, 279-80

and technology, 14-15, 169-97, 199-206

Euthanasia, in Nazi Germany, 25-26, 29, 84

Evans, Donald, 61

Evil, concept of, 28-30, 32-34, 57, 83-84

Evolution and ethics, 207-21, 247-53

Fackenheim, 72

Frankena, William K., 60-63, 66, 76, 81

Freedman, Monroe, 263-70, 274

Freud, Sigmund, 251

Fried, Charles, 268, 273

Fotion, N., 69-70

Germany, Nazi and medical ethics, 25-26, 48, 76-77, 86-87

Gide, André, 164, 168

Goebbels, P.J., 38

Gorovitz, Samuel, 299, 308, 310, 312, 317-18, 341, 343

Guiccardini, F., 39

Gustafson, J.M., 243

Hare, R.M., 53, 81

Haurerwas, Stanley, 11-13, 17, 22-23, 116, 153-56, 162, 166, 168, 343

Heelan, Patrick, 13, 16-17, 228

Heidegger, Martin, 36, 173

Hegel, Frederich, 42, 86, 125, 193

Heine, H., 32

Herder, Johann, 42, 86

Heydrich, Reinhard, 38

Himmler, Heinrich, 38

Hippocrates, 71-72, 275, 315

Hitler, Adolph, 29, 72, 77

Hoess, 38

Holton, Gerald, 263

Holzel, F.D., 29

Hosea, 70

Hucheson, Francis, 71

Hume, David, 80, 155

Hutcheson, Francis, 172

Huxley, Julian, 247

Huysmans, J.K., 159-60

Interdisciplinarity, 20-21, 321-23

logic of, 324-47

psychology of, 355-61

Iphigenia, 39

Isaiah, 103

Isaac, 39, 68

Jacob, 68

Jantsch, Eric, 327

Jonas, Hans, 13-15, 17, 22, 72, 105, 200-04, 206

Judaism and ethics, 59-60, 62-68

Kant, Immanuel, 1, 7-8, 9, 14, 16, 27, 30-42, 46-49, 51-58, 71, 75, 84, 109, 113, 153, 155, 161, 167-68, 172-74, 193, 234, 237-38, 241-43, 333, 338-39, 360

Kierkegaard, Soren, 44, 53, 72, 77

King, Lester, 333, 335

Knowledge, search for, 1-5

Kohlberg, Lawrence, 253

Kovesi, Julius, 119

Kuhn, Thomas, 11, 22

Ladd, John, 332-35

Language, and moral narrative, 119-22

Lappé, Marc, 339-40
Lawrence, D.H., 150
Lawyers, and ethical codes, 263-68
Layzer, David, 215, 217, 220
Leibniz, G.W., 6
Lejeune, Jerome, 228
Lessing, G.E., 53, 77
Levinas, 347
Lewis, C.S., 45, 50
Lewis, R.W.B., 164
Lincoln, Abraham, 70
Linguistics, 235-37
Livy, 39
Lorenz, Konrad, 238
Luther, Martin, 55

MacIntyre, Alasdair, 7-9, 13, 17, 44-58, 63, 71-72, 79-93, 105, 299, 308, 310, 312, 317-18, 333, 341, 343
Malinowski, Bronislaw, 230
Mandelbrot, Benoit, 233
Marcel, Gabriel, 166
Marx, Karl, 38, 120, 193
Medawar, Peter, 214
Medical ethics, 117-18, 139, 254-77, 295-309, 310-19
Michaud, D.G., 326, 328
Mill, J.S., 28, 31, 34, 38-39
Milgram, Stanley, 33
Monod, Jacques, 2-3, 208
Moore, G.E., 4
Montague, 107
Morality, 1-5
   and religion, 100-09
Moral narratives, 11-13, 39-41, 86, 111-41, 153-68
Morgan, G.W., 327, 329
Morgenstern, Christian, 231
Mozart, W.A., 175

Nagel, Thomas, 18-19
Niebuhr, Reinhold, 45
Nietzsche, F., 26, 172-73, 192
Nixon, Richard, 262

Ogden, Schubert, 109
Oman, John, 105
Oppenheimer, Helen, 64

Pareto distributions, 232-34
Parzival, 2, 5, 23
Pellegrino, Edmund, 13, 23, 334
Philo, 80-84
Piaget, Jean, 253
Piccolomini, Max, 93
Pincoffs, Edmund, 115
Plato, 34, 172, 192, 219
Polanyi, Michael, 161
Poliakov, 25-26
Prichard, H.A., 30-31, 35
Professional ethics, 18-19, 254-77, 279-80

Quine, W.V., 50

Ramsey, Paul, 7-9, 75-78, 80-83, 85-90, 94
Rationality, moral, 112-15, 122-24, 153-68
Rawls, John, 122
Religion, and morals, 100-09 (SEE ALSO Theology)
Responsibility, moral, 14-15, 169-97, 199-206
   dimension of future in, 186-90
   natural and contracted, 177-78
   object of, 180-81
   parental and political, 183-86, 204-05
   parent-child relation, 193-97, 200, 204